AIDS, MACROBIOTICS, AND
NATURAL IMMUNITY

AIDS, Macrobiotics, and Natural Immunity

By Michio Kushi
and Martha, C. Cottrell, M.D.
with Mark N. Mead

Japan Publications, Inc.

Note to the reader: Those with health problems are advised to seek the guidance of a qualified medical or psychological professional in addition to qualified macrobiotic teacher before implementing any of the dietary or other approaches presented in this book. It is essential that any reader who has any reason to suspect serious illness seek appropriate medical, nutritional or psychological advice promptly. Neither this nor any other related book should be used as a substitute for qualified care or treatment.

Published by JAPAN PUBLICATIONS, INC., Tokyo and New York

Distributors:
UNITED STATES: *Kodansha International/USA, Ltd., through Farrar, Straus & Giroux, 19 Union Square West, New York, 10003. Fitzhenry & Whiteside Ltd., 195 Allstate Parkway, Markham, Ontario, L3R 4T8.* BRITISH ISLES: *Premier Book Marketing Ltd., 1 Gower Street, London WC1E 6HA.* EUROPEAN CONTINENT: *European Book Service PBD, Strijkviertel 63, 3454 PK De Meern, The Netherlands.* AUSTRALIA AND NEW ZEALAND: *Bookwise International, 54 Crittenden Road, Findon, South Australia 5007.* THE FAR EAST AND JAPAN: *Japan Publications Trading Co., Ltd., 1-2-1, Sarugaku-cho, Chiyoda-ku, Tokyo 101.*

First edition: May 1990

LCCC No. 86–81560
ISBN 0–87040–680–9

Printed in U.S.A.

May peace be bestowed upon the spirit of those who have suffered and passed away from Acquired Immunodeficiency Syndrome and related diseases.

May glory be in heaven and may health and peace, compassion and love be realized on earth.

Preface

This book is divided into four parts plus a section including a number of appendices. The first is a general discussion of the macrobiotic approach to AIDS that I prepared with the assistance of Alex Jack, the director of the Kushi Institute in Becket, Mass., and author of several books; Donna Cowan, my administrative assistant; Lois Thompson, macrobiotic senior; and Carolyn Heidenry, senior macrobiotic teacher and author.

The second part includes supporting medical and scientific information and analysis prepared by Martha C. Cottrell, M. D., the Director of Student Health at the Fashion Institute of Technology in New York, with the research and editorial assistance of Mark Mead, a macrobiotic researcher and author.

The third part is a selection of recipes and home-care guidance based upon the teachings of my wife Aveline Kushi, the leading teacher of macrobiotic cooking and way of life. This section I prepared with the assistance of Wendy and Edward Esko, macrobiotic senior teachers and authors.

The fourth part includes personal accounts of several men with AIDS or AIDS-related conditions who have benefited from the macrobiotic dietary approach. These accounts were compiled and edited by Mark Mead.

This book grew out of macrobiotic educational activities related to AIDS beginning in 1983. Since then, Aveline, our macrobiotic teachers and associates, and I have met with hundreds of people who have suffered from AIDS, ARC or *AIDS-related Complex*, and other infectious disorders. Regular guidance has been offered in various ways—personal advice, group discussions, lectures, seminars, and cooking classes. These meetings have taken place in New York, Boston, Miami, Los Angeles, Amsterdam, London, Switzerland, and the People's Republic of the Congo in Central Africa.

Besides the contributors mentioned above, teachers who have participated in these events include Marc Van Cauwenberghe, M. D., macrobiotic senior teacher; Evelyne Harboun, senior cooking teacher and guidance counselor; Masao Miyaji, senior cooking teacher; and other dedicated teachers and guidance counselors.

Medical and scientific researchers who have initiated and carried out research on the macrobiotic dietary effects on people with AIDS and *Kaposi's sarcoma* include Elinor M. Levy, Ph. D., J. C. Beldekas, Ph. D., and P. H. Black, M. D., from the Department of Microbiology of Boston University's School of Medicine; and Lawrence H. Kushi, Sc. D., previously from the Division of Epidemiology, University of Minnesota and currently from the Fred Hutchinson Cancer Research Center in Seattle.

Administrative efforts have also been provided by the Kushi Foundation for One Peaceful World in Brookline, Massachusetts; the New York Macrobiotic Center; HEAL, a group in New York that helps AIDS sufferers; the Ministry of Health in the People's Republic of the Congo; and macrobiotic educational centers in Miami, Amsterdam, France, Switzerland, and other places around the world.

Behind this book, these wonderful people, and many others, have tirelessly and unselfishly given their time and energy. There are also many health-care professionals, and friends with AIDS who have given their assistance to develop a greater understanding about the nature of AIDS and AIDS-related disorders.

Aveline and I are sincerely grateful to all these people and many other friends. We also extend our heartfelt thanks to Japan Publications, Inc. for their full cooperation in making this book available for the benefit of modern society. Together we can find a healthy and enduring solution to the challenge of AIDS and ensure humanity's continued biological and spiritual evolution for endless generations to come.

MICHIO KUSHI
Brookline, Massachusetts

Introduction

AIDS (Acquired Immunodeficiency Syndrome) first appeared in 1979. In the beginning, the problem of AIDS was confined almost exclusively to the gay community. By the early 1980s, homosexual behavior was condemned by the majority of the public, and many people considered AIDS as God's punishment of gay conduct. The medical and scientific community mobilized to deal with this new epidemic, but the initial euphoria that a vaccine could quickly be developed faded. Medical statements turned increasingly pessimistic and offered no clear solution or relief. AIDS sufferers remained in despair. Rumors and panic swept through the media. Landlords evicted people with AIDS, employers fired them, and churches turned them out. Police officers wore masks and gloves in the gay quarters in San Francisco and other cities. Many public bathhouses were closed. Modern society started to treat people with AIDS as if they were untouchables.

During the summer of 1983, my office and the office of the Kushi Foundation for One Peaceful World in Brookline, Massachusetts, began to receive visits from AIDS sufferers seeking guidance amid this climate of fear and hopelessness. The Wipe Out AIDS group in New York City requested that I visit and encourage men with AIDS by giving lectures and guidance. These educational presentations began in August, 1983, at the Gay and Lesbian Community Center and have continued in New York until the present. Macrobiotic cooking classes and personal guidance have also been continuously offered to people with AIDS at the Kushi Foundation in Brookline; the New York Macrobiotic Center; the Miami Macrobiotic Center; and other places under the orientation of Aveline, myself, and senior teachers and guidance counselors. In the spirit of public service, many of these activities have been carried out without charge.

This encouragement gave many of the men suffering from AIDS hope for the first time. In Aveline's cooking classes, tears streamed down the cheeks of many young men. They began to eat whole grains, beans and their products, fresh vegetables prepared in various ways, sea vegetables, and non-aromatic condiments and beverages, with the occasional consumption of fish and seafood, in order to recover their natural immunity through improved blood and lymph quality. Within the macrobiotic community, these young men were called AIDS friends.

However, as this educational activity began, the following problems had to be solved:

1. There was concern within the gay and lesbian communities that the macrobiotic way of life might share some of modern society's prejudice against homosexuals. This was a misconception, but initially some AIDS friends were hesitant to improve their dietary habits. To overcome these reservations, we had to make special efforts.

2. Because most AIDS friends, especially in New York, were living in separate apartments and had fast-paced life-styles, they tended to eat out often and to eat irregularly. This may have involved taking some undesirable food and drink. In order to provide uniformly high-quality cooking and a calm, harmonious environment, we approached several hospitals and religious establishments in 1983 and 1984 to make their facilities available to AIDS friends. But these efforts were unsuccessful, mostly because these institutions were afraid of adverse publicity and the spread of panic among their usual clientele.

3. Because society at large needed to be educated about the benefits of the macrobiotic approach to AIDS, it was necessary, together with educational activities, to conduct scientific and medical research to measure the effects of improved dietary practice and life-style on the AIDS friends who had changed their way of eating. For this, funding was necessary. Applications for grants were submitted to several funding sources, but all were rejected or ignored.

As in the case of heart disease twenty years ago and of cancer a decade ago, the medical and scientific community was generally unable to recognize a possible connection between AIDS and diet and between AIDS and other life-style factors. Official attention was focused almost exclusively on developing a vaccine against the AIDS virus or on stimulating the immune system by artificial means. However, several individual researchers felt dietary and life-style studies were warranted and initiated such medical tests at their own cost and donations of time and energy. These medical friends included Martha Cottrell, M.D., in New York; P.H. Black, M.D., Elinor Levy, Ph.D., and John Beldekas, Ph.D., of Boston University School of Medicine; and Lawrence Kushi, Sc.D., of the University of Minnesota at that time (currently of Fred Hutchinson Cancer Research Institute in Seattle, Washington).

In spite of these difficulties, many AIDS and ARC friends have demonstrated remarkable improvement in their blood and lymph quality, physical vitality, and mental outlook. Although some AIDS friends could not recover their immunity—probably because the degree of immune deficiency was too low at the time of beginning the dietary improvement or because their dietary practice was irregular and inconsistent—those who did stabilize over the next two to three years experienced, on the average, the following improvements:

1. Their lymphocytes continuously increased.

2. Their T4 cells did not change, but the percentage of T8 cells appeared to decrease.

3. The quality of their mental and psychological outlook and life-style improved remarkably.

4. Their average life span after diagnosis became longer in comparison to other men with AIDS who had not changed their way of eating and life-style.

In the event AIDS friends maintain their residence at a place where well-prepared food can be consumed daily, and active physical exercise is performed, the results will be much more satisfactory.

Since 1985, the preliminary results of these continuing scientific and medical tests have been reported by the researchers in international medical journals and conferences. They have also been presented on many occasions at educational forums and public programs that we have conducted, including meetings at the United Nations and World Health Organization, a medical conference in Central Africa sponsored by the Ministry of Health of the People's Republic of the Congo and the Kushi Foundation in Brazzaville, at medical seminars in Britain, France, and the Netherlands, and at a medical conference sponsored by the government and medical society in Yugoslavia.

A comprehensive overview of the macrobiotic approach to AIDS and AIDS-related infections is outlined in the following chapters. Practical guidelines for dietary improvement are also presented, along with suggested menus and recipes and home cares. Medical and scientific information related to AIDS and immunity in general is also introduced with a hope that the approach presented here may help prevent and possibly help relieve AIDS and its related conditions. With the purpose of creating an AIDS-free planet and a happy, healthy, peaceful world for endless generations to come, this book is presented to every individual and family in modern society.

Contents

1

The Natural Approach to AIDS through Diet and Life-style

Michio Kushi

1. The Challenge of Modern Civilization

Modern technological civilization reached a height in the late twentieth century. However, amid unparalleled material and technological development, the human race on this planet began to experience widespread sickness and disorder. The spread of modern civilization has been accompanied by degeneration of human life at all levels—the physical, mental, psychological, social, ideological, and spiritual. This deterioration is so extensive that the quality of human life has changed completely when compared to that of even one century ago.

Modern civilization, especially in the late twentieth century, has been unable to cope with these degenerative tendencies, including heart disease, cancer, mental and psychological illness, and AIDS and other immune-deficiency diseases, in addition to decline of the family, loss of traditional values, increasing crime and social disorder, environmental pollution, and war.

Rather than being healthy, sound, and positive, civilization is defensive, protective, and negative. Advances in communication and transportation have contributed to uniting different continents, races, cultures, and customs, and may be considered relatively positive and unifying. But many other factors of modern life are dualistic and polarizing and may be considered relatively negative and disruptive. These negative symptoms and factors include:

1. Increasing numbers of hospitals and health-care facilities as well as the growing number of health-care professionals to deal with the sharp rise in the rates of degenerative disease.

2. Increasing complications in the judicial system, including the development of legal and informational technologies as well as the growing number of legal professionals to deal with the spread of crime and wild and anti-social behavior.

3. Increasing psychiatric, psychoanalytical, and psychological training, programs, and facilities as well as the expanding number of professionals to deal with increased mental and psychological disorders.

4. Increasing insurance, investment, and mutual-security systems of various kinds, including public and private agencies and enterprises as well as government welfare and social systems, to deal with weakened social solidarity and the decline of individual and family ability to take responsibility for their own destiny.

5. Increasing defense powers in the form of police at the domestic level and the military at the international level, including the development of destructive weapons and star-war facilities to deal with spreading distrust among people in communities, states, and nations.

6. Increasing chemicalization and artificialization of the drinking water and daily food supply as well as the development of an industry related to these factors in an attempt to protect the human species from the weakening and sheltering effects of living in modern, artificial society.

7. Increasing belief systems including school and university education, the publications industry, the mass media, and many kinds of religious institutions to cope with prevailing human mental and spiritual instability.

These seven major aspects, along with many others, and the associated enterprises, industries, installations, and systems that service them, now compose the larger part of modern civilization. If humanity regained its natural health and developed a calm, peaceful, compassionate mind and heart, almost 90 percent of the activities associated with modern civilization would become obsolete. However magnificent modern life appears to be in the realms of material wealth and technological sophistication, it is collapsing from sickness, negativity, and distrust on the inside. The time left to reverse this trend is running out.

The Spread of Degenerative Disease

The following figures give a statistical profile of the current biological and social decline of modern society, as represented by the United States. They are derived from the most recent reports of the American Heart Association, the American Cancer Society, the Centers for Disease Control, and other national medical and public health organizations. The U.S. population is about 235 million.

Aches: 73 percent of Americans suffer from occasional headaches, 50 percent from aches of the back, muscles, and joints, and 27 percent from dental pain.

Alzheimer's Disease: This degenerative disease of the brain cells affects an estimated 1 million persons, usually between the ages of 40 and 70. There is no current medical treatment.

Arthritis: 50 million Americans (about 1 in 4) are affected by arthritis. This includes 7.3 million crippling cases, mostly rheumatoid arthritis. Osteoarthritis, or degenerative joint disease, affects 97 percent of all people over 60. About 250,000 children also suffer from some form of this disease.

Birth Defects: 12.7 million Americans have birth defects. In the last 25 years, the number of children reported born with physical abnormalities, mental retardation, or learning defects has doubled, jumping from 70,000 in the late 1950s to 140,000 in 1983, including about 25,000 babies born each year with congenital heart defects. This represents a jump from 2 percent of babies born with defects to 4 percent.

Cancer: The second leading cause of death in modern society, cancer claims about 440,000 Americans each year. In addition, 850,000 new cases will develop along with another 400,000 cases of usually nonfatal skin cancer. At the turn of the century, the cancer rate was about 1 in 25 persons. By 1950 it had risen to about 1 in 8, and today it will affect nearly 1 in every 3 Americans now living. Lung cancer is rising the most rapidly, while breast cancer will develop in 1 of every 11 women. About 1.5 million biopsies are performed each year.

Cardiovascular Disease: Heart attacks, stroke, and other circulatory disorders are the No. 1 cause of death in modern society, taking 1 in every 2 lives. This has climbed from about 1 death in 9 due to heart and blood vessel disease in 1920. Today 58 million people have high blood pressure, a major risk factor. Each year about 1.5 million Americans have a heart attack, and 550,000 of them will die. Another half million will suffer a stroke, about one third of which are fatal. Surgically, 1.6 million circulatory operations and procedures are performed each year in the United States, including 159,000 bypass grafts, 177,000 pacemaker operations, and 414,000 cardiac catheterizations.

Cerebral Palsy: An estimated 750,000 Americans have this disorder, about 1 in 300.

Diabetes: 11 million Americans currently have diabetes, about 1 in 20. Members of some Indian tribes are 7 to 10 times as likely as non-Indians to contract the disease.

Epilepsy: 2.1 million Americans have epilepsy, about 1 in 100.

Hearing Loss: About a half million Americans are totally deaf. Severe hearing loss in infants appears to have increased dramatically in the early 1980s. The number of cases of profound hearing impairment reported in babies under 18 months rose almost five times between 1982 and 1983.

Kidney Dialysis: Between 1972 and 1982 the number of kidney dialysis patients rose from 10,300 to 82,000.

Mental Illness: At any given time, 29 million Americans—nearly 1 in 5 adults—suffer psychiatric disorders ranging from mildly disabling anxiety to severe schizophrenia. About 5 million of these people seek medical treatment every six months.

Multiple Sclerosis: About half a million Americans have this disorder, about 1 in 450.

Natural Death: More than 70 percent of the population die in modern hospitals. In contrast, at the turn of the century, most people died at home.

Osteoporosis: About 25 percent of all women over 60 will break a bone, due primarily to the degenerative thinning of the bones, which makes them more susceptible to fracture.

Parkinson's Disease: About 1.5 million Americans have this disorder, about 1 in 150.

Polio: Although polio appeared to be wiped out by vaccine in the 1950s, *Post-Polio Sequelae* (Syndrome) is beginning to appear a generation later. 75,000 polio sufferers, representing about 25 percent of those who recovered three decades ago, are now suffering loss of strength in their arms and legs, aches, and exhaustion, and in many cases have had to return to ventilators.

Reproductive Disorders: 1 out of every 5 American couples is infertile. Sperm count in men has dropped 30 to 35 percent since 1920. More than 20 percent of sexually active males are estimated to be sterile. An estimated 40 percent of women have Premenstrual Syndrome (PMS), including 3 percent with severe cases. Forty percent of women have fibroid tumors. Five of the ten most frequent operations are now performed on the female reproduction organs. These 4.2 million operations include nearly 700,000 hysterectomies and 500,000 operations to remove the ovaries, so that by age 60 over half of American women have had their wombs or ovaries removed. Caesarean sections tripled in the 1970s to about 1 in 5 births. The rate of adverse pregnancies among women working at VDTs (video display terminals) increased by 50 percent in the early 1980s.

Sexually Transmitted Diseases: An estimated 30 to 40 million Americans have herpes or other new STD. The number is expected to increase geometrically, with no effective medical prevention and relief at the present time. Syphilis, gonorrhea, and other older venereal diseases affect slightly over 1 million people.

Sterilization: 18 percent of couples of childbearing age avoid pregnancy through voluntary sterilization of either partner, making it the most popular form of birth control. Between 1965 and 1982, female sterilization rose from 7 to 26 percent, while male sterilization rose from 5 to 15 percent.

Surgery: In 1981, 25.6 million medical operations were performed, a 62 percent increase over the previous decade.

Transplants: Each year about 6,000 kidney transplants are performed, 200 pancreas transplants, 175 heart transplants, and 165 liver transplants.

As for viral and bacterial infections, carriers of the herpes virus may well exceed 30 percent of the current adult population in the United States, and cases of older venereal diseases, including syphilis and gonorrhea, are increasing rapidly. Tuberculosis is also rising dramatically. New types of viral diseases such as *Epstein-Barr virus,* which affects an individual's vitality and strength, are spreading rapidly, especially among the younger generation.

The increasing rates of physical and mental disorders of modern civilization have coincided with changing dietary patterns and life-styles. All other major factors, such as the motion of the earth, the movement of the solar system, and other celestial and terrestrial cycles have remained basically unchanged for thousands and perhaps millions of years. The seasons change, day and night cycle, and the ocean currents and tides ebb and flow pretty much the same as they have since human life first began on this planet. In comparison to these large, relatively constant natural factors, humanity's traditional way of eating and way of life have drastically changed, especially during the past several centuries coinciding with the industrial revolution. This change has continued to accelerate during the past seventy years, particularly after the Second World War. These dietary changes are so dramatic that humanity's biological, psychological, and spiritual condition has fundamentally altered, for better or worse, over the last several generations.

The following table summarizes some of the changes in our modern way of eating, according to data collected by the U.S. Department of Agriculture.

Food Changes, 1910–1976
(Per capita annual consumption in pounds unless otherwise noted.)

Food	1910	1976	Change
Egg	305 whole	276 whole	−10%
Meat	136.2	165.2	+21%
Beef	55.5	95.4	+72%
Poultry	18.0	52.9	+194%
Fish	11.4	13.7	+20%
Canned Tuna	.2	3.1 (1974)	+1,300%
Grains	294.0	144.0	−51%
Wheat	214.0	112.0	−48%
Corn	51.1	7.7	−85%
Rice	7.2	7.2	none
Rye	3.6	0.8	−78%
Barley	3.5	1.2	−66%
Oats	3.5	3.5	none
Buckwheat	2.1	0.05	−98%
Beans, Peas	13.0	7.0	−46%
Fresh Vegetables	188.0	144.5	−23%
Fresh Cabbage	23.2 (1920)	8.3 (1965)	−64%
Sweet Potato	22.5	4.4	−80%
Fresh Potato	80.4	48.3	−40%
Frozen Potato	6.6 (1960)	36.8	+457%

Food	1910	1976	Change
Tomato Products	5.0 (1920)	22.4	+348%
Canned Vegetables	12.6 (1920)	53.0	+320%
Frozen Vegetables	.57 (1940)	9.9	+1,650%
Fresh Fruit	123.0	82.0	−33%
Processed Fruit	20.5	134.6	+556%
Grapefruit	1.0	9.0	+800%
Frozen Citrus	1.0 (1948)	117.0	+11,600%
Frozen Foods	3.1 (1940)	88.8	+2,764%
Dairy	320.2	354.3	+11%
Whole Milk	29.3 gal.	21.5 gal.	−27%
Low Fat Milk	6.8 gal.	10.6 gal.	+56%
Cheese	4.9	20.7	+322%
Ice Cream	1.9	18.1	+852%
Frozen Dairy	3.4	50.2	+1,376%
Yogurt	.5 (1967)	2.0	+300%
Margarine	1.5	12.5	+733%
Sweeteners	89.0	134.6	+51%
Corn Syrup	3.8	32.7	+761%
Sugar	73.7 (1909)	94.8	+29%
Soft Drinks	1.1 gal.	30.8 gal.	+2,638%
Saccharine	2.0 (1960)	8.0	+300%
Tea	1.0	0.8	−20%
Coffee	9.2	12.8	+39%
Alcohol	2.69 gal.	2.69 gal.	none
Food Colors	.03 oz. (1940)	.34 oz. (1977)	+995%
Total Food	4.4 per day	4.1 per day	−9%
Calories	3,490″ ″	3,380″ ″	−3%
Protein	102 gms.	103 gms.	+1%
Fat	124 gms.	159 gms.	+28%
Carbohydrate	495 gms.	390 gms.	−21%

Source: U.S. Department of Agriculture statistics summarized in *The Changing American Diet*, published by the Center for Science in the Public Interest and adapted for this chart. Figures do not measure quality, whether organically grown, or naturally processed. For example, the USDA makes no distinction between whole wheat or white refined bread (included in Grain and Wheat categories).

Life-style Changes ─────────────────────────

Among aspects of life-style that have also drastically changed in the modern era, the following artificial factors directly imposed on the human body and mind should also be considered in understanding the background to AIDS:

1. Food and agricultural products have changed in quality from more whole and natural to more refined and partial. In the traditional way of eating, people received fiber, bran, protein, carbohydrates, fat, vitamins, minerals, enzymes, and other nutrients as part of a well-balanced daily diet. Now they receive much of their nourishment in the form of pills, supplements, powders, and extracts and in food that has been fortified with additives or synthetic ingredients. In addition, most modern agricultural products are grown with chemical fertilizers, sprays, and pesticides and treated with additives, preservatives, and other artificial ingredients. Most recently, irradiation of food products has been introduced, further weakening the energy and nutrients of the foods we eat.

2. Cooking sources have shifted from wood, charcoal, coal, gas, and other natural forms of heat to electricity and microwaves.

3. Chemicals produced artificially have become a major part of daily life in food and drinks, cosmetics, cleaning materials, wrapping materials, carpeting, and building and decorative materials that compose exterior and interior environments.

4. Clothing materials have shifted from more natural cotton or vegetable fibers to more synthetic materials used in everything from underwear to outerwear garments.

5. Media have changed from simple daily news materials made of paper to proportionately more use of radio and television, which now encircle the globe and produce a more unnatural, artificial electromagnetic environment.

6. The modern synthetic living environment, especially in cities and other urban areas, has become densely fortified with concrete, metals, and insulation that separates us from the earth and sky and other natural forces that have supported the human race for millions of years.

7. Inoculations and vaccinations, as well as the overuse of various types of drugs and medicines of which the majority are made of artificial chemical materials, have spread throughout modern society. These include the frequent use of antibiotics, X-rays, and routine operations to remove such vital glands and organs as the tonsils, appendix, ovaries, and uterus.

8. To support these extensive changes of life-style, modern education has also shifted toward developing more technicians, experts, intellectuals, and specialists. Knowledge in general is limited only to certain areas of sensory measurement and intellectual development. Modern education has lost the view of humanity as a whole and has become separated from a rich heritage of natural health and well-being, intuitive consciousness and instinctive understanding.

9. Family life has also changed from a natural bond of love and attraction based on biological and spiritual unity to a contractual agreement based on rights, concepts, and legal protection.

Dramatic life-style changes, including but certainly not limited to, the examples listed above, have extensively influenced modern life and consciousness, including prevailing physical and mental conditions. Without understanding the special characteristics of modern civilization that are shaping humanity's biological and spiritual evolution, we cannot discuss any issue affecting present-day human status including health and sickness, happiness and unhappiness, harmony and conflict, compassion and prejudice, peace and war.

The drastic changes of life-style and dietary patterns in modern civilization have contributed to the loss of humanity's natural adaptability to the natural planetary environment, including changes of climate, weather, temperature, humidity, wind, and other atmospheric and celestial influences. They have also accelerated the weakening of humanity's biological and spiritual quality, which is necessary for survival and for continued evolution. Modern civilization—including its life-style and dietary patterns—has undeniably contributed to the possible extinction of the human species on the planet.

In the case of viral and infectious diseases, there is a definite possibility that the majority of the world's population could be wiped out within several decades. If the present trend continues without a revolutionary change of life-style and dietary practice and without deep reflection on the value of modern civilization and our personal way of life, human life as we have known it for thousands and possibly millions of years will come to an end. Various viral activities in our bodily system are directly influenced by our physical, mental, and spiritual condition. Viral activities are especially sensitive to changes in our internal environment —conditions within the body—especially our digestive, respiratory, and circulatory systems.

Like other viral and bacterial infections, the AIDS-related virus is rapidly spreading through modern society. Every year the number of people infected is doubling. And in the urban areas of certain geographical regions which are more suitable for viral activities—those with higher humidity and higher temperatures—the transmission of the virus may double twice a year. Approximately every six months the AIDS virus is doubling in urban regions of Central Africa and in similar environments. This increase is not arithmetic, but either geometrical or logarithmic.

Although estimates vary, it is generally thought by the medical profession that about 2 to 3 million people in the United States now carry the AIDS virus (*HIV* or *Human Immunodeficiency Virus*). In the last several years, it has been demonstrated that the virus can be acquired through heterosexual as well as homosexual contact. The rate of increase is not precisely known. Initial estimates indicated that the number of virus carriers was doubling every year. At this rate, the entire population of the United States would be infected by the end of this century. Of course, the actual situation may not follow this estimate precisely. The speed of increase of the affected number of people may start to curve down in a few years as a result of various factors. These influences may be natural and climatic changes or social and life-style changes, and some portion of the population—possibly less than 30 percent in the case of the United States—may still retain enough natural immunity not to be affected by the virus following exposure.

However, even with conservative estimates, a majority to three-quarters of the population would be infected with the AIDS virus by the end of the twentieth century. Possibly one-third of this number would die within five to seven years after they were infected, and the remaining infected population would gradually succumb in a further five to fifteen years. In other words, the United States, as the representative of modern civilization, could end around the beginning of the next century if current trends continue. During this period, modern social and institutional systems would be seriously affected by the increasing number of infections. Business would collapse, governments would become paralyzed, organizations would dismantle, families decompose, and churches and congregations would disappear. All modern political, economic, social, and cultural systems and functions would inevitably end in chaos. This includes medical and health-care systems because their staff would also be affected.

The tendency toward disaster in the United States would be followed by all other modern countries, including the Soviet Union, Europe, Japan, and Australia, as well as urban areas of Latin America, Africa, the Middle East, and Asia, though there may be a different rate of transmission in each country owing to different natural and social factors. The catastrophe will be particularly severe in some areas, such as the central region of Africa and regions with similar environments and conditions. There the entire population may vanish from one country after another within two to three decades.

On a planetary scale, it can be estimated conservatively that at the present rate, about one-third of the world population may come down with AIDS or an AIDS-related condition and may die out in the early decades of the twenty-first century. In short, we are facing the fall and end of modern civilization and its social and cultural heritage, including all modern intellectual and technological structures and functions. Whatever has a beginning has an end. Medieval civilization declined after the Black Death killed an estimated one-third of the population in Europe. Modern industrial civilization faces a similar collapse.

Are there ways to prevent this vast disaster or any measures to at least avoid the total destruction of modern civilization by controlling the speed and degree of viral infection, which is now spreading unchecked? To answer this question, we must discover why AIDS and related viral and bacterial actions have become active in recent years.

2. Humanity's Natural Immunity

Everything in the universe is constantly appearing and disappearing. It is a basic premise of macrobiotics that there is an order and pattern to this change. All phenomena, without exception, are governed by two primary forces: centrifugal and centripetal energy, expansion and contraction, decomposition and composition, yin and yang.

The universal principles governing all phenomena can be summarized as follows:

1. Everything changes.
2. Changes take place between two antagonistic and complementary forces or tendencies.
3. To maintain the existence of every phenomenon, both forces or tendencies always coexist in harmony.
4. Opposite forces or tendencies tend to attract each other.
5. The same or similar forces or tendencies tend to repel each other.
6. To maintain its existence, if one force or tendency in a phenomenon becomes larger, the opposite force or tendency also becomes larger. If it becomes smaller, the opposite also becomes smaller.
7. When a certain force or tendency becomes extreme, a phenomenon changes its existence and produces the opposite force or tendency.

In the relative world, these universal principles of balance and harmony govern all natural occurrences as well as all biological phenomena, including human affairs and physical, mental, spiritual, social, cultural, and philosophical matters. This means that to maintain and develop humanity on this planet, there are natural limits to human life-style and behavior within any given natural environment. In the event human life-style and behavior exceed this natural limitation, then humanity's existence necessarily changes. The natural limitations encompassing human existence and development take two forms. For example:

1. Either extreme activity or no activity causes cessation of existence.
2. Either extreme overconsumption of food or prolonged fasting causes cessation of existence.

3. Either extreme high temperature or low temperature causes cessation of existence.

4. Either extreme stress or absence of stimulation causes cessation of existence.

5. Either extreme mental activity or absence of mental activity causes cessation of existence.

There are many other natural limitations or boundaries that serve to maintain existence and achieve continuous development of humanity on this planet.

From this view of natural limitation, we reach an understanding that beings living in modern society have exceeded natural limitations and lack comprehensive awareness of the factors and conditions necessary for continued existence. Because viral and bacterial infection—or natural immune deficiency—is a biological phenomenon, not a social phenomenon like war or group violence, there must be some human factors violating this biological order.

Factors supporting the biological status of humanity can be divided into two broad groups.

1. External environment and stimuli
   A. *Natural:* Movement of the universe, galaxies, and solar systems, and the planet earth. Natural atmospheric and oceanic influences; seasonal and climatic changes including temperature, humidity, and pressures; and other natural influences.
   B. *Human-made:* Civilizational and cultural influence, social structures and conditions, economical and community influences, human relations, occupational and professional stimuli, technological and artificial influences, transportation and communications stimuli, and all other human-made surroundings and their stimuli.
2. Internal environment and stimuli
   A. *Natural:* The various systems and functions of the body and mind including the digestive system, the circulatory system, the nervous system, the excretory system, the skeletal and muscular system, the *meridians* or pathways of natural electromagnetic energy, and all other organs, glands, and channels associated with our physical, mental, and spiritual constitution. The food, drink, waves, rays, and other incoming substances and vibrations that are received, digested, absorbed,

transmuted, and discharged by the above systems and functions.

B. Human-made: Physical, mental, psychological, spiritual, and social images, thoughts, actions, influences, and other impulses and movements generated from within and governed by our higher consciousness centers or autonomic nervous system.

What the human body takes in from the external environment changes and is transformed into the internal environment. Energies coming from the universe and atmosphere are running through meridians—channels of electromagnetic energy in the body—and are distributed to every cell. Conscious images are also carried through the meridians and charge each cell. What we eat and drink forms our cells and nourishes them with various nutrients and natural electromagnetic energy. This nourishment is carried through the digestive and circulatory systems and is distributed to all cells.

This internal environment, though its sources come from outside in the external environment, is largely shaped and controlled by personal freedom. What kind of food, how it is prepared, and how much is consumed all depend on personal choice. Except during times of extreme scarcity or other unusual conditions, free consciousness is exercised completely in respect to what we eat and drink. Accordingly, the internal environment differs among individual people, while external environmental stimuli are more or less common to everyone.

Among the factors supporting humanity on this planet, individual differences—physical, mental, spiritual, and social—are largely dependent upon factors producing the internal environment, especially what we eat and drink daily, upon which everyone exercises his or her free consciousness. Accordingly, to solve the problem of why a certain group of people can be easily infected by an infectious virus or bacterium, while another group is not easily affected, we have to review differences in dietary practice. Of course, we must consider whether the way of eating in any given environment is suitable for existence and development under the prevailing external conditions and stimuli. Certain dietary practices may be more suitable than others, while others may not be suitable for sustaining and supporting life at all.

The macrobiotic view of dietary practice, which considers food as a natural means of adapting, maintaining, and developing humanity, observes the following principles:

1.   Respect for traditional dietary practices followed by many genera-

tions in a given area because these have been securing, maintaining, and developing humanity in that particular natural setting for thousands of years.

2. Respect for the traditional way of preparation and cooking which has been exercised for centuries in a particular natural environment for similar reasons.

3. Respect for the food, ways of natural preparation, and cooking that developed in natural environments and climates similar to our own. This concept enables us to avoid exceeding natural limitations, which are violated when we adopt too much food or drink, ways of preparation, or cooking methods from environments and climates different or opposite to our own.

If we review modern dietary practice, especially in the latter part of the twentieth century, we find that the above principles are constantly violated. These violations may be summarized briefly as follows:

1. Abandonment of whole food through refining, milling, and other processing techniques.

2. Adoption of artificial, chemicalized agriculture and abandonment of naturally and organically grown food.

3. Overconsumption of simple sugars with a decrease in the consumption of complex sugars.

4. Overconsumption of animal-quality protein with decreased consumption of vegetable-quality protein.

5. Overconsumption of saturated fat, largely of animal quality, and decreased consumption of unsaturated fat of vegetable quality.

6. Lack of natural vitamins resulting from the increased refinement of naturally grown products and the waste of edible and traditionally consumed parts of vegetable foods.

7. Lack of consumption of natural dietary fiber due to food processing, including refining and milling.

8. Disorderly consumption of minerals by the refining of salts and other food products, as well as the overuse of chemical fertilizers, insecticides, preservatives, and colorings.

9. Disorderly use of natural enzymes by artificially altering traditional methods of food processing, including fermentation and pickling.

10. Shift from family cooking to the industrial and commercial preparation of food, which also standardizes the way of eating and preparation regardless of regional, seasonal, climatic, and personal differences.

Together with these characteristics of modern dietary practice, various kinds of degenerative diseases have spread throughout modern society. These include cardiovascular disorders, cancer, allergies, arthritis, diabetes, hypoglycemia, skin diseases, osteoporosis, obesity, reproductive and gynecological problems, and many other physical illnesses as well as schizophrenia, paranoia, depression, stress, anxieties, and many other mental and psychological disorders.

To change dietary practice in a more healthy direction, one that is in harmony with the natural environment, the following guidelines may be observed:

1. Food should be more naturally and organically grown, avoiding or minimizing various artificial chemicals in production, cultivation, and processing.

2. The majority of food is to be grown and produced in the same climatic and geographical region where the people who eat it are living. In the event transportation of food from a distance is necessary, this food should come from similar climatic belts and natural environments.

3. Food is to be consumed in whole form as much as possible except for the inedible portion which may be set aside. Refining of food is to be avoided. Whole food secures more balance of nutrients, including fiber, minerals, vitamins, and other necessary components, than food that is processed or consumed in parts.

4. The majority of food is to be vegetable quality rather than animal quality, except for dietary practice in the poorer regions of the world or in cold climates in temperate or polar regions. The main source of food is to originate from the plant kingdom.

5. Animal food, if consumed, is to be lower in hard, saturated fat and cholesterol, and amount to less than 15 percent of total daily food consumption. In poorer or colder regions the percentage may be slightly higher.

6. Carbohydrates are to be taken more in the form of complex sugars (such as those found in whole cereal grains) rather than simple sugars (such as those found in dairy products, fruits, and sweeteners).

7. Protein is to come from more vegetable and plant sources and less from animal sources.

8. Fat should come more from vegetable and plant sources and be more unsaturated in quality and less from animal sources and be less saturated in quality.

9. Minerals should be consumed as a part of whole-food items. In addition, naturally processed unrefined sea salt, which consists of many trace minerals beside sodium chloride, should be used in cooking.

10. Vitamins should be consumed as a part of whole foods and not be taken separately as a supplement.

11. Enzymes should be consumed as a part of daily foods including fermented and pickled food and not be taken separately as an enzyme supplement.

12. Beverages are based upon natural spring or well water and non-stimulant, nonaromatic beverages traditionally and widely used.

Guidelines for the Preparation and Cooking of Food ———

In processing food from its natural form to an edible form, observe methods traditionally practiced over centuries using more natural energies. The natural energies applied to food processing include:

1. Drying under the sun or in the shade without direct exposure to solar energy.
2. Soaking in natural water.
3. Applying pressure and weight.
4. Pickling with sea salt.
5. Smoking by wood fire or charcoal.

6. Fermenting under natural atmospheric conditions, for hours, days, weeks, months, and in some cases several years depending on the kinds of food products and the strength desired.

7. Milling by motion of natural stone or hardwood.

8. Pressing with comparatively low temperatures.

9. Cooking with natural water and fire made of wood, charcoal, or gas.

10. Roasting slowly with a moderate fire produced by wood, charcoal, or gas.

These natural food-processing methods are found in most parts of the world and have been perfected over the centuries by many traditional civilizations and cultures. They all avoid the use of destructive, explosive energies and quick energetic and molecular change of food components such as we find in modern food processing techniques and in electrical and microwave cooking. Moderate transformation of food quality using more natural forces is the essential principle of traditional, healthy, natural food processing. In order to maintain a food's integrity—including its genuine energy, quality, and balance of nutrients—traditional methods of food processing are far superior to quick processing techniques utilizing high technology and applying highly unnatural, violent forces.

Considering the above guidelines, it is recommended that the actual dietary practice in the temperate regions of the world—including most of North America, the southern part of South America, Europe, the Far East, most of Central Asia, Australia and New Zealand—be as follows:

Daily Dietary Recommendations

1. *Whole cereal grains.* At least 50 percent by volume of every meal is recommended to include cooked, organically grown, whole cereal grains prepared in a variety of ways. Whole cereal grains include brown rice, barley, millet, oats, corn, rye, wheat, and buckwheat. Please note that a small portion of this amount may consist of noodles or pasta, unyeasted whole grain breads, and other partially processed whole cereal grains.

2. *Soups.* Approximately 5 to 10 percent of your daily food intake may include soup made with vegetables, sea vegetables (wakame or kombu), grains or beans. Seasonings are usually miso or tamari soy sauce. The flavor should not be too salty.

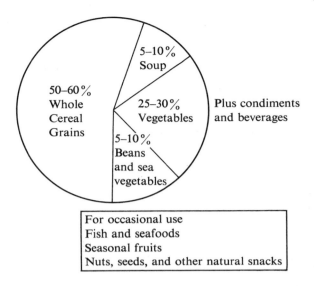

For occasional use
Fish and seafoods
Seasonal fruits
Nuts, seeds, and other natural snacks

3. *Vegetables.* About 20 to 30 percent of daily intake may include local and organically grown vegetables. Preferably, the majority are cooked in various styles (e.g., sautéed with a small amount of sesame or corn oil, steamed, boiled and sometimes prepared using tamari soy sauce or light sea salt as a seasoning). A small portion may be eaten as raw salad. Pickled vegetables without spice may also be used daily in small volume.

Vegetables for daily use include green cabbage, kale, broccoli, cauliflower, collards, pumpkin, watercress, Chinese cabbage, bok choy, dandelion, mustard greens, daikon greens, scallion, onions, daikon, turnips, acorn squash, butternut squash, buttercup squash, burdock, carrots, and other seasonally available varieties.

Avoid potatoes (including sweet potatoes and yams), tomatoes, eggplant, peppers, asparagus, spinach, beets, zucchini, and avocado for regular use. Mayonnaise and other oily dressings should be avoided.

4. *Beans and Sea Vegetables.* Approximately 5 to 10 percent of our daily diet includes cooked beans and sea vegetables. The most suitable beans for regular use are azuki beans, chick-peas, and lentils. Other beans may be used on occasion. Bean products such as tofu, tempeh, and natto can also be used. Sea vegetables such as nori, wakame, kombu, hijiki, arame, dulse, agar-agar, and Irish moss may be prepared in a variety of ways. They can be cooked with beans or vegetables, used in soups, or served separately as side dishes, flavored with a moderate amount of

tamari soy sauce, sea salt, brown rice vinegar, umeboshi plum, umeboshi vinegar, and others.

5. *Occasional Foods.* If needed or desired, 1 to 3 times per week, approximately 5 to 10 percent of that day's consumption of food can include fresh white-meat fish such as flounder, sole, cod, carp, halibut or trout.

Fruit or fruit desserts, including fresh, dried, and cooked fruits, may also be served two or three times a week. Local and organically grown fruits are preferred. If you live in a temperate climate, avoid tropical and semi-tropical fruit and eat, instead, temperate climate fruits such as apples, pears, plums, peaches, apricots, berries, and melons. Frequent use of fruit juice is not advisable. However, occasional consumption in warmer weather may be appropriate depending on your health.

Lightly roasted nuts and seeds such as pumpkin, sesame, and sunflower seeds, peanuts, walnuts, and pecans may be enjoyed as a snack.

Rice syrup, barley malt, amasake, and mirin may be used as a sweetener; brown rice vinegar or umeboshi vinegar may be used occasionally for a sour taste.

6. *Beverages.* Recommended daily beverages include roasted bancha twig tea, stem tea, roasted brown rice tea, roasted barley tea, dandelion tea, and cereal grain coffee. Any traditional tea that does not have an aromatic fragrance or a stimulating effect can be used. You may also drink a moderate amount of water (preferably spring or well water of good quality) but not iced.

7. *Foods to Eliminate for Better Health.* Meat, animal fat, eggs, poultry, dairy products (including butter, yogurt, ice cream, milk, and cheese), refined sugars, chocolate, molasses, honey, other simple sugars and foods treated with them, and vanilla.

Tropical or semi-tropical fruits and fruit juices, soda, artificial drinks and beverages, coffee, colored tea, and all aromatic stimulating teas such as mint or peppermint tea.

All artificially colored, preserved, sprayed or chemically treated foods. All refined and polished grains, flours, and their derivatives. Mass-produced industrialized food including all canned, frozen, and irradiated foods.

Hot spices, any aromatic stimulating food or food accessory, artificial vinegar, and strong alcoholic beverages.

8. *Additional Suggestions.* Cooking oil should be vegetable quality only. To improve your health, it is preferable to use only unrefined sesame or corn oil in moderate amounts.

• Salt should be naturally processed sea salt. Traditional, non-chemicalized *shoyu* or tamari soy sauce and miso may also be used as seasonings.

• Recommendable condiments include:

—Gomashio (12–18 parts roasted sesame seeds to 1 part roasted sea salt)

—Sea-vegetable powder (kelp, kombu, wakame, and other sea vegetables)

—Sesame sea-vegetable powder

—Umeboshi plums

—Tekka

—Tamari soy sauce or shoyu (moderate use, use only in cooking for mild flavoring).

—Pickles (made using bran, miso, tamari soy sauce, salt), sauerkraut.

• You may have meals regularly, 2–3 times per day, as much as you want, provided the proportion is correct and chewing is thorough. Avoid eating for approximately 3 hours before sleeping.

The Importance of Cooking. Proper cooking is very important for health. Everyone should learn to cook either by attending classes or under the guidance of an experienced macrobiotic cook. The recipes included in macrobiotic cookbooks may also be used in planning your meals.

Special Advice.

• The guidelines presented above are general suggestions. These suggestions may require modification depending on your special condition. Of course, any serious condition should be closely monitored by the appropriate medical, nutritional, and health professional.

• Along with beginning to change your diet, we invite you to attend any of our regular study programs or seminars and to meet personally with a qualified macrobiotic counselor as well as attend cooking classes.

These guidelines are intended to supplement your consultation with a medical or nutritional professional or personal guidance received from a qualified macrobiotic teacher.

In the case of semitropical and tropical regions—including Central America, the northern part of South America, the central part of Africa, the Middle East, India, South Asia, and most of the Pacific Islands—the actual dietary guidelines can follow those recommended in the *Message to the Government Aids symposium in Brazzaville, People's Republic of the Congo*, prepared by Michio Kushi.

YIN Energy Creates:	*YANG Energy Creates:*
Growth in a hot climate	Growth in a cold climate
More rapid growth	Slower growth
Foods containing more water	Drier foods
Fruits and leaves, which are more nurtured by expanding energies	Stems, roots, and seeds, which are more nurtured by contracting energies
Growth upward high above the ground	Growth downward below ground
Sour, bitter, sharply sweet, hot, and aromatic foods	Salty, plainly sweet, and pungent foods

Plant Growth According to Yin and Yang

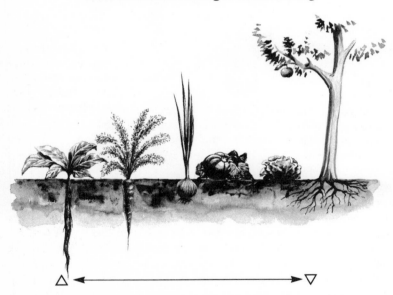

Natural order governs the plant kingdom. Foods that are condensed and grow below ground such as burdock, carrot, and other root vegetables are yang, those that are expanded and grow on the ground such as onion and squash are more balanced, and those that grow above ground such as kale are yin. Fruits that grow high above the ground are even more yin.

Seasonal Diet

Summer: More corn, long-grain rice, more greens, summer fruits, bitter tasting foods.

Spring: Slightly more greens; more wheat, oats, barley, sour tasting foods.

Less salt

Summer

Shorter cooking

Spring   Seasonal Diet   Autumn

Longer cooking

Winter

More salt

Autumn: More round and root vegetables, more short grain rice and millet, autumn fruits, sweet and pungent tasting foods.

Winter: More root vegetables, buckwheat and rice more often, and easily stored and dried fruits.

These dietary recommendations not only satisfy modern nutritional requirements but they are also effective in helping to prevent and lower risk factors associated with major degenerative diseases including heart disease, hypertension, cancer, allergies, arthritis, diabetes, hypoglycemia, and many others, as well as reproductive and gynecological problems and various types of mental, psychological, and emotional instability.

Further, these dietary guidelines may also be helpful in recovering and developing natural immunity against viral and bacterial infection. The reason why viral and bacterial infections spread within a single body, in addition to being transmitted from one body to another, is that the person or persons involved already have weakened natural immunity. Immune factors do not exist separately from comprehensive health conditions. Immune factors are the result of the healthy functioning of all major organs, glands, blood, lymphatic body fluids, hormones, digestive liquid and enzymes, together with sound skeletal, nervous, muscular, and skin functions of the entire body.

Strong immunity to disease—including protection against viral and bacterial infection—is a natural function of a healthy physical and mental human condition, and deficiency of natural immunity is the result of an unhealthy, degenerative human condition. Accordingly, any approach focusing exclusively on isolating a certain virus or bacterium cannot solve the problem of AIDS and related symptoms, though they may be affected temporarily by suppressing infectious agents. The solution lies within a comprehensive approach to recovering total health, including physical mental, and spiritual health and well-being. It is achieved by correcting modern life-styles and dietary habits that are in violation of natural limits or natural order and by changing toward a more natural and healthy way of life and way of eating.

Humanity's Natural Immunity

The purpose of the immune system is to maintain personal existence and to develop an individual's biological and spiritual quality under ever-changing environmental conditions. Natural immunity is the function most directly connected with exercising universal principles of natural order. It works constantly according to laws of attraction and repulsion. It also works with expansion and contraction, decomposition and composition, the process of evolution and the process of degeneration, and the process of forming and the process of decaying.

Human natural immunity includes the following functions:

1. Adaptation to the environment.
2. Maintenance of existence.
3. Continuous biological and spiritual evolution, especially involving the quality and scope of consciousness.

To secure these functions, human natural immunity has an eight-fold constitution. This includes:

1. *Intuition and Instinct.* When a new factor is introduced into our environment, intuitive and instinctive judgment are the primary levels that immediately act or react to this influence. They do so by adapting to the new factor by changing ourselves, or by rejecting and avoiding the new factor. Intuitive and instinctive judgment are constantly at work in

the selection of our place of residence, our partners and friends, our occupations and habits, and numerous occasions and conditions of daily life. Avoidance of danger, caution of abrupt, dramatic change, and seeking a middle way between extremes are all manifestations of intuitive and instinctive judgment. Without these functions, human life cannot be maintained and developed, and human identity would vanish.

2. *Consciousness.* Human consciousness includes several levels, namely, the sensory, emotional, intellectual, social, and ideological levels. In the exercise of this consciousness, and levels work through the processes of discrimination, selection, and attraction or repulsion. For example, consciousness functions to make distinctions in the following ways:

A. The sensory level—pleasure and pain.
B. The emotional level—love and hate.
C. The intellectual level—reason and unreason.
D. The social level—harmony and disharmony.
E. The ideological level—justice and injustice.

Through the exercise of this judgment, natural selection involving attraction or repulsion, and absorption or expulsion, are constantly being made for certain tendencies, objects, behaviors, or persons. As long as these levels of consciousness are working, extremes can be avoided without exposing us to danger.

3. *Autonomic Response.* In addition to the central nervous system, which mainly serves to produce and exercise consciousness, autonomic nerves—sympathetic and parasympathetic—function to react immediately to surrounding stimuli. Depending upon the kind of stimulus, sympathetic nerves control the immediate contraction of certain organs and glands as well as parts of the body. For an opposite type of stimulus, parasympathetic nerves produce an opposite reaction causing certain organs and glands to expand. For example, the pupil dilates in darkness and it contracts in bright light through this autonomic nerve response.

When the sympathetic nerve operates, the stomach expands and the connected sphincter contracts, while the parasympathetic nerve acts to contract the stomach and expand the sphincter. Through autonomic control, the necessary balance and harmony with the stimulus can be maintained for preserving and supporting the life of the organism.

4. *Body Surface Protection and Reaction.* For physical and chemical invasion and stimuli, the skin functions to protect the inner environment and reacts by contraction and expansion according to the nature of the stimuli. In cold temperature, for example, the skin becomes dry and shrinks, while in warmer temperature it becomes more moist and expands. When a physical shock is given to a certain part of the body surface, immediate reaction is experienced on the skin. More blood, especially white-blood cells and lymphatic liquid, gathers, often resulting in swelling of that portion of the skin. Further, slightly salty alkaline moisture secreted by sweat glands protects the body from invasion of acid poison. The body surface also acts to expel toxins and unnecessary energies from the inside of the body to the surface. These discharges often appear as various types of skin disease and discolorations, as well as skin cancer.

5. *Internal Liquid Protection.* Through digestive functions, alkaline liquid and acid liquid are alternatively secreted in the body in the form of digestive liquids. First food is subjected to the action of saliva (alkaline) in the mouth. Then stomach liquid (acid) is secreted, followed by liver and gallbladder biles and pancreatic juice (alkaline). Finally, metabolized foodstuffs are readied for absorption in the small intestine by intestinal juice (acid). These digestive liquids minimize and neutralize poisonous chemical and biological factors, including the undesirable action of microorganisms, in addition to normal food decomposition and digestive functions. Proper chewing facilitates the immune process. The more we chew, the more saliva is produced. Saliva accelerates these protective functions, enhancing other digestive secretions and related nervous activities.

Further, immunoglobulin A (IGA) existing in the internal fluids secreted throughout the digestive system (and in other systems such as the reproductive system) as well as in intercellular fluids can act as a protective agent from poisonous substances that have entered from outside the body or that have been produced inside the body. The protective functions of IGA in the mouth cavity together with saliva and in the wall surface around and in between numerous villi in the small intestine are especially active in neutralizing and minimizing the undesirable activities of viruses, bacteria, and other microorganisms.

6. *Blood and Intercellular Fluid Protection and Reaction.* Within the bloodstream, there are constant balancing mechanisms and buffer actions to neutralize strong toxic acid compounds, changing them to weak acids through the mobilization of minerals in the body. These minerals

are normally supplied in the daily diet, but if additional minerals are required for this buffer action, stored minerals are used. As a result, weakening of the bones often arises following the consumption of excessive amounts of acid-producing foods such as meat, dairy, and sugar. In children, this is the chief cause of tooth decay. In older people, chronic weakening of the bones from improper diet can lead to a potentially crippling condition known as osteoporosis.

Further, white-blood cells act as protection from undesirable viral and bacterial invasion. White-blood cells known as *lymphocytes* have various kinds of cells, such as B-cells and T-cells. These cells coordinate the maintenance of normal conditions by either neutralizing or harmonizing the poisonous effects of invading viruses or other microorganisms. Among their functions there are antagonistic-complemental relations constantly working as well-known helpers and suppressors. Among the group of T-cells, antagonistic-complemental relations between T4 cells and T8 cells are one of the balancing and harmonizing activities relating to undesirable viruses and microorganisms.

Because lymphocytes can exist within the body's intercellular fluids— that is, outside the bloodstream—these actions also arise within this location.

In addition, when foreign substances such as undesirable viruses or bacteria enter the blood and intercellular fluids, antagonistic and complementary factors can naturally be produced. These are called antibodies. The purpose of antigen production is to balance and harmonize foreign substances and maintain continuous body functions. Accordingly, the presence of antibodies can be an indication of the activity of undesirable viruses or other microorganisms within the individual.

7. *Lymphatic Protection.* After the blood and intercellular fluids nourish various body cells, they are collected in the lymph system. A great number of *lymph nodes* form a network throughout the body for cleaning undesirable wastes. If the collected fluids contain a great amount of undesirable poisonous wastes, various kinds of minerals are mobilized into the lymph nodes to make drastic action or cleaning. This action often results in the swelling of the lymph nodes. If such poisonous effects continue for some period, chronic swelling of lymph nodes and the spleen and ineffectiveness in the function of the lymphatic system arises as in the case of lymphoma.

In connection with this function, the surgical removal of some important lymph nodes such as the tonsils also directly contributes to the inefficiency of lymphatic functions and a general weakening of the natural immune system.

8. *Cellular Protection.* Each cell of the human body has its own protective function to maintain its identity and existence. *Cell membranes* act for direct protection from undesirable physical stimuli and chemical invasion. Firm bondage of several elements in DNA and RNA are not easily impaired unless the power of foreign substances and stimuli far exceeds the protective mechanism. Cell membranes and intercellular fluids also serve to protect the nucleus of the cell.

Each cell is constantly rejuvenated by the energy and nutrients that are being supplied through blood and intercellular fluids. Accordingly, if the quality of blood and intercellular fluids changes substantially, the quality of cells also inevitably changes. Such changes arise not only in the cell membrane and intercellular fluids, but also possibly in the nucleus of the cell.

These eight aspects of natural immunity do not function completely independently. Each acts to ensure its integrity, and yet all are inter-related and united as a whole. The decline of natural immunity—or AIDS—is not the result of a sudden failure, defect, or ineffectiveness in one or more of these immune functions. It is the result of partial or total failure or decay of all of them, usually over a period of time.

The primary origin of natural immune deficiency is cloudiness in intuition and instinct. The decline of intuitive and instinctive judgment causes us to observe abnormal life-styles and dietary practices that exceed the natural limitations of our environment, climate, constitution, or condition. Adopting imbalanced ways of life and eating, in turn, results in the further decay and weakening of other levels of the natural immune system.

While the primary origin of immune deficiency is the decline of intuitive-instinctive response, the biological cause of natural immunity is improper dietary habits. In other words, when intuitive-instinctive judgment is not exercised naturally in our daily eating, the decline of our natural immunity begins, and harmful viruses and bacteria in our environment can easily affect either some or all of the systems of the body.

The energy and nutrients of the food we eat day to day creates, nourishes, and governs the quality and volume of blood and intercellular fluids, the quality of lymphatic fluids, and the quality of organs, tissues, and cells as well as their functions. Daily food largely shapes and determines our destiny in life. It is the major factor determining whether our natural immunity to infectious disease remains strong or weakens and decays.

3. The Dietary Causes of Natural Immune Deficiency

To understand the dietary cause of natural immune deficiency, it is convenient to classify food and modern eating habits into two general groupings:

1. *The Yin Category.* Foods that produce a result or tendency toward expansion, decomposition, softening, loosening, and other similar effects of the muscles, tissues, organs, glands, and their functions.

2. *The Yang Category.* Foods that produce a result or tendency toward contraction, composition, hardening, gathering, and other similar effects of the muscles, tissues, organs, glands, and their functions.

The following chart illustrates examples from the vegetable and animal kingdoms.

Yin and Yang in the Vegetable Kingdom

	Yin ($\triangle$) Centrifugal	Yang (∇) Centripetal
Environment:	Warmer, more tropical	Colder, more polar
Season:	Grows more in spring and summer	Grows more in autumn and winter
Soil:	More watery and sedimentary	More dry and volcanic
Growing direction:	Vertically growing upward; expanding horizontally underground	Vertically growing downward; expanding horizontally above the ground
Growing speed:	Growing faster	Growing slower
Size:	Larger, more expanded	Smaller more compacted

	Yin (△) Centrifugal	Yang (▽) Centripetal
Height:	Taller	Shorter
Texture:	Softer	Harder
Water content:	More juicy and watery	More dry
Color:	Purple—blue—green—yellow—brown—orange—red	
Odor:	Stronger smell	Less smell
Taste:	Spicy—sour—sweet—salty—bitter	
Chemical components:	More K and other yin elements	Less K and other yin elements
	Less Na and other yang elements	More Na and other yang elements
Nutritional components:	Fat—protein—carbohydrate—mineral	
Cooking time:	Faster cooking	Slower cooking

Yin and Yang in the Animal Kingdom

	Yin (▽) Centrifugal	Yang (△) Centripetal
Environment:	Warmer and more tropical; also in warm current	Colder and more polar; also in cold current
Air humidity:	More humid	More dry
Species:	Generally more ancient	Generally more modern
Size:	Larger, more expanded	Smaller, more compacted
Activity:	Slower moving and more inactive	Faster moving and more active
Body temperature:	Colder	Warmer
Texture:	Softer, more watery and oily	Harder and drier
Color of flesh:	Transparent—white—brown—pink—red—black	
Odor:	More odor	Less odor
Taste:	Putrid—sour—sweet—salty—bitter	

	Yin (▽) Centrifugal	Yang (△) Centripetal
Chemical components:	Less sodium (Na) and other yang elements	More sodium (Na) and other yang elements
Nutritional components:	Fat....Protein........Minerals	
Cooking time:	Shorter	Longer

YIN Energy Creates:	YANG Energy Creates:
Growth in a hot climate	Growth in a cold climate
More rapid growth	Slower growth
Foods containing more water	Drier foods
Fruits and leaves, which are more nurtured by expanding energies	Stems, roots, and seeds, which are more nurtured by contracting energies
Growth upward high above the ground	Growth downward below ground
Sour, bitter, sharply sweet, hot, and aromatic foods	Salty, plainly sweet, and pungent foods

Of course, all foods are composed of both yin and yang characteristics but in different proportions. This categorization is a general rather than an absolute one, and varies depending upon the environment. In the modern way of eating, foods producing extreme yin or yang tendencies are customarily served or prepared together. Though they make a rough balance, they are often too extreme for daily eating. Examples include:

Poultry and sweets
Meat and potatoes
Meat and black pepper and other spices
Turkey and cranberry sauce, herbs, and gravy
Lamb and mint jelly
Ham and pineapple and cloves
Beef and garlic
Clams and horseradish
Hamburger and catsup and raw onions
Hotdog and mustard

Eggs and mayonnaise and raw onions
Shrimp and tomato sauce
Fish and lemon and oil
Lobster and escargo and butter and garlic
Cheese and tomatoes
Cheese and wine
Bacon and eggs and citrus fruit and citrus juices

In general overconsumption of animal food attracts sweets, stimulants, spices, oils, soft drinks, fruit and fruit juices, as well as *nightshade plants* such as potato, tomato, eggplant, and green and red peppers. Similarly, baked flour products attract sweets, oily spreads, and aromatic beverages, as well as more liquid including milk and beer.

These attempts to harmonize extremes often cannot achieve comprehensive balance and harmony in the long run and inevitably lead to disease and disorder at many levels. On the other hand, a macrobiotic way of eating based on a traditional diet centered around whole cereal grains and vegetables, supplemented with beans and legumes, fresh vegetables prepared in various ways, sea vegetables, and occasional consumption of fish and seafood, seasonal fruits, seeds and nuts, as well as nonstimulant beverages, can easily achieve more comprehensive harmony of nutrients, energies, and other factors contributing to physical health, mental well-being, and spiritual development.

Food can further be categorized into two groups of *acid-producing foods* and *alkaline-producing foods*. Examples include:

Acid-Producing Food	*Alkaline-Producing Food*
Food containing more simple sugars, protein, and fat	Food containing more complex sugars, less protein and fat
Food containing less fiber and minerals in general	Food containing more fiber and minerals in general
Food containing more water-soluble vitamins	Food containing more alcohol-soluble vitamins

A daily diet composed of rich animal meat, dairy food, sugar, fruits, refined products, and oily, greasy food, together with frequent consumption of tropical fruits, soft drinks, and aromatic, stimulant beverages —in other words, the modern way of eating—produces a more acidic condition within the body. On the other hand, traditional dietary practice consisting of whole unrefined grains, cooked vegetables, beans and their products, sea vegetables, and other natural foods seasoned with sea-salt-based condiments and accompanied by nonstimulant beverages tend to produce a more alkaline condition in the body.

Weakened Organs Contributing to Immune Deficiency ——

According to our careful observation since the beginning of the AIDS epidemic, people who have weakened their natural immunity and are susceptible to the activity of viruses and bacteria share the same general dietary tendencies. These tendencies are:

1. Consuming a great amount of sweets, including food containing sugar, chocolate, carob, honey, and chemical sweeteners.

2. Consuming a great amount of fruits and fruit juices, including such tropical fruits as banana, papaya, mango, avocado, kiwi fruit, and others.

3. Consuming a great amount of dairy products, especially milk, yogurt, cream, butter, ice cream, and food products containing them.

4. Consuming refined flour products, including refined white flour, yeasted bread, and other baked products.

5. Frequent consumption of nightshade plants such as tomato, potato, eggplant, and peppers, as well as plants that originated in a tropical climate.

6. Consuming a great deal of oily and fatty food products, including salad dressing, spreads, sauces, and deep-fried foods.

7. Frequent consumption of soft drinks and sparkling carbonated waters.

The items in these seven categories all fall more within the category of extreme yin foods and beverages. They produce expanding, decomposing, loosening, and weakening results in various organs and glands and their functions. At the same time, these foods generate overwhelming acid-producing conditions in the body.

Because of the chronic consumption of these foods in excessive amounts, the following physical disorders arise:

1. *Intestinal Weakness.* The intestinal tract tends to become expanded and loose. Stagnation of bowel movements and sometimes constipation, but often diarrhea, and gas-formation occur. Associated symptoms, such as colitis, may also appear, causing discomfort and suffering. Further, the activity of microorganisms in the intestines becomes chaotic, and their natural synthesizing function of necessary nutrients, including the important vitamin-B group, becomes deficient. A lack of the vitamin-B group further creates various disorders in body functions, including loss of clear judgment.

Further, weakened intestines cannot absorb food molecules effectively through the villi. This results in the deterioration of blood components including lymphocytes and other elements of the immune system. In addition, these extreme foods make the condition of the inside of the intestines abnormally acidic and leads to the formation of excess mucus and fatty acid. Parasites and other undesirable microorganisms including harmful viruses and bacteria thrive in this weakened internal environment and multiply rapidly.

2. *Liver Infection, Hepatitis, and Mononucleosis.* At some point, with or without conscious awareness, a liver infection occurs, often accompanied by fever. Chronic weakness of the liver and its various functions often continues for a long period despite medical treatment. When the liver is impaired, its primary function of storing excess nourishment in the form of *glycogen* and supplying stored nourishment to the bloodstream when required cannot work well. As a result, overeating becomes more frequent. Foods rich in sweets and easily digested foods are especially craved.

3. *Lymphatic Disorder.* In coordination with intestinal disorders and weakened liver function, the function of the spleen and its related lymphatic network tends to become chaotic. Spleen functions become weak, and the organ tends to enlarge. Lymph nodes also become swollen, and their function of cleansing poisonous waste from the lymphatic stream remains impaired. Because of the lack of minerals resulting from excessive consumption of the above mentioned foodstuffs, malfunction of the lymphatic system occurs. The symptoms of *lymphoma*— a cancerous condition of the lymphatic system—are often produced as a result.

4. *Weakening of Respiratory Function.* Weakening of the respiratory function results from the excessive consumption of foods in the extreme yin category and acid-forming foods. Sound respiratory functions become hindered. These foods also produce mucus, and fatty acid also gathers in the lungs. Symptoms of pneumonia or similar feverish disorders tend to occur occasionally or chronically. Breathing difficulties with accompanying fever are also often present.

Weakening of respiratory function interferes with the smooth supply of oxygen (O_2) to the red-blood cells and the proper elimination of carbon dioxide (CO_2). Disorders in blood components, including red-blood cells, white-blood cells, blood platelets, and blood plasma can result from respiratory disorder or from impairment of the intestinal, liver, and lymphatic functions. In any case, the condition of the blood and intercellular fluids worsens.

5. *Pancreatic Disorders.* One of the primary reasons for craving sweets, fruits, and other soothing foods in excessive amounts is due to chronic pancreatic disorder. The pancreas secretes two hormones, *insulin* and *anti-insulin.* Impairment in insulin secretion can lead to diabetes, while impairment in anti-insulin can lead to *hypoglycemia*, or chronic low blood sugar. Hypoglycemia results in frequent cravings for simple sugars or food rich in simple sugar including fruit and alcohol, as well as food rich in fatty acid. This condition of the pancreas is caused by excessive consumption of dairy fats, including cheese, as well as frequent consumption of poultry and eggs. In modern society, especially in the Western world, the consumption of these foods begins in early childhood and continues in adulthood, The fat from these foods is gathered in the pancreas and hinders the secretion of anti-insulin, which works to elevate the level of blood sugar. This results in a craving for simple sugar and wild, erratic changes in emotions when the body's blood sugar levels drop, especially in the afternoon and evening. The majority of adults in modern Western society suffer from hypoglycemia to a varying degree.

6. *Weakness of Bones.* Because of the excessive consumption of acid-producing foods, including simple sugar, the pH factor of the blood tends to become more acidic, producing a tendency toward acidosis. To prevent this dangerous condition, the body's mineral reserves (especially stored calcium in the bones) are mobilized, to maintain a weak alkaline condition in the blood stream.

This buffer-action changes strong acid to weak acid and then further breaks it down to water (H_2O) and carbon dioxide (CO_2). The minerals required for this buffer-action must be supplied in a daily diet that includes land and sea vegetables and other traditional foods high in vitamins and minerals, as well as moderate use of good-quality traditional, unrefined sea salt. Otherwise, the body will draw upon reserves in the bones, which results in a gradual weakening of the skeletal frame and degenerative conditions such as osteoporosis.

7. *Skin Disorders.* Because of the excessive consumption of simple sugar and fatty acid, body metabolism cannot support the active elimination of this dietary excess in most cases. Accordingly, the surface of the face and body becomes more milky in color with a red-pinkish shade. The milky texture is due to excessive consumption of dairy food, as well as oily, greasy food. Red-pinkish shades are due to expansion of the blood capillaries beneath the surface of the skin, resulting from over-consumption of foods in the extreme yin category, especially sweets, fruits, and others. In some cases, however, elimination of excessive dairy fats may appear on the skin in the form of white-yellowish patches. In other cases, the surface skin may not show these discolorations because fat layers are formed immediately below the skin which prevent elimination at the surface.

8. *Skin Cancer—Kaposi's Sarcoma.* In some but not in all cases, the elimination of excess fat and protein, combined with excessive simple sugar, especially refined cane sugar, chocolate, honey, and others, is actively made in the form of skin cancer. As in the case of malignant melanoma, which is caused chiefly by excessive fat mainly from poultry, eggs, and cheese, and the case of skin cancer, mainly caused by excessive oily, greasy food, *Kaposi's sarcoma* is formed as a process of elimination toward the surface of the body by an undesirable combination of fat, protein and simple sugar. In many cases, excessive animal-quality protein may combine with these substances.

Kaposi's sarcoma appears in the form of dark, brownish-black marks and may spread all over the skin. They continuously appear and spread as long as excessive fat, protein and simple sugar remain within the system beyond the capacity of normal eliminatory functions, especially respiratory and urinary elimination. Kaposi's sarcoma can also appear in the inner lining of the oral cavity and gums, as well as inside the respiratory tract, the digestive tract, rectum, and anal region.

Following a change in dietary practice, Kaposi's sarcoma may still continue for some period until the accumulation of fats caused by long-time consumption of oily, greasy food, dairy fats, and sugars, is eliminated. But thereafter, the sarcoma would gradually dry up, and the dark discolorings would change to a lighter shade. However, it may take several years until the lesions completely disappear—unless radiation or medical treatment is specifically applied—provided physical metabolism and other body functions have been restored to normal healthy conditions.

9. *Reproductive Organ Disorder.* Because of overconsumption of foods in the extreme yin category and of acid-producing foods, fatty acid and mucus gather in the reproductive organs such as the prostate and testes and the uterus and ovaries. In males, the condition may appear as a skin rash, as a red and white skin discoloring, and sensitivity at the time of urination. Other abnormal conditions may also appear. In females, this condition may manifest in a similar way and also in the form of vaginal discharge and vaginal and other localized infections.

The internal fluid in these regions becomes more acidic with various acid chemical compounds, including fatty acid, uric acid, sulphur compounds, and others. This condition creates a state easily receptive to viral growth and supports their activities. The degree of susceptibility to infectious viruses and bacteria such as those associated with gonorrhea, syphilis, herpes, and HIV differs according to the strength of the individual's natural immunity and dietary habits.

10. *Nervous Sensitivity.* Because of the excessive consumption of foods from the extreme yin category, the peripheral nerves become more expanded and sensitized. Physical and chemical sensations and stimuli tend to produce overreactions. It becomes difficult to tolerate cold weather or withstand strong physical pressure or stress. Moving to a warmer climate in the winter, avoiding hard physical labor, and seeking relations only with similar types of people are typical life-style changes associated with this condition.

On the other hand, this tendency also sensitizes the nervous system, often creating a liking for delicate matters. Aesthetic appreciation of the arts and culture is often highly developed, producing a preference for certain types of occupations such as designing, furnishing, decorating, art work, music, hairdressing, and others activities that require more refined aesthetic sensitivity.

11. *Mental Indecision.* Overconsumption of foods in the extreme yin category and acid-producing foods gradually leads to the develop-

ment of general indecisiveness, lack of clarity, and self-indulgence. Daily life tends to lack clear direction, and the person's ability to persevere in the face of difficulty and the ordinary vicissitudes of daily life declines.

Procrastination, timidity, and cowardice often develop, interfering with the person's overall direction in life and weakening their ambition, dream, and vision. Tenderness and kindness in human relations are demonstrated, and yet there is a general tendency for a lack of clear decision, resolution, and order.

A subconscious tendency to depend upon other people and circumstances arises. This mental tendency often results in a chaotic life-style lacking self-discipline, responsibility, and direction, as well as individual isolation or withdrawal into an exclusive group with those who share similar tendencies.

By improving eating habits in a more healthy direction, this mental tendency gradually changes toward more self-discipline, responsibility, ambition, and a positive and creative spirit and life-style.

12. *Receptivity toward Infectious Viruses and Bacteria.* In people who share the above physical and mental tendencies and life-styles, infectious viruses and bacteria can be easily transmitted and multiply within the body. These microorganisms thrive in more acid-producing environments where excessive fat and mucus have accumulated, such as in the reproductive organs, the intestinal tract, and even the mouth cavity if an acidic condition arises. When these parts of the body make direct contact with an infected person or fluid carrying viruses and bacteria, the microorganism can be easily transmitted and may spread quickly.

If a dietary change takes place toward healthier eating practices, this receptivity to infectious viruses and bacteria would gradually decrease. As an overly acidic condition of fat and mucus is reduced, a more normal condition develops, and natural immunity may gradually be restored.

Natural immune deficiency develops in accordance with the physical and mental disorders and changes in life-style outlined above. These conditions develop gradually over a period of many years. The modern way of eating is a primary cause of natural immune deficiency. Dietary influence is not limited to childhood and adulthood. In some cases weakened natural immunity has already begun to develop during the period of pregnancy. During the embryonic period, energy and nutrients that support the formation of the body and associated functions are supplied through the placenta and the embryonic cord. If the mother's eating habits consisted largely of foods from the extreme yin category and acid-producing foods—including excessive consumption of animal protein and fat, dairy foods, simple sugars, fruits and fruit juices, soft drinks, chemicalized food and beverages, and others—a baby developing in the mother's womb may be born with a tendency toward natural immune deficiency. This orientation may manifest in symptoms of AIDS, especially if improper foods continue to be consumed after birth throughout the growing period.

4. Life-style and Natural Immune Deficiency

In addition to improper diet, many aspects of modern life promote and encourage the development of natural immune deficiency. Modern living is oriented toward satisfying sensory pleasure and emotional comfort through material prosperity. It largely sacrifices physical health, mental strength, and spiritual development. The problems of modern living are often treated symptomatically through technical applications emphasizing speed, convenience, and efficiency, ignoring a more comprehensive view that takes into account humanity's biological and spiritual nature. Various aspects of modern life-styles and technology produce harmful effects that imperil the existence and continued development of humanity on this planet.

Some of the harmful aspects of modern life that promote natural immune deficiency can be outlined as follows:

1. *Biological Orientation in the Embryonic Period.* During pregnancy, from the time of conception to the time of birth, the human embryo increases in weight approximately 3 billion times. Formation of systems, organs, glands, and their related functions establish the human physical and mental constitution. Primary orientation for this development is made by hereditary genes such as DNA, but the quality and capacities of the human constitution are primarily developed through the energy and nutrients received through the placenta. The mother's eating habits largely shape and determine her baby's destiny. If the mother's way of eating is imbalanced, deformities may be produced including harelips, missing fingers or toes, multiple or transposed organs, retardation, and other abnormalities. At the same time, the quality and functional ability of systems, organs, and glands are also influenced.

In addition to dietary influence, parental consciousness—especially that of the mother—strongly influences the subconscious mind of the child. A mother with a calm, peaceful mind tends to produce a child with a peaceful orientation, while a mother with a disorderly, chaotic mind passes that attitude to the subconscious of her child.

The modern way of life tends to produce a child that is weaker physically and mentally than children in the past. The size and weight of children today tend to be larger and heavier than necessary. Physical and mental response tends to be duller.

On the average, natural immunity is stronger in a smaller, thinner, and shorter child and weaker in a larger, fatter, and taller child. Compared with children from a few generations ago, modern children are weaker in their physical and mental resistance, endurance, and response in general. This means that modern newborns are also weaker in natural immunity than a few generations ago. This weakness prevails especially among children who were born after about 1950. At that time, dietary habits began to change dramatically with the use of chemicals in the production and processing of food, and food itself became more highly refined.

Following several years of social and economic reconstruction after World War II, the modern diet, including large amounts of meat, poultry, eggs, dairy food, and other animal products, along with sugar, soft drinks, canned and frozen food, white bread and white flour, and other highly processed foods, began to spread throughout society. At the same time, the trend toward economic depression and material sacrifice that preceded and followed the Second World War was followed in the 1950s and early 1960s by a conscious quest for physical comfort, sensory gratification, and mental pleasure.

2. *Weakening of Natural Immunity at Birth.* Because increasing numbers of newborns are physically larger and heavier and many mothers have weak contracting power during delivery, Caesarean surgery has tripled in modern society, accounting for about one in every five births. In addition, the use of forceps, drugs, and other emergency measures to assist in delivery has become more widespread.

If the newborn does not experience passing through the natural birth canal with strong repeated contractions, the child tends to be weaker in physical endurance and resistance in general.

At the same time, nursing is often intentionally stopped, and artificially produced formula is substituted for mother's milk. During the first few days after delivery, the mother's breast secretes a yellow fluid, called *colostrum*, which has ample immune factors. Throughout the next period of breastfeeding, as regular mother's milk is produced, the newborn continues to receive essential natural immune factors. These include antibodies that resist the growth of undesirable viruses and bacteria, provide immunity against infectious disease (especially against rickettsia, salmonella, polio, influenza, strep, and staph), promote strong white-blood cells, and produce *B. bifidum*, a unique type of healthy bacteria found in the intestines of babies that creates resistance to a large variety of microorganisms.

These immune factors decrease as time passes. It is more difficult for the newborn to develop natural immunity if it has not been breastfed. Further, during these first few days, the newborn loses weight, contracting itself in order to acquire strength for adaption to the new environment.

The period of breastfeeding is very important in strengthening natural immunity. Upon birth, the newborn's living environment changes from the world of water in the uterus to the world of air on land. Naturally, the newborn is exposed to many kinds of new influences in the surrounding environment, including solar and celestial radiation, cosmic rays, and other influences of the universe, as well as the movement, pressure, temperature, and humidity of the atmosphere and many physical, chemical, and vibrational factors. Therefore, it is important for the newborn to develop natural immunity as smoothly as possible as a means of adapting to the environment and to resist undesirable factors including harmful viruses, bacteria, and other microorganisms as well as physical and chemical invasion and other adverse stimuli.

All mammal species depend upon breastfeeding directly from their mother. Breastfeeding supplies not only energy and nutrients but also confers immunity. If breastfeeding is replaced with artificial formulas which are produced for chemical and nutritional composition without careful consideration of natural immunity, the newborn may appear to grow satisfactorily, but it tends to be weaker, and its ability to adapt to its changing environment is diminished. Such a child may experience such undesirable symptoms as frequent colds, indigestion, diarrhea, skin rashes, allergies, complaining, oversensitivity, and other problems.

Though breastfeeding is desirable, circumstances may not always allow the mother to nurse her child. In such cases, food for the newborn should be carefully considered, including the quality and proportion of carbohydrate, protein, fats, vitamins, enzymes, and especially minerals. Until a few generations ago, it was common practice for newborns to be breastfed by other mothers as substitutes when a mother could not nurse the child herself.

In undeveloped societies, newborns who could not develop natural immunity sufficient for adapting to the new environment in the world of air would, in many cases, not survive to the age of three years. In modern society, health care, including improved sanitation, protects the newborn even when it does not develop sufficient immunity. However, this only postpones the problem to a future date. The child with weak immunity may well continue to survive if he or she is well-protected from the natural environment, like a plant growing in a hot house. Or if properly nourished, the child can develop natural immunity during the growing period.

3. *Weakening of Natural Immunity During the Growing Period.* In modern society, every individual faces many influences and occasions which weaken natural immunity. These include:

A. *Change of Dietary Habits.* Modern dietary habits have drastically changed, especially since the 1950s when a high-protein and high-fat diet became standardized in the United States and most of the industrialized world. Chemical agriculture replaced organic farming, and grain and flour products were increasingly refined. Commercially prepared fast food replaced home cooking, and modern advertising elevated sensory appeal and satisfaction, along with packaging, over such basic concerns as food quality and wholesomeness. This vast, fundamental change in the modern way of eating has naturally altered the biological, mental, and spiritual status of human beings, contributing to degenerative disease and the weakening of natural immunity. The lack of whole grains and natural minerals in fresh vegetables has particularly contributed to the decline of natural immune functions.

The cooking methods favored by modern food technology—electricity and microwave—have also changed food quality. Cooking by wood, charcoal, gas, and other natural fuels maintains the harmonious unity of foods, while electricity, microwave, and other highly refined forms of heating tend to decompose food molecules, creating chaotic energy and a disorderly vibration.

Microwave cooking has now spread from many public establishments to private homes. About 80 percent of all American families report having a microwave oven, and a majority use them regularly. Growing up, every person today is exposed more or less to this type of food, and their natural immunity may naturally be weakened as a result.

B. *Abuse of Medication.* In modern daily life, the use of drugs and pills is nearly universal. Sleeping pills, digestive pills and aids, aspirin and pain killers, tranquilizers and sedatives, and other medications and drugs are widely used as a normal part of daily life in the majority of families. The use of over-the-counter and prescription drugs and pills has constantly grown over the past several decades. However, many of them produce a very acidic condition in the body, which directly contributes to the weakening of natural immunity.

C. *Removal of Tonsils and Other Glands.* The majority of adults in modern society have had their tonsils and adenoids surgically removed during childhood to prevent tonsilitis. However, this is based on a deep misunderstanding of the nature and function of these glands. *Tonsillitis* (inflammation of the tonsils) does not occur because of the existence of the tonsils. It occurs because of excessive consumption of food rich in simple sugars and fat. The tonsils are one of several important immune glands that serve to cleanse toxins, excess mucus, and other substances from the lymph system. Chronic swelling and inflammation show that they are doing their job of localizing and neutralizing dietary excess. The way to relieve tonsilitis is not to take out the tonsils but to stop the intake of improper foods and drinks that are overburdening the lymphatic system. If the tonsils are removed, infectious diseases can spread more easily.

D. *Exposure to X-Rays.* Unlike our ancestors, the overwhelming majority of people in modern society have been exposed to X-rays on various occasions such as during medical and dental examinations. Frequent exposure to X-rays may increase the risk of certain kinds of cancer, including leukemia and lymphoma. It also weakens natural immunity.

E. *Exposure to Other Radiation.* In modern life, daily exposure to artificial electromagnetic radiation is often experienced, including that from television, especially color television, computers, and other electronic equipment. Furthermore, throughout the atmosphere and underground, some regions of the earth have been exposed to large amounts of undesirable radiation caused by the use of nuclear energy and nuclear explosions. Because radiation—both ionizing and non-ionizing, though to differing degrees—gives yin, expansive, decomposing, and in some cases freezing effects, it contributes to the decline of natural immunity. Irradiation of food may also produce similar effects over an extended period of time. Further, the loss of ozone in the earth's atmosphere has increased humanity's exposure to potentially dangerous ultraviolet radiation. Ultraviolet damage to the surface of the skin weakens natural immunity and may result in the increase of infectious diseases. Ozone loss is caused primarily from *chloroflurocarbons* (CFC) used in aerosol sprays, plastics, computers and electronics, and other industrial applications.

F. *Drug Abuse.* The use of drugs has soared since the 1960s, especially among older adolescents and young adults. These include marijuana, mescaline, LSD, and other hallucinogenic substances; amphetamines and barbituates; and heroin, cocaine, and other narcotics. These drugs give more yin, expanding and decomposing effects to physical and mental conditions and have the effect of dulling the functions of the nervous system. The overall result contributes to the weakening of natural immune functions.

G. *Abuse of Medical Treatment.* In modern society, medical treatment has become the standard method of treating sickness. Because degenerative disease is so prevalent and modern people experience so much physical and mental decline, medical treatment has sometimes been overused. Removal of the appendix without the actual occurrence of appendicitis causes unnecessary weakening of the intestinal functions in many cases. Similarly, the excessive use of medication and surgical operations causes the decline of natural immunity. Chemotherapy and other strong drug applications, although they may be required in some cases, tend to weaken natural immunity by changing the quality of the blood, including decreasing the number of white-blood cells.

H. *Overuse of Antibiotics.* Antibiotics have been employed successfully for the past several decades to deal with viral and bacterial infections. However, the use of antibiotics tends to change and weaken the activities of microorganisms in the digestive system, especially in the intestines. This causes disorders in the digestive functions and contributes to the decline of natural immunity. In general, the use of drugs to weaken or suppress viral and bacterial activities may also cause the deterioration of normal healthy microorganisms which, in turn, further contribute to the decline of natural immunity. Moreover, in recent years, new strains of microorganisms have developed that are resistant to ordinary doses of antibiotics. They require ever-stronger drugs to control, further weakening natural immunity.

I. *Environmental Pollution.* Despite more public awareness of industrial and chemical pollution, much of the planet's land, water, and air has been polluted. Acid rain damages crops, forests, and biological life in rivers and lakes. Nuclear wastes and radioactive substances are contaminating the atmosphere, water, and ground, endangering life at all levels. Chemicals and toxic wastes dumped into lakes, rivers, and oceans are destroying marine life, while pesticides and other chemical sprays used on fields and forests are killing wild animals and birds.

In metropolitan areas, pollution from automobiles, airplanes, and industry is also poisoning the atmosphere. Abnormal electromagnetic influences from power plants, high-voltage power lines, and communication facilities are also damaging human health and the environment. Apart from pollution in the external environment, overly insulated modern houses often pollute interior environments through use of synthetic building materials and other artificially treated substances.

As a result of worldwide environmental pollution, all animal life, including human life, is under threat of deformation, weakening, degeneration, and even possible extinction. Environmental pollution may also be a significant risk factor in the weakening of natural immunity and the spread of infectious disease.

J. *Promiscuous Sexual Behavior.* Due to the weakened natural immunity of modern people, viral and bacterial infections can be easily spread, especially among those whose life-style includes promiscuous sexual behavior. Since the sexual revolution of the 1960s, the incidence of *sexually transmitted diseases* (STD), including herpes and others, has risen dramatically.

From early childhood, most young people today have been exposed to sexually explicit material in books, magazines, on television, in films, and in the home, school, and community. As society's attitude toward sexual behavior has become more permissive, many of them have begun to have sexual encounters at an earlier age. As a result, there is a tendency among modern people not to select sexual partners carefully. Together with decline of spiritual intuition and biological instinct, the ability to choose an appropriate partner has declined, and promiscuous sexual behavior has increased. Compared to the recent past, the potential number of carriers of infectious viruses and bacteria has soared.

In the case of heterosexuals, physical contact with prostitutes is one of the major potential sources of infection. In the case of homosexuals, sexual activity is often accompanied by hallucinogenic drug use. Also, among various forms of sexual intercourse, oral and anal intercourse have a higher risk of lowering natural immunity than vaginal intercourse, because semen contains acid-forming compounds, along with sulphur, ammonia, and uric acid, in addition to simple fatty acids, which contribute to an overall acidic internal environment. In the case of seminal fluid, the yin decomposing power of sperm and male reproductive follicles is roughly one hundred times greater than simple sugar or other extreme dietary yin. Frequent anal or oral sex, in which semen is absorbed into the blood and lymphatic stream through the digestive system, would have the overall effect of lowering natural immunity.

5. The Virus and Biological Revolution

To understand AIDS and AIDS-related syndromes, as well as other disorders related to infectious viruses, bacteria, and other microorganisms, we need a comprehensive overview of biological evolution. The medical and scientific community has approached the epidemic from a microscopic point of view aimed at isolating certain viruses (HIV-I and HIV-II, in the case of AIDS) and destroying their activity through chemical, pharmaceutical, or other means. This approach may provide temporary relief in some cases, but it cannot solve the underlying problem of AIDS. Regardless of the type of chemical or physical therapy employed, the symptomatic approach to eradicating a specific virus eventually produces a weakening effect to the metabolism as a whole. The more effective such an application is in the short run to check a certain virus, the more harmful it proves to be in the long run for the well-being of the whole body and its harmonious functions.

Biological life on this planet began an estimated 3.4 billion years ago. The earth itself was gradually formed approximately 4.5 billion years ago. During the process of the earth's formation, whirlpool gaseous states gradually created a center, which later became more solidified. A liquified heavy atmospheric layer covered the solidified core. Within this environment, the first primitive life forms developed. They had a very simple chemical structure. Thus the world of *viruses* began.

For a period of possibly one billion years, viruses ruled the earth. During this period, however, these simple-structured viruses gradually evolved into more complex-structured biological organisms—*bacteria*.

As time passed, the condition of the earth changed, and three distinct layers formed: a solidified core at the center, a liquid mantle above that, and a gaseous atmosphere. Together with this process, bacteria developed and transformed into more complex units—the first *single-cell organisms*.

In the liquified layer, or surface water, of the premordial earth, the single-cell organisms further evolved and developed into *multi-cellular organisms.* This process probably took place over a period of from 500 million to 800 million years and occurred while the earth's surface water gradually increased its content of minerals such as sodium (Na), magnesium (Mg), calcium (Ca), and others. Multi-cellular organisms formed a group of species called *invertebrates.*

Thereafter, in the surface water—the ancient ocean which was becoming richer in salt and mineral content—softer multi-cellular organisms transformed and evolved into harder shell-forming multi-cellular organisms. At first they absorbed minerals on the surface of their bodies, developing into *crustaceans.* Later they gathered minerals from the sea into the center of their bodies, forming a skeletal structure and evolved into *vertebrates.* This process continued over a span of approximately 500 million years. Vertebrates further developed into various branches in accordance with changing environmental conditions, and many species appeared.

Sea-vertebrate evolution continued until land was formed over the surface of the ocean approximately 400 million years ago. As the land emerged, some species shifted their living environment from the ocean to the ancient muddy land. They began to adapt to the new air environment and acquired the ability to live in both water and air. *Amphibians* appeared.

As the earth's condition continued to change, the land became more solidified, although the atmosphere still retained a relatively high humidity. Amphibians evolved into ancient *reptiles* and *birds.* As the climate of the earth warmed, giant species developed, culminating in the *dinosaurs.* Then after several millions of years, owing to a change in celestial cycles, the climate started to cool, and a new evolutionary line of animal species began. Giant reptiles and birds disappeared, and *warm-blooded animals* emerged about 60 million years ago. They are biological ancestors of present-day mammals.

From that time, the earth's dominant climate has continued to grow cooler. Among plant species, fruit trees, nut trees, and other seed plants developed. Together with the change of environment and eating habits, *monkeys* and *apes* appeared among the mammals.

As the cooling trend continued, seed plants contracted, forming wild cereal grains. The species that began to eat these free-standing upright grains as a central part of their daily food developed into *human beings.* By eating grains, they began to stand erect and developed more advanced brains and central nervous systems.

The earth continued to grow colder. Humanity has experienced at least four major ice ages in the last one million years. In order to adapt to this climatic change, the human species began to apply fire to food to energize and vitalize it. In addition, minerals such as salt and various ways of processing natural food started to be used. The art of cooking developed as a method to adapt to the changing environment and to vitalize physical and mental activities. Thus, through food cultivation, selection, and preparation, humanity became more intellectual and active, and culture and civilization arose.

The macrobiotic view of biological evolution can be summarized as follows:
1. Biological transformation has been made:
   A. from elements and compounds to viruses
   B. from viruses to bacteria
   C. from bacteria to single-cell organisms
   D. from single-cell organisms to multi-cellular organisms
   E. from multi-cellular organisms to simple skeletal organisms
   F. from simple skeletal organisms to complex skeletal organisms, and
   G. from complex skeletal organisms to present human beings.

2. During a period of over 3 billion years of planetary evolution, environments for biological life have progressed:
   A. from a gaseous state
   B. to a liquid state with a few minerals
   C. to a liquid state with more minerals
   D. to an atmosphere with high humidity
   E. to an atmosphere with lower humidity
   F. to the present atmosphere polluted by chemicals, nuclear radiation, and various artificial electromagnetic energies.

3. The climate for biological life has also alternated between a higher temperature and a lower temperature. However, as a whole, the temperature of the environment has changed from a higher to a lower one, though it has fluctuated between the two many times during the process of biological evolution.

4. According to these larger environmental changes and trends, biological life changes its forms, structures, and functions. These changes have been characterized by relative expansion and contraction, softening and hardening, decomposing and composing, dispersing and gathering —in other words, between yin and yang. However, as a whole, the

evolutionary process from simple to more complex life forms has taken place through the composing, condensing, and gathering process—a yang development.

5. The food consumed by each species during the entire period of biological evolution has changed, as a whole, from a compound of simple molecules to a compound of complex molecules, for example, from simple sugar to complex carbohydrate, from amino acid to protein, and from simple fat to more complex fat. Minerals consumed have also changed, as a whole, from few minerals to a greater variety of minerals and from lighter minerals to heavier minerals.

From this perspective, we can understand that biological degeneration represents a reversal of the evolutionary process. When human beings stop eating predominantly whole cereal grains and cooked vegetables as their main food, they can no longer adapt to their changing environment and begin to lose their human condition and quality.

Biological degeneration can transform multi-cellular organisms to single-cell organisms, and single-cell organisms revert back to bacteria and viruses. In the human body, individual cells that are not properly nourished can degenerate into more primitive stages of life. Such cell degeneration would possibly occur more easily in less-developed cells such as blood cells, especially white-blood cells and reproductive follicles, than in well-developed body cells.

Such degeneration could arise if the body's internal environment reproduced environmental conditions similar to the primordial conditions of the earth when bacteria and viruses flourished. If the blood, lymph, body fluid, and interior of the intestines, as well as reproductive organs, increase their content of fatty acids, sulfur compounds, uric acid, ammonium compounds, methane gas and other gaseous conditions, and decrease their content of minerals, white-blood cells and other more primitive human cells may weaken and degenerate into viruses. In other words, AIDS may not in all cases be transmitted virally from the outside through sexual or other contact with someone who is infected. AIDS may arise, in some cases, internally from the long-time degenerative effects of dietary and environmental imbalance. We must emphasize that this hypothesis—based on the macrobiotic understanding of the Order of the Universe—requires further study. It may explain, however, why AIDS-related symptoms have appeared in some individuals who have not been exposed to HIV-I or HIV-II through sexual contact or other known means of transmission.

Even if future research shows that such degeneration of primitive cells does not occur within the body, the acid condition of the body's internal environment which simulates the primordial earth could easily receive, activate, and spread harmful microorganisms. The viruses known as HIV-I and HIV-II belong to the primary viruses that may have existed from the beginning of biological evolution. We can assume that they may have existed in a dormant state in the external and internal environment for billions of years. When environmental conditions suitable for their life developed, they may have been reactivated. HIV-I appears to be more prevalent in people who have been consuming various acid-producing foods but at the same time including animal sources such as meat, dairy food, and so on in their diet. On the other hand, HIV-II appears to be more common in people who have been consuming almost exclusively vegetable sources of acid-producing food including excessive consumption of sugar, chocolate, fruit, vegetable oils, and the like, without much animal food.

According to recent scientific observation, the AIDS virus appears to be exceptionally capable of hiding in the various parts of the human system. These parts include intestinal tissues, cervical tissues, the interior of the uterus and vagina, as well as the male reproductive organs. *Macrophages*, which are special sacks inside large cells, appear to become laden with AIDS viruses and carry them to rectal cells, cervical cells, vaginal fluids and semen. If the environment of these cells and fluids changes and becomes more suitable for the activity of viruses, they will be released and become more active. Furthermore, it appears that these viruses overcoat their protein surface with sugar molecules which protect the surface of the viruses from attack from antibodies. This scientific observation may suggest that viruses may be produced through decomposition of large cells. Regardless, dietary habits rich in acid-producing factors and overconsumption of foods rich in simple sugars appear to reserve, protect, and activate AIDS virsues. As noted above, a weakened internal environment is produced by various extreme and undesirable factors of modern life, especially improper dietary habits which result in more fat, mucus, and acidic conditions in the blood and body fluid, the intestines, and the reproductive organs. Therefore, return to a more balanced way of life and dietary practice is essential to prevent AIDS and other infectious.and communicable diseases.

Factors That Support Viral Activity ━━━━━━━━━━

As we have seen, viral infection and communication are activated by more yin tendencies—expansion, decomposition, dilution. Loss of energy arising from these tendencies also stimulates viral activities.

This view helps us understand the incidence and spread of AIDS and AIDS-related viral infections. The sociological profile that emerges is as follows:

1. Viral infections tend to arise and spread more in warmer climatic regions than in colder ones. Practically speaking, tropical and semi-tropical areas would be affected more than northern areas and areas closer to the polar regions.

2. Viruses would be more active in the summer and less active in the winter in temperate regions. For example, in central Europe or most parts of North America, there would be a more rapid increase of viral activity in late spring, summer, and early autumn and a slower increase in late autumn, winter, and early spring.

3. There would be more viral activity in a humid environment than a dry one. There would be more activity in a rainy season than in a dry one.

4. There would be more viral activity in cities with large populations than in rural areas with smaller populations. Urban regions would suffer more than villages and towns.

5. Viral activity would be greater where sanitary conditions are lacking.

6. Infection would be more likely among social sectors that consume larger amounts of food rich in animal protein and fat, including dairy food; food rich in simple sugar such as refined cane sugar, chocolate, honey, ice cream, and soft drinks; and fruit and fruit juice, especially of a tropical and semitropical nature. Viral activity would also be greater among people who consume large amounts of acid-producing food, including the above mentioned items, vegetables of the nightshade family, and oily, greasy food.

7. Infection would be greater in communities that depend more heavily upon the transportation of food from a different climatic region, especially a hotter and more humid zone.

8. Infection would be higher where drug abuse is prevalent and where promiscuous sexual activity is practiced.

9. In temperate regions, males would be affected more frequently than females because they are more easily weakened by yin acid-producing food such as simple sugar, fruit, and alcohol. However, in hot tropical regions, both males and females would be affected about equally.

10. There is a greater risk of viral infection among the population born after 1950.

11. The risk of viral infection would be greater among people engaged in sexual relationships with multiple partners rather than monogamous relationships.

12. Viral infections would be more common among homosexual men than homosexual women because risk factors as noted above are more predominant among males than females.

From this pattern, it would be possible to draw a map projecting the future development and spread of AIDS and AIDS-related viral infections. At the same time, this pattern would help epidemiologists and other scientific and medical researchers investigate possible counterbalancing dietary and environmental factors that could help prevent or slow epidemic trends in different regions of the world.

Means of Transmitting Viral Infections ——————————

In spite of possible production of viruses, including AIDS-related viruses, within the body, especially in the blood, body fluids, in the interior of the intestines, and within the reproductive organs, through degeneration of primitive cells, the transmission of viruses from one person to another is currently a major means of spreading AIDS and other viral infections.

Since each person has a different degree of natural immunity and receptivity to viruses, the current health or already existing degenerative condition of a person is the underlying factor that determines whether he or she is infected and to what degree. Even if exposed to harmful microorganisms, the metabolism of a healthy body harmonizes or neutralizes the undesirable viruses and bacteria by naturally producing antibodies.

The possibile means of transmitting infectious viruses are generally as follows:

1. *Sexual Intercourse.* In the event a partner carries an infectious virus, it could be transmitted to another partner during sexual intercourse. Transmission is made more easily through blood and bodily fluids high in acid, fat, and mucus, and fluid that is rich in nitrogen, sulfur, and ammonium compounds, uric acid, methane gas and other gaseous states, and others. Accordingly, primary means of transmission include:

A. Vaginal intercourse
B. Anal intercourse
C. Oral intercourse

In the case of oral intercourse, the risk of transmission is higher for the male receiver than the female receiver.

Although the act of kissing exchanges fluid, the possibility of transmitting the virus remains small. The strong yang alkaline condition of the saliva helps neutralize the yin acid nature of the viruses.

2. *Physical Contact.* Simple physical contact such as shaking hands, touching, hugging, and caressing will not transmit viruses. However, if the skin's surface has an open wound, ulcerated rupture, cancerous condition, or allergic rash, transmission may occur through these sites.

3. *Blood Transfusion.* Viruses can also be transmitted through contaminated blood. A blood transfusion is frequently needed for those who have lost a substantial amount of blood by accident, injury, or any other reason including hemophilia, leukemia, or malnutrition.

The blood used for a transfusion, in most cases, is blood collected from donors and stored in a blood bank. There is a possibility that some of this blood carries viruses, especially that of donors who have abused drugs, engaged in promiscuous sexual activity, or practiced chaotic eating habits. The viruses in stored blood can be eliminated by heat treatment, but this treatment may not have been applied in some cases.

The safest measure of blood transfusion is to collect blood from a member of the immediate family, relative, or close friend who has the same blood type and whose blood has been tested for safety prior to the transfusion.

4. *Blood Supplements.* Consumption of blood in the health-care field has greatly increased over the past several decades. In addition to blood transfusions, blood is utilized in the form of various tablets taken to boost energy and restore vitality. These tablets are also used for hemophilia, leukemia, and in cases where there has been a loss of blood. Until 1984, no precautions were taken to test such forms of blood for AIDS-related viruses. Blood supplements in tablet form have been distributed by manufacturers and they have been consumed by great numbers of people primarily in modern industrial societies. Accordingly, users of such supplements may be at higher risk for AIDS-related conditions.

5. *Eating and Drinking.* If harmful viruses are present in the food and water supply, there is a possibility of their reaching our digestive system and bloodstream. Recently, discoveries have revealed that some animal foods, such as meat and dairy products, may have AIDS-related viruses, as well as some water in rural areas in hot climates, especially those with high humidity and stagnant conditions. When we take these foods and water without proper processing, such as cooking with high temperature and the addition of salt or minerals, transmission could occur.

6. *The Use of Needles and Instruments.* The AIDS virus may also be transmitted by contaminated hypodermic needles and other unsterilized medical instruments. Needles are often used to inject chemicals or nutrients in the blood, lymphatic stream, and into the tissues. Needles are also used in acupuncture treatment and other therapies. Among drug users, the needles are often circulated among a group without proper sanitation or sterilization.

Furthermore, invasive instruments are often used in the cases of intraveneous injections, surgery, dental treatment, abortion, chemotherapy, and others. Unless these instruments are properly sanitized prior to their use, there is a possible risk of infection through these means.

7. *Embryonic Transmission.* In the event that a mother carries AIDS-related viruses in her body fluids, though she may not have any apparent symptoms herself, it is quite possible that her baby could be infected through the umbilical cord, as well as through the fluids directly

contacting the fetus. As the AIDS epidemic spreads, there will be increasing numbers of newborn infants who already carry viruses at birth. This degenerative trend alone gravely threatens humanity's continued existence, especially toward the beginning of the next century when the logarithmic increase of this number begins to become apparent.

8. *Transmission by Insects.* In tropical regions, it is well documented that mosquitos can transmit malaria and other diseases. There have been suspicions that AIDS-related viruses may also be transmitted by mosquitoes, cockroaches, lice, and other insects. Medical researchers have found no evidence to date of transmission from this source. However, such transmission remains a theoretical possibility and may require further investigation. Even if transmission by insects does not occur, infection caused by insects may serve to lower natural immunity.

These factors, each a potential means of transmitting viruses, have been experienced by many people in the modern world. It is essential that everyone know that a healthy life-style, proper diet, and a more disciplined approach to sexual relations are necessary precautions to prevent the further spread of AIDS and AIDS-related viral infections. These precautions can also serve to prevent other communicable diseases and to promote general health and happiness.

The Symptoms of AIDS and AIDS-related Infections ——

After contracting AIDS-related viruses, the symptoms of infection start to show up in various ways and degrees. They may appear within two months or they may not appear for several years. At the same time, the nature and degree of the symptoms are different and varied.

These variations are due to the individual's life-style and dietary habits, as well as the degree to which a person might have lowered his or her natural immunity prior to contracting the virus. However, the common symptoms are generally as follows:

1. *General Fatigue.* Both mentally and physically, the individual gradually loses his or her vitality. Ambition, endurance, and ability to meet challenges, as well as positive and optimistic attitudes, all decline. As a result, the person grows more inactive and seeks more comfortable situations and surroundings.

2. *Development of Colds and Infections.* Because of natural immune

deficiency, viral and bacterial infections can easily occur. Such individuals often suffer from colds and infections accompanied by light fevers.

3. *Skin Rashes.* Similar to allergic infections, red and white rashes appear in some cases on the skin. These result from the elimination of infectious material on the surface of the skin together with excessive fatty substances.

4. *Intestinal Disorders.* Such individuals often suffer from gas formation, constipation, and frequent diarrhea. In the case of diarrhea, parasites may also be involved.

5. *Feeling of Nausea.* Some individuals frequently experience the feeling of nausea. Usually it occurs after eating or drinking. However, actual vomiting does not often arise.

6. *Irregular Appetite.* Appetite is often disturbed. At times people with AIDS or related symptoms may have a great appetite for food, but at other times they may have almost no appetite. Furthermore, they may favor certain types of food such as sweets or fruits. Food preferences may also change frequently.

7. *Night Perspiration.* During sleep, especially at night between midnight and early morning, abnormal perspiration may occur in some cases. It may be associated with a light fever and shivering.

8. *Chronic Hypoglycemia.* The individuals usually experience symptoms associated with hypoglycemia, including a tendency to be more mentally depressed, irritable, and pessimistic, particularly in the afternoon. Feelings of exhaustion occur during the night even while sleeping. Peripheral parts of the body such as the hands and feet are colder than normal in temperature. Cravings for simple sugars are also strong.

9. *Liver Infection.* Weakness of liver functions often appears. It may take the chronic form of hepatitis, mononucleosis, and other similar infections.

10. *Swelling of Lymph Glands.* The lymph glands, especially in the groin, armpit, neck and chest area, often become swollen in order to cope with viral activity. These conditions may develop to lymphatic cancer—lymphoma.

11. *Abnormal Balance of Blood Components.* Within the blood-stream, the white-blood cells tend to continuously decrease, but lympho-cytes in particular decrease markedly. The ratio of immunity-related cells such as T4 and T8 cells changes. The number of T4 cells progres-sively decreases, and the ratio between the two becomes less than 1.0 and may even reach 0.1 or lower, which is one of the indications of very low immunity.

12. *Pneumocystis Carinii.* Some individuals may develop pneumo-cystis carinii accompanied by a state of chronic fever in which the body temperature tends to rise more in the evening and night than in the daytime. A chronic low-temperature fever, however, may continue over several months. As the situation develops, difficulty in breathing may tend to arise.

13. *Kaposi's Sarcoma.* In some cases, though not all, the individuals develop Kaposi's sarcoma, which is cancer appearing on the skin. In the beginning, it may appear as a simple dark spot of small size. Gradually the number of spots may cover various body surfaces. The sarcoma may also arise in the cavity of the mouth, especially in the upper region, and in some cases around the anus. These spots are dark black or brown in color and semi-soft in texture. They are the result of the active elimina-tion of excessive protein, fat, and simple sugars on the surface of the body, though in some cases this may happen within the interior of the digestive vessel and the respiratory tract.

There are many other symptoms which may appear in relation to AIDS-related viral infections. Strictly speaking, the symptoms are different according to the individual, but on the average the ability to adapt to the environment and to resist undesirable conditions within the environment declines. Ultimately, the condition will deteriorate to the point that basic life activity as a human being can no longer be sustained.

Conclusion: The Necessity of Biological and Spiritual Transformation

Every modern individual and family, as well as every community, every country, and the world as a whole is facing the epidemic spread of AIDS and related viral infections. In addition, other communicable diseases can be expected to increase rapidly by the mid-1990s. Everyone may have a close friend or family member who will suffer from one or another of these viral infections.

To cope with this grave threat to the continued existence and development of humanity on this planet, a revolutionary transformation in our view and way of life is urgently required.

The principles underlying this transformation include the following points:

1. It should be understood that the order of the universe and nature is endless, governing all phenomena, including human life.

2. Self-reflection and evaluation should recognize that modern industrial civilization has weakened the natural immunity of human beings to the extent that the future of humanity is imperiled.

3. It should be clearly understood that modern society's symptomatic approach to AIDS is limited and does not offer a lasting solution.

4. It should be understood that viral and bacterial infection is the result of degenerative conditions involving the disorders of major organs and functions of the human body.

5. It should be further understood that the solution for degenerative diseases and viral and bacterial infections, including AIDS and related disorders, does not deal only with symptoms or with certain micro-organisms alone, but involves a comprehensive approach to reconstructing the total health of people living in modern society.

6. It should be understood that the total reconstruction of human health cannot be made by present medical treatment or health-care technology, though, in some cases, they can help slow the epidemic and relieve suffering. What is needed is a revolutionary change of view, life-style, and dietary habits that respect the universal traditions of humanity and the natural environment. AIDS and the whole challenge of biological degeneration can only be met by a biological and spiritual transformation of humanity.

7. It should be understood that for this biological transformation to take place, all spiritual, religious, philosophical, and scientific communities and orientations must cooperate. East and West, North and South

must meet. Ancient traditions and modern technologies must work together to create one healthy, peaceful world.

8.   It should be understood that the headquarters for this biological and spiritual transformation of humanity is the kitchen in every home and the eating place in every community. In most cases, the leaders of this transformation will be women who take responsibility for preparing the daily food for their family and nourishing their children. Everyone— male and female—is encouraged to learn to cook and should actively participate in some aspect of food cultivation, production, or preparation.

9.   It should also be understood that this transformation will affect all political, economical, cultural, and social systems. These will inevitably be transformed toward a planetary system which will secure the maximum possible health of humankind and peace in the world.

10.   It should be recognized that the AIDS epidemic, disastrous as it is, offers humanity an opportunity to self-reflect and begin a new civilization on this planet.

Scientific and Medical Evidence

Martha C. Cottrell, M.D.

with

Mark Mead

1. The Biological Basis of Immunodeficiency

> Medicine has separated the sick human being into
> small fragments, and each fragment has its specialist.
> When a specialist, from the beginning of his career,
> confines himself to a minute part of the body, his
> knowledge of the rest is so rudimentary that he is
> incapable of thoroughly understanding even that
> part in which he specializes.
>
> —Alexis Carrel, *Man the Unknown*

The Healthy Immune Response

The human body is composed of a variety of organ systems, each designed to carry out specialized functions. The heart and blood vessels, for example, make up the *cardiovascular system* which serves to pump and circulate blood. The stomach, pancreas, liver, and intestines make up the *digestive system* which serves to break down and absorb food into the bloodstream and transform it into usable energy. The lungs, nose, and throat comprise the *respiratory system* which serves to bring oxygen into the bloodstream and to nourish all cells, tissues, and organs. The nervous system and circulatory system—which carries oxygen, nutrients, hormones, immune cells and other substances throughout the body—link all systems together in an intricate communications network which enables the body to function as an integrated whole.

Like other systems, the *immune system* is composed of various cells, tissues, and organs, each contributing in some way to certain specialized functions. The overall function of this system, simply speaking, is to maintain peace and order in the body. This function has two dynamic components: (1) to *recognize* substances which are foreign to the body, and (2) to *react* to them in ways which ultimately lead to their removal from the body. Foreign substances, or *antigens*, may consist of anything which is not biologically part of the human body, for example, food additives, cow's-milk protein, synthetics, animal dander, pollen, cigarette smoke particles, bacterial toxins, viruses, and cancerous cells that arise within one's body.

Antigens are, in a sense, the biological reason for the immune systems' existence. The body is incapable of recognizing what is intrinsically dangerous or toxic; instead it has learned to distinguish *self* from *nonself*, inner world from outer world. Things are designated as "foreign" (antigenic) because they do not belong in the body. Of course, some substances, such as nutrients, hormones, and enzymes, do belong and would necessarily be accepted by the immune system. Over the course of evolution, the body has learned to distinguish what is essential from what is non-essential to its biological integrity. In accord with this natural economy, the immune system responds by discarding that which is not essential to the body's overall functioning.

A central role of the immune system is to provide protection against infectious diseases. In ordinary daily life, the body is constantly exposed to various kinds of infectious microorganisms such as viruses, bacteria, protozoa, and fungi. These microbes can lead to a variety of diseases, some relatively common and usually not serious, and others less common and more serious. For example, most people experience a number of "colds" or "flus" each year that are triggered by various kinds of respiratory viruses. Other viruses can bring about severe liver infections (*hepatitis*) or brain infections (*encephalitis*). Common bacterial infections among Americans include strep throats and certain ear infections (*otitis*). A bacterial infection becomes more serious when it affects the brain (*meningitis*) or involves the bone (*osteomyelitis*). From a macrobiotic perspective, when an infectious virus or bacterium penetrates to the deeper or more yang areas of the body—the liver, heart, bones, or brain—the resultant condition can be very dangerous.

Even though we may be exposed to microorganisms several times a day, most of us rarely develop any immediate signs or symptoms of infectious disease. Whether the infection involves a virus or a bacterium, whether it is relatively harmless or relatively dangerous, whether it is in the throat or the brain, the immune system is responsible for protecting the individual against the related microorganism. A healthy immune system gives us the ability to neutralize and eliminate the microorganism, limit or prevent the spread of infection, and recover from disease before it progresses too far. By contrast, an unhealthy immune system is unable to fully counter an invading microorganism. The infection may spread and, in some instances, lead to death. The immune system in a person with AIDS, for example, is so weak that the individual is extremely susceptible to infection by microbes of all kinds. If people with AIDS choose to enhance their immune functions through a health-promoting life-style, the infections occur with diminishing frequency over time. If people neglect their immune systems, the infections tend to be frequent and increasingly severe over time.

The immune system's cells and chemical constituents are found in virtually every part of the body, providing far-ranging protection from infectious organisms, toxins, or other foreign material. It is by far the most diffusely organized system, with key components concentrated in the blood, lymph nodes, thymus, spleen, tonsils, adenoids, bone marrow, lungs, liver, intestines, and even the appendix. When an infection starts in a location that has relatively few immune cells, such as the skin, signals are sent throughout the body to call forth a large number of immune cells to the site of infection. In addition, the immune system's functions are closely integrated with those of the nervous, excretory, and *endocrine* (hormonal) systems. This complex integration compels us to think of immunity—and our approach to immune-related diseases—in dynamic and holistic terms.

Many immunologic tissues are located in and around the sinuses, lungs, and intestines, which serve as portals of entry for microorganisms, chemical toxins, and other antigenic material from the outside world. Some foreign substances are airborne, some are introduced through our food and water, while others enter by various kinds of human and animal contact. Some are controllable while others are virtually beyond control. Food additives, dairy proteins, prescription and illicit drugs, cigarette smoke, synthetic fibers, and so on, all pass through these entry points, which constitute the body's first line of protection. A heavy antigenic load may overwhelm the immune mechanisms localized in these areas and eventually deplete the reserves of these and other specialized immune cells and substances. This type of "immune overload" may be the major starting point for the development of immune-related diseases such as cancer and AIDS.

The immune system is composed of a diverse array of cell types and proteins, each designed to perform a specialized function aimed at either recognizing antigens or reacting to them. For some components, recognition of a material as foreign to the body is their only function. Other components function primarily by reacting to the antigens, while still others function by both recognizing and reacting against the foreign material. Altogether, these cells and substances comprise a highly intricate communications network which ensures the effectiveness and efficiency of the immune response. Since the functions of the immune system are so critical to our survival, nature has designed the system to utilize more than one component for carrying out recognition and reaction. Thus, if one component of the whole system is lacking or functioning poorly, another component can be called forth to take over some of its functions. If these back-up mechanisms are also overwhelmed, then one becomes more vulnerable to serious infections and cancers.

The body's initial protection against microbes is afforded by what immunologists call *natural immunity*, which consists of a diverse array of general mechanisms for immediate protection against infection and toxificity. This area of immunity involves substances which are not specifically designed for the particular chemical configurations of foreign substances, toxins, or microorganisms. If this system should be unable to eliminate some potential threat from the environment, the body has another, more subtle form of immunity termed *acquired immunity*. This involves the highly specific or selective modes of action of small lymphocytes and certain proteins, notably the antibodies. In acquired immunity, the body produces lymphocytes and antibodies of the desired specificity for recognizing and reacting to a particular antigen. If the antigen persists in the body, or is re-introduced at some later time, the lymphocytes have acquired "memory" of the previous exposure and are ready to respond.

The terminology used here to distinguish the two fundamental facets of immunity, natural and acquired, is somewhat misleading. From a microscopic view, the *acquiring* of immune cell memory involves a kind of biological learning at the cellular level. From a macroscopic perspective, however, the meaning of acquired takes on a more expanded dimension whereby *acquire* means "to gain through one's own efforts." By this broader definition, we acquire the integrity of specific immune mechanisms (lymphocytes and antibodies) by eating a balanced diet and generally taking care to reduce our exposure to toxins. We acquire a more competent immune system—including so-called natural immunity —through a health-promoting mode of living. Similarly, one may question the intended meaning of *natural immunity* to describe those systems involved in the body's first line of defense. What exactly is the distinction here? Why should the immune system's more general mechanisms be considered any more natural than the specific mechanisms of acquired immunity? Just as the integrity of both types of mechanisms is acquired, so also is this integrity natural. Indeed, every mechanism in the body is natural. In this sense, the conventional terminology is both superfluous and fallacious.

It is interesting that medical science has designated these general mechanisms as "natural" when this is the part of the immune system involved in the earliest phases of the disease process, even before symptoms manifest. In treating immune-related disorders, modern medicine tends to focus on the more specific components of the immune system— the small lymphocytes and antibodies—which usually represent the final phases of immune breakdown. It is almost as if the distinction between natural and acquired implicitly supports modern medicine's sanctioning of powerful pharmacologic drugs, most of which are directed toward the more specific mechanisms of acquired immunity. Modern immunology's delineation of *acquired* and *natural* therefore reflects an overly divisive and microscopic conception of the nature of health. It would seem more appropriate to categorize so-called acquired mechanisms under *specific immunity* and so-called natural immune mechanisms under *general immunity*. These are the terms we shall emphasize henceforth in this chapter.

Mechanisms of General Immunity

Let us now consider the two complementary areas of the immune system in more detail. General immunity, as we have said, encompasses all systems responsible for dealing with the initial exposure to toxins and microorganisms, as well as for maintaining biochemical equilibrium and stability in general. The mechanisms of general immunity include intact skin and mucous membranes, mucus and iron-binding proteins, phagocytic cells, salivary secretions, indigenous microflora, and many physiological systems often taken for granted in the maintenance of health. These nonspecific host defenses may be described as follows:

1. *Skin and Mucous Membranes* The mechanical barriers of intact skin and mucosa prevent most microorganisms from entering the general circulation, and various secretions minimize the survival chances of potentially infectious agents. As the body's largest organ, the skin is the body's main physical barrier to all kinds of infection, serving as both a passive and an active protective covering. (Note: The active protection also involves numerous specialized cells in skin which have interacting roles in the specific immune response and are implicated in skin malignancies, for example.[1]) Sweat and sebum contain acidic antiseptic substances which inhibit bacterial growth; and saliva, mucus, tears, urine, semen and vaginal secretions all possess natural antibacterial properties.

Mucous membranes are very thin, moist tissues located around openings and passages in the body; they are found in the mouth, on the inner eyelids, inside the nose and air passages leading to the lungs, the vagina, the anus, in the stomach and much of the digestive tract. The essential function of these membranes is to provide "front-line" protection against incoming environmental irritants, toxins, and microbes. Mucus can trap bacteria and may inhibit viruses from attaching to mucosal cell surface receptors for a key enzyme called *neuraminidase.* Ciliary movements, together with coughing and sneezing, promote expulsion of foreign pathogens and potentially toxic materials. Most of these secretions contain *lysozyme,* the enzyme which has also been found to exhibit bactericidal activity. Mucus and saliva together keep the surrounding tissues moist, which in turn promotes the movement of foreign particles along these passages. The maintenance of mucosal surfaces along the digestive tract is largely ensured by the salivary glands (see saliva, number 7 below).

Although bacteria are usually eliminated by intact mucous membranes, some viruses can travel through the membranes to enter the bloodstream. For example, the flu virus can pass through the mucous membranes of the eyes and mouth, and therefore is transmissible by casual forms of physical contact. Whether or not Human Immune-deficiency Virus (HIV), the AIDS virus, is able to traverse the mucous membrane is unknown, although the virus is not usually found around mucous membranes. While the flu virus can thrive in the lungs, throat and sinuses, the AIDS virus is most concentrated in the blood, primarily targeting cells of the immune system. HIV is rarely present in the saliva and *sputum* (the viscous substance expelled by coughing or clearing the throat), and then only in very low concentrations.

2. *Interferons* Certain immune cells infected by viruses release *interferons,* protein molecules which prevent invasion of uninfected body cells by the same virus as well as by other viruses. Natural chemicals such as *interleukin-2* can stimulate the production of interferon. Interferons seem to play an important role in fending off prolonged infectious conditions and thereby may aid in the process of recovering from viral illness. Interferons are also potent agents in the body's protection against abnormal cells or cancer. In either case, whether a potential viral infection or tumor development, human interferon serves to arrest the replication of the threatening virus or cancer cell. Some research suggests that vitamin C and other nutrients may be capable of promoting interferon activity in the body.

3. *Iron-binding Proteins* Iron is an essential nutrient for the growth and multiplication of all microorganisms with the exception of lactobacillus. Too much iron in the system can encourage bacterial growth and may even increase the risk of cancer (see chapter 8). One protein called *transferrin* can bind iron and thereby sequester it from pathogenic microorganisms. Increased susceptibility to bacterial infections may involve low serum transferrin levels or iron-saturated transferrin in the blood. The latter case may occur from taking iron supplements or eating an excessive high-iron diet, such as too much red meat. An analogous situation may involve molecules produced by the body which bind or interact with other nutrients that promote bacterial or parasitic growth.

4. *Phagocytes* A large part of the immune system's first line of defense is carried out by *phagocytes*, or *phagocytic cells*, which are literally "cell-eaters." These abundant white blood cells can engulf and digest foreign cells and toxins, as well as debris left over from other immune cell encounters. They contain a host of enzymes and other substances which break down the ingested antigenic material. As integral components of the immune surveillance system, phagocytes may circulate throughout the entire body to consume and help eliminate anything foreign; they are our body's clean-up experts.

Phagocytic cells consist of two types: *neutrophils*, non-dividing cells that are produced in enormous quantities and provide the primary barrier against certain kinds of bacteria; and *macrophages*, monocytes important in dealing with intracellular microorganisms and parasites. Neutrophils are required to ingest the bulk of incoming foreign material. Their phagocytic capacity is limited to one antigenic encounter, after which they die and release toxins that are picked up by the macrophages. The macrophages thus serve as a kind "fail-safe" or back-up system for the dying neutrophils.

Macrophages are relatively large cells which deal with antigens in highly versatile ways. They may engulf an antigen and process it so that it is easier for other white blood cells and antibodies to recognize it as foreign. Macrophages send out signals to *T helper cells* (where *T* stands for thymus, the organ where these cells mature), to attract the helper cells to the site of immune activity. The T helper cells then stimulate the production of antibodies from other white blood cells. The macrophages can then break up the entire antigen-antibody complex, and eventually carry their ingested contents to the intestinal and bronchiolar (lung) lumen for excretion from the body. When encountering viruses or other microbes, macrophages secrete a chemical which can produce a rise in body temperature, or fever. The elevated temperature makes it difficult for most microorganisms to survive.

The rate of production of both neutrophils and macrophages is relative to the demand imposed by toxins and pathogenic microorganisms. When demand exceeds the supply of these phagocytes, other aspects of the immune system must compensate by working harder. Once the phagocytic cells are overburdened, however, the body's protective mechanisms are to some degree compromised. Macrophages, in particular, are needed as messengers to the more specific cells, the *T* and *B lymphocytes*. Without a full set of macrophages, the functions of these other cell populations are diminished. Proper nutrition serves to maintain the supply of all phagocytes and thus helps to avert immune overload.

5. *Complement Proteins* The *complement system* is composed of 18 serum proteins which function in an integrated fashion to help protect against infection and produce inflammation. Some of these proteins are produced in the liver, while others are produced by certain phagocytic cells, the macrophages. Complement proteins have the ability to *lyse* (split or dissolve) cells and foreign bodies which are coated with antibodies. One of the proteins of the complement system coats microorganisms to make them more easily ingested by phagocytic cells, while other complement proteins send out chemical signals to stimulate antibody production and attract phagocytic cells to sites of infection. They also support the activity of lysozyme, a circulating polysaccharide that dissolves certain bacteria. Conversely, some polysaccharides (derived from dietary carbohydrates) directly support the activity of complement proteins.

Complement proteins thus play an important part in our protection against bacterial and viral infection. If a foreign bacteria or virus stimulates an antibody response and becomes coated with antibody, the complement contained in body fluids can cause the microbes to lyse, thereby leading to their rapid elimination from the body. Because these proteins are capable of interacting with virtually all antigen/antibody complexes, their multiple functions are termed nonspecific.[2] Many of the so-called immunodeficiency-related disorders—including *systemic lupus erythematosus-like syndrome*, *dermatomyositis*, *glomerulonephritis*, *angioedema* and others—appear to involve some defect in the complement system.[3]

6. *Gastrointestinal Flora* The precise role of the human microbial flora has been controversial ever since Louis Pasteur hypothesized that

they were essential to life.[4] A multitude of bacteria, fungi (yeast), protozoa, and other microbes are represented among the "normal" or indigenous flora of most mammalian species, including humans. Many of these live within us and derive benefit without injuring or upsetting our internal milieu. Others, such as the fungus, *Candida albicans*, can become pathogenic if not kept in check by neighboring microflora. Results from rodent studies indicate that cholesterol synthesis, bile acid metabolism, and modification of various polyunsaturated fatty acids are influenced by the intestinal flora under certain conditions.[5]

Production of a natural antibiotic called *bacteriocin* is likely to be the principal means by which indigenous bacteria of the bowel and lower urinary tract suppress potential pathogens that are attempting to colonize these two sites.[6,7] Degradation of bacterial toxins is a means by which normal flora may prevent disease caused by certain toxin-producing microorganisms.[8] In addition, the sheer density of normal microflora inhabiting gastrointestinal surfaces suggests that *steric hindrance* (interference with potential binding sites or portals of entry along the intestinal mucosa) may be another means by which the adherence of undesirable microbial newcomers is prevented.

Aside from these direct mechanisms for inhibiting potential pathogens, our normal microflora may accomplish the same result indirectly by stimulating the immune system. Animals lacking their natural microbial flora typically show a variety of immune deficiencies when exposed to foreign microbes. The significant deficit in immune responsiveness shown by germ-free animals is rapidly eliminated upon reestablishing the normal microbial flora in these animals.[9]

Various synergistic relations between the normal flora of the digestive tract appear to be important in inhibiting the growth of a variety of common pathogens.[10,11,12] The role of resident microorganisms in protecting against infection through the body's mucous membranes may therefore comprise an essential aspect of the body's first line of defense. According to epidemiological studies, our indigenous *lactobacilli* exert a protective effect against infection by *N. gonorrhoeae*, the bacterium linked with gonorrhea.[13] (Lactobacilli are very concentrated in *miso*, the fermented soybean paste used as soup base in regular macrobiotic dietary practice.) The possible role of human gut microbial flora in protecting against viral infection remains to be determined.

7. *Saliva* The important immunologic role of human saliva has only recently been recognized by medical science. However, the salivary glands were considered integral to the body's disease resistance even as

far back as ancient Greece. In fact, until the early nineteenth century, many physicians believed in Galen's premise that disease was a morbid state of the four "principal humors" (phlegm, blood, yellow bile and black bile) and employed salivation as one of their therapeutic strategies. Lack of saliva is often accompanied by a dry or sticky throat, sore mouth, difficulty in eating, and poor digestion. Although human beings can manage without saliva, its loss results in multiple miseries, mainly discomforts at mealtime, but also increase susceptibility to infections and blood toxicity.[14]

Human saliva has two major functions: (1) *digestive*, in helping break down the carbohydrate content of thoroughly masticated food, in preparing food mass for proper digestion, and in enhancing the perception of taste (the longer you chew fibrous, starchy foods, the sweeter they become); and (2) *protective*, both in protecting the teeth and oral soft tissues, in maintaining bacterial flora, and in various localized immunologic functions. Saliva plays a key role in maintaining the ecological balance in the oral cavity through direct antibacterial activity, normal pH balance, and other mechanisms. Various salivary proteins—lysozyme, *lactoferrin*, and *lactoperoxidase*—destroy harmful bacteria and prevent excessive bacteria growth.

Saliva also possesses antifungal and antiviral capacities, including protection against both candidiasis and herpes simplex.[15,16] Most of saliva's antimicrobial properties are significantly enhanced by interaction with the mucosal antibody called *secretory IgA*.[17] Children who are malnourished show lower levels of IgA and other proteins in their saliva, and also experience heightened susceptibility to infectious diseases.[18] Other studies have found depressed IgA levels under various conditions of psychological stress such as college exams.

Mastication and certain nutritional factors can directly affect salivary secretion and composition: less chewing leads to less salivary flow, and poor nutrition leads to reduced levels of salivary proteins. These mechanisms may, in turn, compromise the various salivary defense systems and increase susceptibility to infectious disease. Since low-fiber, animal-quality diets require virtually no chewing, they fail to adequately stimulate the salivary glands. Over the long run, such dietary practices may cause gradual atrophy of these glands along with reduction in salivary flow rate and in the antimicrobial protein output.[19] Similarly diets high in simple sugars (honey, maple syrup, fruits, fruit juices, refined flours, etc.) tend to depress the salivary system and may thereby contribute to compromised immunity.[20] In other research, the salivary content of partially digested foodstuffs appeared to reduce the level of bile acids in the duodenum. Excessive levels of bile acids are thought to indicate increased risk for developing cancer. Thus it seems that the more we chew, the lower our risk of cancer and other immune-related problems.

According to a 1988 study reported in the *Journal of the American Dental Association*, human saliva does contain protective substances that prevent the AIDS virus from infecting lymphocytes. Dr. Philip Fox, who headed the study for the National Institute of Dental Research (NIDR), says this could be the reason AIDS is not transmitted orally. Fox and his research team took saliva from the glands and mouths of three healthy men and then exposed the samples to HIV. Though the NIDR researchers could not determine what, precisely, the protective factor might be, they found the saliva 100 percent effective in blocking the virus from infecting lymphocytes. It is of interest, however, that saliva did not stop transmission and incubation of the less fragile Epstein-Barr and hepatitis B viruses.

As mentioned before, saliva plays a key role in maintaining the integrity of mucous membranes in the upper gastrointestinal tract. These membranes must be kept moist for proper physiological functioning, and the mucin content of saliva serves as natural "water proofing" in this regard. *Salivary mucins* affect the permeability of mucosal surfaces, providing an effective barrier against penetration by viruses, fungi, and other microorganisms, as well as by chemical irritants, carcinogens, toxic dietary elements, and potentially hazardous agents from tobacco smoke and other sources.[21] During an oral inflammatory reaction (e.g., *periodontitis*), the integrity of mucous membranes can be seriously altered by substances called *proteases*, which are generated by active immune cells. They may also be linked with oral cancers. Protease activity is partially inhibited by the mucins in saliva and by a substance called *Cystatin S*, which is mediated by other enzymes present in the salivary glands.[22]

8. *Basic Back-up Systems* Biologic protection of general immunity is also afforded by seven important "back-up" or reinforcement systems. These provide ways of dealing with disease organisms and toxic substances which in turn tend to reinforce the more specific responses of the immune system.

(a) **Stomach:** This organ produces powerful acids which destroy undesirable microorganisms (including HIV) and break down proteins into more digestible form.

(b) **Liver:** This organ carries out metabolic detoxification of many potentially harmful chemical compounds, including drugs and food additives, and ensures that nutrients are properly metabolized.

(c) **Intestines:** The large and small intestines must function smoothly to excrete toxic fecal matter and ensure proper absorption of essential nutrients.

(d) **Kidneys:** These organs help maintain blood alkalinity, mineral-salt and fluid balance, and overall blood quality through highly versatile filtering mechanisms. The sodium proportion of the blood plays a key role in preventing harmful microbes from infecting the body.

(e) **Lungs:** These organs maintain blood alkalinity and oxygenation through the respiratory action of the lungs (most foreign bacteria are unable to survive in an oxygen-rich environment).[23]

(f) **Reticuloendothelia System:** The system filters the blood and lymph through the action of specialized cells distributed throughout the circulatory and lymphatic channels.

By constantly maintaining fundamental biochemical balances in the body, these general mechanisms provide essential support to the more specific immune functions. If they should ever become overworked and depleted—perhaps through inappropriate nutrition and stressful lifestyle—the entire immune system stands to be weakened as well. For example, the kidneys are key organs in maintaining sodium/potassium balance, which is also influenced strongly by diet. When the blood and lymph fluids contain ample amounts of sodium, many types of potentially harmful bacteria (e.g. *E. coli*, *Staphylococci*, and *Salmonella*) are unable to propagate.[24] Hence dietary salt content and the physiologic condition of the kidneys may play an important role in maintaining this antimicrobial properties of the blood. The kidneys are weakened primarily by excessive intakes of animal proteins, refined salt, refined sugars, chemical additives, and various drugs and medications.

A diverse variety of specialized immune cells circulate throughout the body via the bloodstream and *lymphatic system*. The *lymphatics*, or lymph channels, function to transport *lymph fluid*—that portion of the blood which leaks out of the circulatory system due to the enormous pressure the blood is under. The lymph is a clear fluid which accumulates in the tissue spaces between cells and blood capillaries, and eventually enters the lymphatic network. Interspersed throughout the lymphatic channels are tight clusters of the cells called *lymph nodes* (glands), which act as primary filters, protecting the bloodstream from numerous foreign and toxic substances. Each node contains scavenger cells—macrophages and reticuloendothelial cells—which help break down toxins and microbes. As said before, macrophages are also important mediators between antigens and lymphocytes.

Specialized immune cells are generally termed *white-blood cells* (WBCs). They exist in a number of varieties and differ among themselves in size, function and appearance. Unlike red-blood cells (RBCs), WBCs are nucleated and non-pigmented, and they are generally larger than RBCs. Most WBCs have the unique ability to leave blood vessels, travel through tissues and between cells of the body, and constantly circulate between the lymphatics and the bloodstream. In this way, they can monitor the entry of foreign entities—such as bacteria, viruses, and parasites—and prevent such microorganisms from multiplying and spreading throughout the body.

Altogether comprising about 25 percent of the body's approximately 100 trillion cells, white-blood cells can be divided into two classes: (1) *granular*, having a nucleus of complicated shape, formed into two or more lobes, and hence also called *polymorphonucleocytes* (PMNs) meaning "nucleus of many forms." These ordinarily make up two-thirds of all leukocytes in blood, and consist of several subsets of cells, the most abundant of which are the neutrophils; and (2) *agranular*, having large nuclei simpler in shape than those of the granular leukocytes. This latter group consists of monocytes (e.g., macrophages), large lymphocytes and small lymphocytes. Among these three subgroups, small lymphocytes play a prominent role in the specific binding of foreign microorganisms. Without their specific binding abilities, the body is rendered vulnerable to the microbial world in which we live.

The Delicate Dance of Specific Immunity ——————

The immune system's high level of integration with other systems makes it a kind of second brain within the body. After the *cerebral cortex* of the human brain, the immune system is the most recent development of mammalian physiology on the evolutionary scale. Its primary function is to "recognize" and "remember" the outer world to which it is continually exposed. The establishment of cellular memory after an initial exposure enables the immune system to immediately recognize something as foreign to the body and to respond in any subsequent exposure.

The ability to recognize and neutralize toxins, foreign organisms, and cancer cells reflects a level of biological intelligence unique to higher, multicellular organisms. Specific immunity involves cellular memory and recognition at the most refined level.

The total number of small lymphocytes in the human body is about two billion.[25] Approximately half of these are a cell type called *T-cells*, the other half are called *B-cells*. Thus the specific immune response can be loosely divided into two types, those involved in antibody formation (*humoral*) and those involved in tissue reactions (*cell-mediated*). The separation between humoral and cell-mediated functions is a bit over-simplistic, however, since the functions of B-cells and T-cells are in fact strongly interwoven. It now appears that the immune response to virtually all antigens involves the cooperation of the two types of lymphocytes.

B-cells. The *B-lymphocytes* are specialized cells whose major function is to produce antibodies (also called *immunoglobulins* or *gammaglobulins*). B-cells arise from primitive cells in the bone marrow and then reach maturation in the spleen, lymph nodes, liver, and some parts of the intestines. When stimulated by antigen, B-cells respond by changing into *plasma cells*. The plasma cells are then capable of producing *antibodies*, which find their way into the bloodstream, respiratory secretions, intestinal secretions, and even tears. These tiny globular proteins are designed to combine specifically with a particular foreign substance, such as the outer surface of a virus or bacterium. When antibodies recognize a microorganism as foreign, they physically attach to it and set off the complex chain of integrated reactions that eventually destroys and eliminates the microorganism.

Antibodies consist of five major classes of immunoglobulin (Ig), each varying with respect to their specialized functions in the body:

1. **IgM** are rapidly produced in response to infection and thereby afford important protection during the first few hours or days of an infection; they trigger the action of complement proteins.

2. **IgG** are formed in large quantities and can travel from the bloodstream to the tissues; they are the major class of antibodies to cross the placenta and pass on immunity to the newborn; they also stimulate complement proteins.

3. **IgA** are abundantly produced near mucous membranes; as important components of saliva, mucus, tears, and bile, these antibodies may strongly protect against infection in the respiratory and intestinal tract.

4. **IgE** are key participants in allergic or hypersensitivity reactions, and may play a role in protecting the body against parasites.
5. **IgD** are still incompletely understood, but may help in the differentiation of B-cells.

Once antibodies bind to the surface of a foreign microorganism, they can protect the host against infection by various means. Antibody-coated bacteria are easier for the phagocytic cells to ingest than bacteria which are not coated by antibody. The complement system is also more effectively activated in the presence of antibodies. In addition, viruses and certain microorganisms must attach to body cells before they can cause an infection, but antibody on the surface of a microorganism can interfere with its ability to adhere to the host cell. By these and other means, antibodies serve to prevent viruses and other microbes from entering cells and tissues where they can produce serious infections.

Theoretically, B-cells have the ability to produce antibodies of unlimited variety—that is, against virtually all possible antigens in the environment. They do this not only with great specificity, but with great power. A single activated plasma cell can synthesize and pump into the blood some two thousand antibodies per second. By the same token, a group of active plasma cells may produce approximately one hundred million trillion (100,000,000,000,000,000,000) antibodies per second! One of the greatest marvels of human biology is that such tremendous production can occur so consistently and accurately in response to any one of millions of antigens in our environment. Apparently the mechanism behind this amazing versatility involves a rapid translocation of gene segments ("transposons") which code for the protein design of each antibody. No wonder some immunologists sometimes refer to the genetic material as G.O.D., or generator of diversity.

Whenever conditions are right, antibodies can neutralize a foreign microbe. Several studies of people with full-blown AIDS indicate that the levels of neutralizing antibodies to HIV seem to protect against the progression of the disease.[26] Further, some healthy individuals evidently produce antibodies to HIV and later show no presence of antibody. They remain symptomless and typically show improvement in other immune-system parameters.[27] Approximately 5 in 2,000 people who originally test positive for the AIDS virus later show no sign of it in their bloodstream. However, because HIV may hide inside cells for an indefinite period of time, it is unknown whether the absence of antibody indicates that the virus has been entirely eliminated. Other immune components, such as complement and macrophages may play a complemental role to the antibodies. Since antibodies are ineffective against the virus once it has entered a cell, other components of immunity must be called forth to enable people to eliminate the AIDS virus. According to immunologists, this would most likely be accomplished by certain members of the T-cell system.

T-cells. T-cells, another type of specialized immune cell, cannot produce antibodies. Instead, they interact directly with a particular antigen. Just as B-cells can produce an extensive variety of antibodies, the potential variety of T-cells is also extensive and capable of reacting against virtually any antigen. T-cells arise from the primitive stem cell of the bone marrow and reach maturation in the thymus gland, which is located behind the breastbone in the chest. The thymus begins to shrink during the early years of life, but remains somewhat functional in healthy individuals. Mature T-cells leave the thymus to populate other organs of the immune system, such as the spleen, lymph nodes, bone marrow, and blood.

Like the antibodies, T-cells vary with respect to their function. There are three basic kinds of this specialized lymphocyte group.

1. **Killer or effector T-cells.** These *cytotoxic* cells perform the actual destruction of foreign organisms and abnormal cells (cancer). Moreover, they protect the body from certain bacteria and viruses which have the ability to survive and multiply *within* the body's own cells. In this way, they can compensate for the shortcomings of antibodies, which are impotent against viruses hiding inside cells. T-killer cells migrate to the site of infection or perhaps to the location of a transplanted tissue. Once there, they directly bind to the antigenic source and destroy it.

2. **Helper T-cells.** These cells, as their name indicates, have a central role in assisting and even enhancing the functions of many other cells, including the antibody-producing B-cells, the T-killer cells, and even the macrophages. For example, the T-helper cells cause B-cells to produce antibodies more quickly.

3. **Suppressor T-cells.** By contrast, these cells suppress or shut off the function of B-cells and T-killer cells. This is an important function, for without it, the humoral and cell-mediated immune mechanisms would continue along even after an infection had been effectively resolved. Laboratory tests have shown that suppressor cells of healthy individuals may prevent the AIDS virus from replicating in the body.[28] Scientists speculate some chemical is secreted by these cells which inactivates the virus.

Specific immunity is maintained by the intricate interplay of lympho-cytes, hormones, and neural signals. When stimulated by an antigen, T-helper cells turn on the antibody-generating activity of B-cells, where-as T-suppressor cells act to turn off that activity when it has gone far enough. B-cells and T-cells, and T-helpers and T-suppressors, are com-plementary cell populations that collectively serve to keep the immune system in balance. The balance of T-helper and T-suppressor cells com-prises a kind of biological gauge for specific immunity, keeping it turned on to just the right extent, neither too much nor too little. When this dynamic cooperation is upset, however—perhaps due to a combination of improper nutrition, environmental toxins, repeated infections, and various psychosocial stresses—resistance is lowered and disease pro-cesses are potentiated.

The pivotal role played by the T-helper cell is dramatically shown in the case of AIDS, which involves a deficit or functional abnormality in one set of T-helpers, known as *T4 cells*. Without the T4 cells, the immune system cannot respond as well to infectious organisms. This does not mean, however, that the T-helper cells are the central problem to be dealt with. Indeed, the lack of them may only be a symptom. Let us recall that the specific actions of T- and B-cells are largely mediated by the macrophages, which may be affected at an earlier stage of the disease. Abnormalities in B-cell function have also been observed in AIDS, al-though this usually has more to do with defective regulation by the T-cells. Some leukemias, lymphomas, and cancers of the *hematological* (blood-forming) system, seem to result from wild proliferation of defec-tive B-cells in some cases and T-cells in others.

T-cells also produce powerful substances called *lymphokines*, such as interferon and interleukin-2. These chemical mediators help bring various immune cells into action in the body's defense. Medical scientists have been excited by the possibility of accelerating T-killer cell activity by introducing synthetic lymphokines. So far these treatments have had little effect except in some cases of leukemia. It may be naive to assume that by reintroducing one particular component of immunity—in a relatively arbitrary quantity, as far as nature is concerned—we can pro-duce a desired effect without also upsetting the essential balance of other components. The effectiveness of lymphokines undoubtedly depends on numerous co-factors, and this balance should be considered before seek-ing to manipulate one particular facet of the immune system.

Unlike B-cells, which can recognize and ultimately neutralize harmful bacteria and free-floating viruses or other foreign particles, the T-cells are capable of specializing in tumor cells and virus-infected cells. Its receptors must be able to distinguish between self and non-self on the cells to which it binds. In organ transplantation, T-cells will bind to foreign tissues unless powerful immunosuppressive drugs are administered to depress T-cell proliferation. Autoimmune diseases (e.g., rheumatoid arthritis) may involve an inability of the T-cell to distinguish appropriately between self and non-self so the body actually attacks its own tissues. In this case there is obviously some functional abnormality in the T-cell itself.

To ensure that lymphocyte (T- and B-cells) and antibody functions are properly directed, the chemical configurations of the cells' receptors act as keys in a lock-and-key recognition system. When circulating antibodies encounter viruses or other foreign matter with surfaces having an electro-chemical profile that complements the B-cell receptor's, the antibodies can bind directly to them. In one way or another this binding activity puts the virus, toxin or bacterium out of action, eventually leading to their removal from the general circulation. As the immune system normally preserves a memory of any such stimulation, a second intrusion by the same type of virus will be responded to so efficiently that infection never sets in. This is the basis for the practice of vaccination, which is a way to artificially generate such immunological memory in people who have never encountered the natural virus.

Once the immune system has recognized a foreign substance or organism, it proceeds to react in a highly specific and orderly manner, ultimately leading to the antigen's removal from the body. The basic sequence of events goes something like this. When any antigen enters the body, circulating macrophages pick up the signal and relay it to the T- and B-cells, which then determine whether the signal represents self or non-self. If recognized as non-self, the *lymphoid tissues* (concentrated in the thymus and spleen, but also in the liver and intestines) produce mature lymphocytes and antibodies which will specifically bind and neutralize these foreign bodies. The phagocyte and complement systems are then called upon to break down and remove the now inert foreign matter.

One example of the integrated nature of human immunity is the immune response to a tumor. The T-helper cell may recognize tumor cells as foreign and signal B-cells to begin producing antibodies. Macrophages and another type of white blood cell called *natural killer cells* (similar to T-killer cells) descend directly on the cancerous growth and begin devouring and disintegrating the cancerous tissue. Millions of antibodies are elicited to bind to tumor cells, which are further degraded by the body's complement system. When enough antibody has been synthesized and bound to the tumor, a signal is relayed back to the lymphoid tissues, and a second wave of antibodies goes out to bind up residual antibodies from the first wave. (This is now referred to as the *network theory* of immunology). T-suppressors will meanwhile turn off the first wave of antibody production. Finally, phagocytic cells step in to clean up the debris and antibody-bound tumor cells. This demonstrates the complex feedback system within and between the humoral and cell-mediated components.

The activities of T- and B-cells involve a highly complex level of communication whose end product, if all goes well, is the so-called immune response. The specific binding by white blood cells and antibodies to the complementary receptor sites of any foreign entity is the functional basis of immune recognition. Faulty recognition can lead to infection, cancer or other illnesses.

Dietary Fats and Immune Function ──────────────

The immune system's billions of cells must function optimally to prevent major infections and cancers from taking hold. What determines how well the immune cells can recognize foreign matter, communicate with each other, and direct the essential activities of antibodies and various white-blood cells? All forms of cellular recognition and communication are mediated by the *cell membrane*, the fluid coating which surrounds the cell. Various types of natural chemicals and materials are constantly entering and leaving the cell via the cell membrane to participate in physiological processes. This membrane serves as a filter or gatekeeper between the intra- and extracellular environments. Efficient attachment to and transportation across this membrane is essential to the cell's biological integrity.

The cell membrane is made up of a thin, fluid coat of *lipid* (fat) and protein molecules. The organic composition of these molecules is ultimately derived from the food we eat. Compared to the protein content, however, the lipid content of cell membranes is more readily altered by dietary changes. Too many saturated fats in the diet will render the cell membrane more rigid and less permeable, and this would tend to alter exchanges between the cell's internal and external environments. Conversely, unsaturated fats such as *linoleic acid* (a plant oil obtained from many seeds, nuts, grains, and vegetables) tend to make the membrane more fluid, thereby promoting a smooth flow of essential materials into and out of the cell.

The lipid molecules which mediate cell-membrane fluidity are also subject to change by indirect environmental sources. Normally, these lipids have a somewhat crooked, loose shape and are arranged side by side in the membrane. But the lipids can be altered and severely damaged by *free radicals*, those highly unstable and reactive molecules generated primarily by oxidized dietary fats (due to too much oil and fat in the diet, and fried and barbecued foods) and heavy metals (lead, cadmium, mercury, copper, and even iron). Contact with free radicals causes *peroxidation* of the membrane lipids—they become straight and rigid, no longer functioning in their normal capacity as dynamic filters. The cell membrane then allows unwanted, toxic material into the cells. Free-radical damage to the membrane lipids ultimately leads to premature cell death.

Many environmental sources of free radicals are difficult to avoid, such as the heavy metals in our air, food, and water, or other pollutants which tend to cause excessive oxidation in the body. But when we consume an excess of fatty or oily foods we are actively promoting free-radical damage and cell degeneration. Particularly harmful are those foods that have been fried or barbecued, or foods cooked in commercial "supermarket" oil, which are processed by a heat-extraction process. We should therefore eat less fats in general, and favor only moderate amounts of cold-pressed vegetable oils, seeds, and nuts as our most concentrated sources of fat. Another important aspect of preventing free-radical damage is the consumption of food which contain "antioxidant" nutrients and constituents of "free-radical scavengers." The primary nutrients for this purpose are vitamins E, C, and beta-carotene, as well as the trace elements zinc and selenium—all well supplied by a diet based on organically grown whole grains, legumes, and land and sea vegetables.

The cell membrane also contains millions of tiny molecular gates or *receptors*, made of *glycoprotein* (carbohydrate and protein), which allow nutrients and natural chemicals (enzymes, hormones, interferons, etc.) to enter the cell. These receptors serve as sites of attachment for microorganisms or foreign substances, or for other cells and antibodies which in turn influence the cell's metabolism and immune activities. Immune receptors are found not only in the lymphoid tissues but also in other tissues distributed throughout the body—the spleen (*splenic red pulp*), liver (*hepatic lobules*), kidneys (*renal glomeruli*), lungs (*alveolar* walls), intestines (*villi*), sinuses and other areas. These locations may determine where pathological damage may or may not take place, depending on how well the cells of the immune system are coordinating with each other and properly distinguishing between self and non-self.

Embedded in the fatty membrane, the cell's receptors are three-dimensionally structured proteins whose physical configuration and electrical charge determine the specificity of binding. The receptors themselves are strongly influenced by the surrounding lipids—the phospholipids, cholesterol, and fatty acids located throughout the cell's membrane. As stated above, the proportions and availability of these organic substances is largely determined by our daily diet. With too much saturated fat in the membrane, the receptors may not be replaced as quickly, and their electrical affinity may be altered. Dietary practices may determine receptor availability, specificity, and binding capacity. Excessive quantities of cholesterol in the cell membrane may impede receptor binding and alter the immune system's ability to recognize bacteria, viruses, or malignant cells.[29]

Some of the most fascinating investigations on the influence of dietary fats on the immune system have focused on B- and T-cells, the two central cells involved in specific immunity. In animal studies, saturated fatty acids were shown to suppress the proliferation of T-cells, while B-cells seemed much less prone to these effects.[30] Other studies have shown that T-cells exposed to high levels of saturated fatty acids may die within a relatively short period of time, whereas increasing the unsaturated fatty acid content of the membrane enabled cells to live considerably longer.[31] These effects on the T-cells appear to carry over to other cells with which they interact, such as the antibody-producing B-cells. An increased ratio of saturated to unsaturated fats produces a significant decline in antibody production.[32] In sum, saturated fats could be a major contributing factor in the development of immunodeficiency conditions, including susceptibility to AIDS and cancer.

These and other nutrition studies suggest that it is highly erroneous to consider a single virus as the ultimate cause of AIDS. Like other microbes, viruses are threatening only insofar as the immune system is incapable of responding to them. The success of infection hinges primarily on how well the immune system is functioning at the time of viral exposure. "Immune competence" must involve many cell types, organs, and systems working in harmonious synchrony with one another.

Viral Origins and Dynamics

Viruses are found throughout our environment. Like bacteria and other microbes, most viruses are normally harmless—they rarely if ever produce obvious signs of disease. There are viruses of mammals (humans, apes, dogs, cats, etc.), birds, fish, amphibians, insects, higher plants, algae, fungi and even bacteria. Over the past thirty years, scientists have isolated a large range of viruses in humans. Most of these produce only minor forms of illness. The human intestine and human respiratory tract are now known to harbor on occasion viruses almost as diverse as their bacterial inhabitants. Many viruses are considered as indigenous to the human body, which may carry between 70 and 100 different types at any one time. Yet most of these viruses are harmless because they are continually neutralized by the immune system.

The virus is to biologists what the coyote represented to the native Americans: deceptively simple in appearance yet surprisingly tricky in action. First of all, viruses are extremely small creatures. The average AIDS virus is about 0.00000047 inches long, so literally tens of thousands of them could fit into the period at the end of this sentence. A *virus* is simply a protein-coated bundle of genes (either DNA or RNA) containing instructions for making identical copies of itself. All viruses demonstrate the three interrelated characteristics of living things: *reproduction, variation*, and *selective survival*. However, because they lack the kinds of self-reproductive features carried by cells, biologists are at odds about calling viruses "living" or "organisms." Indeed, they are often referred to as viral *particles* or *virions*—making it sound as if they were of extraterrestrial origin.

Incapable of existing on their own, viruses are *parasitic* in nature. Their functions depend entirely upon the reproductive capacities of other organisms' cells. Once present inside a human cell, the virus's bundle of genetic information merges with our own DNA and begins issuing its own instructions. The cell becomes a factory capable of mass-producing copies of the virus. Eventually these new viruses may rupture the cell, disintegrating it and sending viral clones out to infect nearby cells. Viruses have been linked with many common diseases, such as the common cold, the flu, herpes, mononucleosis, and some childhood illnesses such as mumps and chicken pox. Viruses are also thought to be responsible for certain types of cancer because they are often found in or around malignant tumors.

How did viruses evolve? Where do they come from? Biologists have been pondering these questions for decades, and the answers remain speculative. First, as the simplest of all microscopic creatures, viruses may also be among the most primitive. They may have been derived from similar structures of nucleic acid dating back to the dawn of life. But how, then, did viruses become parasitic? This fundamental question introduces the second and more widely held view that animal viruses probably evolved by a process of parasitic degeneration from larger life forms, such as bacteria. For instance, it appears that bacteria which became highly adapted to a parasitic existence gave rise to the virus-like organisms known as *rickettsiae* and *chlamydiae*. These organisms are now officially regarded as both viruses *and* degenerate bacteria.

The logic behind the theory of parasitic degeneration is expressed by Burnet and White in *Natural History of Infectious Disease*:

> To derive viruses from such [higher] forms we have to press the idea of parasitic degeneration to its absolute limit. There are analogies at higher levels of organization where it is characteristic of many though not of all parasites that the organism will tend to evolve in the direction of losing all unnecessary faculties, not infrequently being reduced until it is little more than a simple mechanism for providing sufficient nourishment to the reproductive cells. . . . If a parasitic bacterium could utilize the cell's metabolic equipment for its own use it could in principle surive the loss of many of its own genes. A corresponding reduction in size would become possible, and . . . such a process might continue until the organism is reduced to the absolute minimum, a fragment of matter still retaining the power of growth and multiplication, and capable of surviving in its own particular biological environment . . . just a single molecule of nucleic acid carrying only enough genes to provide for its replication and for a protective coat of protein needed to convey it safely from one host cell to another.[33]

A third and equally popular theory is that viruses arose from something in the host cell itself—either from a genetic mechanism in the cell's nucleus or something in the organism's protoplasm, liberated from normal control and able to get into other cells to carry on as an independent entity. In other words, viruses may represent the descendants of cell components that have somehow gone astray and turned back on their own host cell. Then, as is the logical outcome for a self-replicating unit, the "mutineering" particle may have become a relatively autonomous participant in the process of evolution. Geneticists have observed fragments of DNA, contained in animal cells, which are not integrated into the main body of chromosomal DNA. To achieve the status of virus, these free genetic fragments would simply need to become encased in protein. It is by this course that bacterial DNA fragments could conceivably be transformed into viral particles.[34] Some believe that retroviruses such as the AIDS virus originated from the DNA of animal species, possibly even of humans.

Perhaps it is best to consider the evolutionary basis of viruses in terms of some combination of the three views expressed above. This integrated perspective requires a very broad frame of reference spanning the subtle energies from which life was formed, through the elemental world, and finally to the molecular realm, which represents the tangible starting point of all biological phenomena. Out of the elements combining together arose mineral salts, peptides, proteins, and other molecular compounds serving as the functional groundwork of all life forms. The beginning of life involved a further refining of the molecular material into the most versatile and fundamental of all biological structures: the *ribonucleic acids*, DNA and RNA—the master and working copies of all cellular blueprints upon which the structural design and operations of the cell depend. As little more than protein-coated nucleic acids, viruses are quite similar to DNA and RNA on the molecular scale of things. Both DNA/RNA and viruses are capable of self-replication, yet both also require cells for completion of their function.

The Order of Life

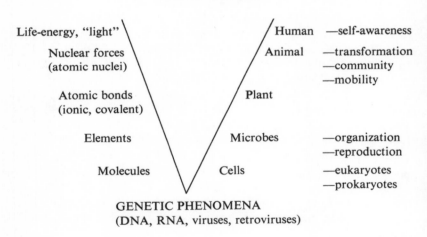

Life-energy, "light"		Human	—self-awareness
Nuclear forces (atomic nuclei)		Animal	—transformation —community —mobility
Atomic bonds (ionic, covalent)		Plant	
Elements		Microbes	—organization —reproduction
Molecules		Cells	—eukaryotes —prokaryotes

GENETIC PHENOMENA
(DNA, RNA, viruses, retroviruses)

DNA, RNA, and viruses represent the most refined development of the molecular realm, the physical basis of life. Both can exist inside the body throughout one's lifetime. Both require cells for the completion of their functioning. Prokaryotes represent the more simple, primitive cell structures whereas eukaryotes are more complex and advanced cell structures.

Viruses which originate within the human body and normally persist throughout one's lifetime are termed *endogenous*, while those which originate from outside the body are termed *exogenous*. HIV may represent a mutant form of an endogenous human retrovirus, perhaps one of the most primitive components of the human genome. How did this mutant arise? Was it somehow spontaneously generated by animal cells, or degenerated from more complex biological structures such as bacteria or fungi? Could modern environmental conditions have anything to with its emergence?

The fact that the AIDS virus has entered our population in a pathologic form now, perhaps after millions of years of benign quiescence, may suggest several possibilities: (1) certain environmental conditions may have contributed to the original mutation of a benign retrovirus; (2) environmental conditions may have caused weakened immunity, which then allowed the virus to multiply and spread; and (3) both conditions occurred together to produce AIDS. It is possible that the AIDS virus originated in humans as a mutation arising from polluted or toxic environmental conditions, including Westernized living conditions, radiation, and excessive use of drugs and medications. Science is now beginning to understand how such mutation could take place.

Retroviruses are peculiar forms of viruses. Whereas most viruses carry their genetic information in the form of DNA—the genetic material found in the center of the nucleus—retroviruses carry theirs in the form of RNA, the intermediary between DNA and protein synthesis, located in various forms throughout the cell's cytoplasm. Retroviruses transcribe their genetic material in a backwards manner, that is, from RNA to DNA, and then integrate it into the host cell's DNA. The endogenous retroviruses are primarily benign and do not have any known function within human cells. They appear simply as fragments of unintegrated genetic material. The odd reversal of the genetic mechanism orchestrated by HIV may reflect something fundamental about the nature of retroviruses and their hosts. Perhaps it reflects something about the integrity and stability of the host's DNA. Are some individuals' DNA more susceptible to retroviral activity than others? In a short time, scientists may be able to answer such subtle questions.

A virus is considered biologically successful when multiplication can take place within the living cells of a susceptible host. Three factors determine success of a virus species: (1) infection, a means by which the viral particles can reach susceptible cells; (2) integration, activation, and multiplication of viruses within these cells; and (3) liberation of the newly manufactured virions into the environment. The specific manner by which these requisites are met varies widely from one virus to another.

If viruses are able to enter cells, there is a "latency period" in which the virus must integrate its genetic material into the hosts' nuclear contents. For HIV and other retroviruses, the latency period can go on for a very long time—perhaps indefinitely—without causing any sign of illness. At any given time, depending on certain biochemical conditions, the virus is activated within the cell nucleus and begins to multiply. Upon multiplying within the cell, liberation of the virus into the environment occurs almost automatically. Polio virus is liberated in the intestine and contained in fecal matter, while yellow fever (spread mainly by the bite of certain mosquitoes) is passed through the blood. Herpes viruses and the AIDS virus are found in free form primarily in the blood, but also in the semen and in vaginal and cervical secretions.

Another aspect of viral success involves the mode of transmission. During an influenza epidemic, such as occurs periodically throughout the United States, viral spread occurs directly from infected to uninfected persons by transfer of airborne droplets. Other viruses, such as those belonging to the herpes family, must be transmitted by direct human contact. However, these viruses only create symptoms in susceptible individuals. The effectiveness of an individual's immune response will differ according to the virus being presented and to the relative condition of his or her immune system. In most cases, it is likely that those people whose immune systems are unable to eliminate the virus upon initial exposure stand a greater chance of becoming afflicted by disease than those who can eliminate the virus before it begins to infect and propagate within the body cells.

Many viruses, such as the AIDS and influenza (flu) viruses, have the capacity to rapidly alter their outer protein coating. This occurs by virtue of mutations in the viral genes. Evidently, the AIDS virus is capable of mutating and thereby changing its outer structure much more rapidly than the influenza virus. For this reason, the immune system may have a harder time trying to eliminate HIV than it would the influenza viruses.

Some viruses are capable of changing so much as to represent entirely different strains. These *mutant strains* elicit the production of antibodies which are entirely different in structure from antibodies produced previously to a similar virus. Under specific laboratory conditions (chemicals, radiation, etc.), viruses can be transformed into a wide range of mutant strains, each bearing some variation in one or another property of virulence. One property may be the ability to target and damage certain kinds of cells, while another may be the ability to survive more effectively in a new medium such as saliva or sweat. Mutations may also arise from recombination of genetic characters between different virus types, such as between bacterial viruses and influenza viruses. Thus infections which take place together could give rise to progeny virus showing some of the characters of each parent virus.

Mutations seem to be important in determining changes in the virulence of certain viral diseases over time. In most cases of mutation, however, a virus is rarely able to change its mode of transmission. The influenza viruses have undergone continual change in their antigenic patterning since their first isolation in 1933, but they are still transmitted by airborne droplets only. A few mutant strains of HIV have been identified, although they seem to be benign and the mode of transmission has remained the same.

To understand how viruses may be affected by the environment at the *micro* level, let us consider the evolutionary process which takes place in the germ world and mirrors the process of adaptation and *natural selection* in the plant and animal kingdoms. Over time, successful or hardy adaptations prevail and thrive while less appropriate adaptations disappear. Viruses have evolved over millenia with ever-more refined strategies for evolutionary success—such as altering their outer physical structure to evade the host's immune system. Of course, individuals with *already* weakened immune systems would be more susceptible to the more versatile viruses. The AIDS virus has adapted so successfully to its micro-environment that it now represents one of the most formidable examples of this family of deadly retroviruses.

Probably due to their remarkable ability to mutate, most disease-associated retroviruses are highly virulent. For example, the *feline T-cell leukemia virus* (FTLV), when exposed to cats, produces symptoms of feline leukemia in some cats and immune suppression and AIDS-like symptoms in others. This finding led Dr. Gallo, of the National Cancer Institute, to speculate that changes in the protein coating of the feline retrovirus could also occur in analogous fashion in HIV. The FTLV observation furthermore suggests that the condition of the immune system among cats—and probably any other organism—varies in response to the virus. Some cats get leukemia, some get AIDS-like symptoms, and most important, *some do not get ill at all.*

After infection with FTLV, some cats show a transient rise in antibodies yet remain healthy. By contrast, others fail to show any substantial antibody increase and subsequently develop leukemia, opportunistic infections, and ongoing infection by FTLV.[35] The same transient antibody response and protective effect has been observed in heterosexuals after exposure to HIV.[36]

A recent study showed a very small number of people—5 in 2,000—who originally tested positive for the AIDS virus later had no sign of it in their bloodstream. This could mean that these individuals have managed to successfully get rid of the virus; alternatively, it could mean they have only temporarily subdued the virus, which is hiding in body cells and undetectable by current tests.[37]

Our study of viral diseases involves the following three aspects: (1) origin of the virus; (2) its ability to mutate in blood of an infected individual; and (3) the immune response to the virus. According to the science of virology, the probability that a mutation in a virus should render it pathogenic is extremely low. On the other hand, the probability that an already pathogenic virus should be able to change its outer protein structure as a function of its genetic variability is quite high. This, again, is a common adaptive feature of viruses toward the environment. HIV in particular is a master of self-transformation. Perhaps this ability to mutate so rapidly depends on the biochemical milieu in which the virus is placed. It is known, for instance, that certain proteins in the blood undergo change at different rates among individuals, some changing very fast while others change more slowly. In this vein, certain protein variants are associated with resistance to AIDS and better survival rates in AIDS patients.[38]

There are several plausible mechanisms for genetic mutation leading to either a pathogenic version of an originally benign retrovirus (low-probability event) or a more changeable retrovirus (high-probability event). These may be presented as follows:

1. *Radiation.* The AIDS virus may have emerged as a mutation due to radioactive fall-out from atomic-weapons' testing above Central Africa during the 1950s. Alternatively, it may have been introduced through mutation arising on some other occasion, possibly even in one of the U.S. nuclear mishaps, or from excessive medical X-rays.

2. *Free radical generation.* These unstable and highly reactive molecules are recognized as a major mechanism for environmentally induced genetic mutations. Free radicals are primarily generated by excessive dietary fats, chemical additives, heavy metals, and immune stimulation by antigens and toxins. (Nuclear radiation generates free radicals, too.)

3. *Glycosylated proteins.* As presented by Cerami and co-workers in the May 1987 issue of *Scientific American*, in an article entitled "Glucose and Ageing," refined or simple sugars may play a major role in the aging and degenerative processes. It has been known for many years that the hemoglobin protein within red blood cells is glycosylated throughout the cells' lifetime—that is, glucose molecules bind on to the protein. Glycosylated hemoglobins have been used as an integrated index of long-term blood sugar regulation. Now it appears that excessive rises in blood sugar level cause increased binding of not only hemoglobin, but of all proteins, including those which interact (cross-link) with the DNA. The binding may render proteins non-functional or may alter their functioning. For this reason, Dr. Cerami suggests that glycosylation (due to excessive refined sugar intakes) may be one of the environmental causes of genetic mutation. This might explain, in part, why people who reduce their sugar intakes begin looking younger quite rapidly.

4. *Synthetic chemicals.* These substances are found throughout the modern environment, including our food, water, and air. Due to their foreign and often toxic nature, they probably make the immune system less competent over time and therefore render the body more vulnerable to infection and malignancies. Some chemicals have been known to induce mutations which alter the integral functioning of viruses and bacteria; others are thought to induce cancer and other disease states. Their effects may occur synergistically with other disease-causing factors and manifest disease only over the long-term in many instances.

It is possible that several of these mechanisms may be involved simultaneously in creating a viral mutant. One could, for instance, conceive of a situation in which fatty acids, refined sugars, and artificial chemicals could *collectively* enhance virulence by creating unusual mutant strains of the virus. A 1986 study reported in *Science* found that immune cells carrying a latent form of the AIDS virus could be induced to produce copies of the virus by treatment with the chemical compound *5-iodo-2'-deoxyridine.*[39] This leads us to speculate whether some of the thousands of other synthetic chemicals permeating our food, water, and air, could have similar activating effects on HIV.

Exactly how the AIDS virus evolved as a disease entity remains a mystery. Although the virus could indeed have originated in African green monkeys, our research suggests this is not necessarily the case. It is also quite plausible that a mutation occurred in one of the human endogenous retroviruses without any monkey business. Whatever the case may be for the origin of the virus, the pertinent issue of today is why this virus is capable of wreaking such destruction on human populations at this time. If understanding HIV's true origin can help us prevent AIDS, then the foregoing discussion may offer some valuable food for thought.

Our viewing of the data on the AIDS virus, its geographic distribution and affinity for certain high-risk groups, leads us to propose two possible mechanisms to account for the origin and etiology of AIDS:

1. *Origin: Western, civilized living conditions induce the virulence of HIV.* This is what may have made the AIDS virus such a formidable foe to begin with. Among the known high-risk groups, the additive and cumulative effects of antibiotics, pharmacologic drugs, and recreational drugs may critically upset the body's internal milieu and alter the structure of the AIDS virus itself, which was originally nonthreatening. Such structural changes could render it pathological and extremely virulent. Furthermore, along with the adverse effects of ionizing radiation, drugs and toxic chemicals, various nutritional imbalances and psychosocial stresses may provide biochemical conditions which further promote mutation of the AIDS virus. In susceptible individuals, this mutant form could then participate in processes identified with the development of AIDS. The disease-causing form of the virus could be produced inside the body and still be transmitted by recognized external means—as long as it is contained in the body fluids.

2. *Etiology: Compromised immunity enables the virus to cause disease.* It is well established that our powerful yet delicate network of immune mechanisms can be weakened by health-negating dietary practices, overuse of pharmacologic and illicit drugs, and psychosocial stress such as dramatic life-style changes, loss of job, academic exams, and marital problems. Repeated use of marijuana, amphetamines, barbiturates, cocaine, and even such common substances as tobacco and alcohol, have been directly implicated in suppressed immunity.[40] Many drugs, food additives, and industrial and agricultural chemicals previously considered harmless, are now thought to be harmful to human health.[41,42,43] By directly impairing the immune system, such stresses could render the individual susceptible to infection by the now pathogenic virus. Individuals with strong, healthy immune systems would be able to deal effectively with this virus. This would place the AIDS virus in the same category as any other opportunistic infectious organism, all of which become pathogenic in the context of an incompetent immune system.[44]

Postindustrialized societies have introduced environmental conditions in which the emergence of a disease entity such as AIDS seemed inevitable. This is simply nature's way of signaling the gradual breakdown of our biological integrity in response to the diminishing quality of our environment. Like all biological systems, the immune system is limited in its capacity to adjust to adverse living conditions. Under these conditions, the body's adaptive strategies eventually become maladaptive, and natural resistance is eventually compromised. While the body is not innately invincible toward potential pathogens (viruses, cancer cells, etc.), we *can* strengthen its natural protective systems by reducing those factors which weaken it and increasing those which strengthen it.

Immunity and Viral Infection

Vulnerability to viral infection is partly a matter of the route of entry. Some viruses, including hepatitis B and the AIDS virus, must get into the bloodstream swiftly because they are so fragile. If exposed to the air, heat, or most common disinfectants, they rapidly lose their power and become inactive. For this reason HIV and hepatitis B are virtually impossible to contract except through the intimate exchange of blood, semen, and possibly saliva. By contrast, the flu and common-cold viruses are airborne and much hardier. They can land on the body's mucous membranes and penetrate the first line of defense to enter the bloodstream.

Another factor may be the degree of exposure to the infectious agent: a substantial concentration of the virus must be present to be truly infectious—that is, to overwhelm the body's natural defenses. This may be the case in people with AIDS, but it is still only part of the overall picture. Even those who have received a heavy dose of HIV may be able to eliminate the virus, provided their immune systems are strong enough. Conversely, many studies suggest that only one exposure to HIV is required for transmission and infection to take place. In this case, the body's relative protection against infectious agents must be considered.

If a virus manages to penetrate or bypass the body's first line of defense, it then enters the bloodstream and encounters other immune mechanisms. If these natural protective mechanisms are sufficiently strong, the virus will be unable to enter (infect) cells. For example, many white blood cells produce interferon. This minute protein substance can readily diffuse through the fluids of the body and into uninfected cells, rendering them resistant to virus damage. Why does one person produce more interferon than another? While genetic mechanisms are likely to be important, behavioral and nutritional factors play an equally important role.

The most prominent antiviral mechanisms center around the T-cell system, and particularly the T-killer cells and natural killer (NK) cells. When these cytotoxic cells are stimulated by foreign particles (viruses), or by antigens on the surface of virus-infected cells, their surfaces become damaged and they liberate a variety of strong chemicals which can be highly damaging to adjacent cells. This has the effect of destroying cells which may be carrying "silent" or latent viruses. The important result is that the cell containing the virus may be entirely disintegrated. When many such reactions occur at once, the cytotoxic cells and viruses become engaged in a vicious cycle by which capillaries become damaged, immune components become depleted, and a leakage of fluid occurs. Certain essential nutrients such as vitamins E, C, and beta-carotene— all abundantly found in a grain-and-vegetable-based diet—are needed to minimize the damage incurred by the immune system's antiviral mechanisms.

Other immune components such as macrophages and antibodies provide additional protection against viruses. Since the virus is inaccessible once it has entered a cell, antibodies are only effective against liberated or free-floating viruses. At the height of most viral infections, one usually finds an unusually large number of plasma cells and antibody being rapidly formed. This is a healthy response, as long as the antibodies formed are properly neutralizing the viral particles. However, the resultant antibody/antigen complexes can be irritating to the tissues, and other processes must then come into play to minimize tissue damage. Macrophages are called upon to clean up the toxic debris left over from these antiviral activities.

In most cases of viral exposure, a virus may produce minor or *subclinical* symptoms of disease. In the presence of large numbers of T-cells, any cell in which viruses are beginning to multiply will almost certainly be destroyed by T-killer cells. At the same time, some sort of rash, blister, or fever may appear. These external manifestations reflect the immune system's normal reaction to viruses. For example, the influenza (flu) viruses may produce mild fever in some individuals, yet severe and even life-threatening fever in others. If the body's back-up immune mechanisms are inefficient, the virus may then enter cells and eventually produce symptoms of infection. Thus the efficiency of cooperation between various parts of the immune system has a direct bearing on the virus's ability to create disease.

Despite great advances in the field of virology, modern science still has little more than a superficial understanding of what determines whether a virus infection—recognizable by the fact that virus is liberated in the blood or antibodies are produced—does or does not produce disease symptoms in an individual. Most viruses that completely destroy cells cultured in the lab are readily restrained in the body by a highly complex array of immune mechanisms.[45] Thus the individual's degree of immunocompetence is important in averting diseases associated with viruses.

Immunocompetence versus Immunodeficiency

Every one of the commonly known infectious diseases has been associated with specific viruses, microbes, or their toxic products. However, the presence of the organism alone is never enough to produce the disease. There must be a breakdown or deficit in the host's immune system in order for the microbe to take hold and produce symptoms. This is why, in the midst of an epidemic, some people remain healthy while others become ill. This is why some people never seem to "catch colds" while others are constantly struggling to fight them off. Combining the immunological view with an ecological perspective, it becomes apparent that there is no single cause—nor a magic-bullet cure—for infectious disease. There is only a context which involves multiple causes, both internal and external, operating in synchrony.

The context of living by which health is maintained entails a high degree of immune *competence* or *immunocompetence*. This term refers to the immune system's capacity to respond appropriately to some foreign organism or potentially harmful entity; it describes the organism's ability to sustain the most versatile protection possible toward the microbial world.

The concept of *disease resistance* has all too often been obviated by modern medicine's exclusive concern with correcting, rather than preventing, disease. In correcting disease, one focuses on symptoms or superficial mechanisms, not on the conditions of internal breakdown which precede the manifestation of symptoms. In allergy treatment, for example, antihistamines may be administered to interfere with inflammation, which is actually only the last link of a chain of events involved in the allergic reaction. The overt illness is obviously in and of itself not the cause, but merely the expression of some fundamental error or breakdown in immunocompetence.

The primary issue is not so much whether one is exposed to a certain microorganism—since this is often unavoidable—but how strong one's overall resistance or immunity is. The relative strength of the immune system is based on a certain economy by which adequate numbers and proportions of cells are maintained. We know that the immune system is constantly being challenged by viruses, bacteria, fungi, and other microbes harbored within the body. To keep these entities at bay, the system must be adequately maintained through a health-promoting way of life. The economy of immunity calls for maximizing the supply of nutrients and minimizing the demand posed by antigens, toxins, and abnormal cells.

The Economy of Immunocompetence

Supply	Demand
Primary factors: ←Human Judgement→Antigens (foreign substance)	
genes, nutrition	chemical toxins, viruses,
	fungi, protozoa, bacteria,
Secondary factors:	food additives, undigested
hormones, enzymes,	milk proteins, drugs, etc.
interferons, lymphocytes,	
antibodies, macrophages	
natural killer cells, etc.	

Mediating factors:
Proper food selection and preparation
Thorough mastication of food
Regular physical exercise
Deep and regular breathing
Relaxation or stress management
Adjunctive therapies: yoga, massage, etc.
Medical treatment for runaway infections
  and overgrown tumors.

According to this model, nutrition provides the primary form of controllable *supply* (raw material) for the production of enzymes, antibodies, white blood cells, and organ systems which support natural immunity. Antigens and toxins comprise the *demand* by which the immune system is continually stimulated and stressed. Health and disease manifest as a balance or imbalance, respectively, of immune supply and demand. If the body is continually stimulated by antigens over time, as is the normal situation, it must be supplied with adequate nutrition and endowed with sufficient genetic strength to keep the balance maintained. In the case of viral infection, a variety of white blood cells, neutralizing anti-bodies and certain natural antiviral chemicals may be missing or some-how defective, thereby allowing infection to take place.

Immunocompetence reflects the vitality of the immune system, in-cluding the amount of energy available to promote and maintain health. All cells have a limited supply of energy, and some cell types run out of energy sooner than others. Neutrophils, for example, are unable to replenish this energy and sustain *phagocytic* (cell-eating) activity. Al-though they may be very active, they are rapidly exhausted and are usually capable of no more than a single phagocytic event.[46] When neutrophils are unable to completely eliminate a foreign entity, macro-phages must be called upon. Macrophages have a more slow-acting and sustained phagocytic activity, so they can compensate for neutrophil deficits when the immune system is challenged excessively.

As noted earlier, macrophages process antigens for recognition by lymphocytes and also participate in removing old, dying, or damaged tissue. Macrophages too have their limits, however. Their lifespan depends largely on the quantity and quality of material they consume. In the lungs, they consume particles of dust and other pollutants that enter, and they can cleanse lungs blackened with the contaminants of cigarette smoke. But too much smoking will overburden the macro-phages and lead to their demise. Similarly, other particles—such as inhaled asbestos particles and certain ingested food additives—are toxic to hungry macrophages. When subsequently released from dying cells, these toxins are promptly eaten up again, producing a cascade of macrophage destruction.[47]

An essential function of these phagocytic cells is to dispose of potential-ly dangerous material, while permitting the free access of nutrients and oxygen to body tissues. What happens when this initial line of defense is overwhelmed or depleted by excessive toxic demand? Obviously, when this occurs, toxins and other foreign materials are allowed to pass throughout the body via the bloodstream, and the burden of dealing with them is given to T-cells, B-cells, and antibodies. In essence, when one part of the system cannot fulfill its protective role, other parts are forced to compensate by working extra hard. Eventually, these other parts may also become overworked and depleted. The result may be transient states of diminished disease resistance followed by a pro-nounced condition of immune deficiency.

This situation is analogous to savings in a bank account. When some-one continually spends more than he or she saves, an empty account results. Common sense dictates that spending should never exceed savings. If savings become low, more money must be deposited to prevent a negative balance. Alternatively, if savings are high, then one can afford to spend a little more freely. The continual maintenance of bank savings is analogous to the body's need to replenish its supply of key organic substances making up lymphocytes and antibodies—particularly when challenged by bacteria, viruses, allergens, and toxins—through appropriate nutrition. The ideal supply of immune components is maintained by balanced proportions of essential nutrients together with reduced intake of harmful food elements. For example, although cow's milk provides much protein, a fraction of these is comprised of indigestible proteins (e.g., casein) that may pass into the bloodstream and pose as a regular source of antigenic stress.

Overburdening of the immune system may occur by various means following entry of foreign substances—chemical additives, foreign proteins, toxic metals, recurrent infections and antibiotics—into the bloodstream.[48,49] In a recent study when laboratory mice were repeatedly exposed to foreign substances, the mice constantly produced antibodies to these antigens. But when the same mice were then injected with a molecule from a bacterium, they produced fewer antibodies than did a control group. Furthermore the ratio of the two types of key immune cells, T-helpers and T-suppressors, decreased. Both the suppressed ability to respond with antibody and the change in the T-cell ratio were exactly like that seen in people with AIDS. The researchers concluded, "Just by manipulating the immune system you can have an AIDS-like effect without even infectious [HIV] particles." They also suggested that repeated infections or exposures to foreign substances could make high-risk group members more susceptible to infection by the AIDS virus.[50]

A macroscopic example of immune overload appears in inflammation of the tonsils and appendix. The tonsils consist of various masses of lymphoid tissue in the pharyngeal area of the mouth. They act as the lymph nodes do: in filtering out bacteria and foreign debris as well as neutralizing toxic substances. When these glands are overworked, they can become inflamed, swollen, and painful. In more extreme cases, their protective function becomes overwhelmed and thus they instead become a source of infection, a condition known as *tonsillitis*. At this point most Western people opt for a *tonsillectomy* (surgical removal of the tonsils). An analogous situation occurs when the concentrated lymphoid tissues of the appendix—one of the key reservoirs of mature B-lymphocytes—become inflamed (*appendicitis*). In either case infection and other stresses have overburdened the detoxification mechanisms; the tissues themselves have reached a critical threshold in their ability to handle antigens, toxins, and bacteria. The problem is not the immunologic structures themselves but the stressful nutritional and antigenic conditions which weaken them and promote persistent infection.

The fact that the AIDS virus itself can severely disrupt the body's immune mechanisms has overshadowed the possibility that weaknesses in the immune system *precede* infection by HIV. In most studies the balance of T- and B-cells has been analyzed *after* the virus has already taken hold. But as discussed in the next chapter, there is ample evidence that the high-risk individuals are likely to exhibit some degree of compromised immunity prior to infection by the virus. For example, repeated use of narcotic drugs (heroin, cocaine, crack, etc.) is associated with increased risk of infectious disease such as tetanus, septicemia, hepatitis, candidiasis, staphylococcal endocarditis, and respiratory infections.[51] Drug abusers typically show an inverted ratio of T-helper and T-suppressor cells as well as abnormal antibody production.[52]

Although more research is needed to determine with certainty the conditions which may set the stage for HIV infection, we do know the general relationships between ecological factors (nutrition, exercise, and mental states) and key immune mechanisms involved in protecting against viruses. When an individual is exposed to the AIDS virus, several possibilities arise for whether one goes on to develop the syndrome. In most cases, if immunocompetence is adequate, the virus probably fails to get past initial antiviral defenses: the macrophages, natural killer cells, and various natural chemicals in the bloodstream.

What about the antibodies against the AIDS virus? Upon first exposure to HIV, antibodies are normally produced and memory B-cells retain the shape of the antibodies they have created for HIV. If more HIV is introduced, or if the first-line protection is insufficient, the B-cells rapidly begin antibody production. In many cases, these antibodies may be able to neutralize the virus and eliminate it from the body. However, if HIV mutates or changes its outer coating, the existing antibodies cannot stop it and new antibodies must be produced. The process of generating new antibodies may take anywhere from three weeks to nine months, depending on the individual's condition of health. Meanwhile, the virus may gain a foothold within cells and begin to multiply.

The real trouble starts when HIV is allowed to get past the body's first line of antiviral protection and reaches the T-helper cell. It is thought that HIV is capable of interfering with the recognition capacity of T-cell receptors—the components which enable T-cells to recognize a foreign entity and to direct the production of antiviral substances (interferons), neutralizing antibody production, and the cytotoxic T-killer cells. Once this receptor is altered, the immune system as a whole becomes increasingly incapable of responding to additional HIV exposure. Once HIV infects the T-cell, the lymphocyte functions gradually begin to decline. Through the process of *reverse transcription*, the HIV establishes part of its retroviral genetic material in the host cell. No obvious harm results, however, until the host T-cell is activated by some antigen. Then, rather than signaling other parts of the immune system, the T-cell manufactures HIV particles. Most likely the activating antigen is not another HIV but some unrelated virus, fungus, parasite, bacterium, or foreign substance.

Perhaps the lack of functional integrity of immune cells and exposure to HIV are two synchronous and interdependent aspects of the genesis of AIDS. In other words, neither one alone causes AIDS; instead, they may operate together as partners in a biological conspiracy. Since HIV can rapidly change its outer surface and thereby fool the antibodies, the immune system's relative ability to counter these changes with sufficient antibody diversity may be one of the pivotal determinants of one's resistance to AIDS. In addition, adequate reserves of macrophages and other components of the body's antiviral defense system must be maintained. Simply stated, HIV's success may result from its ability to capitalize on an incompetent immune system.

Nutrition provides a context for the immune system to function either appropriately or inappropriately in the presence of a potential disease entity. We now have ample evidence that nutritional imbalances may compromise immunocompetence (IC). For example, deficiencies in single nutrients such as zinc and vitamin E may adversely affect immune responsiveness. Excess of fatty acids also contribute. Protein-energy malnutrition is associated with alterations of the T-cell, B-cell and T-killer cell populations that very closely resemble the changes seen in AIDS.[53]

Altered nutritional status may also impede the functioning of other systems which indirectly support the immune response. For example, nutritional imbalances may lead to the liver's inability to neutralize toxic substances in the bloodstream, causing an over-burdening of the immune system. Food antigens from highly antigenic sources such as cow's milk and junk foods may constitute an undesirable stress on the immune system, causing a drain of its natural reserves for biological defense.

The fundamental importance of IC may be grasped by considering signs of greater susceptibility to infectious diseases among the high-risk groups. The male homosexual community and the intravenous drug users have both shown strong tendencies toward multiple infections, including a higher susceptibility to viruses such as hepatitis B, cytomegalovirus, and Epstein-Barr virus, as well as repeated polymicrobial enteric infections. Haitians and Africans evidence a high degree of various parasitic infections. A history of recurrent infectious disease reflects an immune system which is already depressed or compromised. Given the integral relationship between nutrition and immunity, the overall empirical evidence worldwide supports the idea of an immunodeficient state secondary to a combination of imbalanced nutrition and immune-overload in the development of AIDS.

The immunocompetence perspective is less concerned with how viral transmission takes place (e.g., sexual intercourse) and more concerned with why a virus is able to dominate the immune system in the first place. Healthy persons have strong IC and should be resistant to the virus. The observation of the HIV antibody without the presence of HIV in blood samples of some people may suggest sufficient IC to protect these people from the virus.

A primary reason the issue of immunocompetence has been overlooked by most medical professionals is that nutrition, as the biological crux of the matter, is a very controversial field. Moreover, most medical schools do not offer nutrition courses beyond an extremely rudimentary level, if at all. Hence when doctors begin to practice medicine, their practical and theoretical understanding of nutrition and dietetics often extends no further than the now out-dated *Basic Four Food Groups*. This is a seriuous flaw in our system of medical education. The magnitude of the problem is further reflected by the poor-quality foods served to patients in Western hospitals.

Most medical doctors advocate symptomatic drug therapies *after* sickness has already developed. The underlying reason for this practice is that medical science has no definition for immunologic resistance. There is no scientifically legitimate way to define resistance because medical methodology only identifies and diagnoses the problem *after* it has developed. This has profound importance. It means that allopathic medicine's view of disease is confined by its methodological framework, which can only perceive tangible symptoms of a substantially progressed degenerative disorder. It refuses to look at the more primary developmental aspects of disease because, technically speaking, it cannot! Until a working scientific definition for resistance is established, conventional medicine will be unable to provide preventive guidelines which are truly protective without greatly restricting personal freedom.

By contrast with the Western medical view, the view of human health espoused by Oriental medicine is holistic and dynamic, based on the idea that no single part can be understood unless in relationship to the whole. Each diagnosis is based on an overall pattern of symptoms, and patterns will vary according to individual differences. Whereas ten patients in a Western clinic may be diagnosed with one particular disease, the same group of ten would very likely receive ten different diagnoses and treatments in a traditional Chinese clinic. Symptoms are not traced back to ultimate causes but are seen as manifestations of imbalance. When a person is ill, the symptom is only one part of a complete bodily imbalance. In this way, the Chinese doctor is able to detect illness often before pronounced degenerative illness develops.[54] The Chinese have no concept of an immune system *per se*. For them, the whole body constitutes the immune system, the physiological means by which health is maintained despite continual challenges from the environment.

Macroscopic and Microscopic Manifestations of AIDS ——

As we have seen, the *Acquired Immune Deficiency Sydrome* (AIDS) is due to a defect in the person's immune system, which renders him or her more likely to develop severe and usually fatal, opportunistic infections. People with AIDS are easy prey for a variety of viruses, bacteria, protozoans, and fungal pathogens. While we all have *potential* pathogens in our body, for example, herpes virus, chicken-pox virus, candidal fungi (yeast), and even cancer cells, our immune surveillance system normally prevents them from harming us. If our immunity is impaired or malfunctioning, these pathogens seize the opportunity to spread infection or support the development of malignant cancer cells. The immunodeficiency provides the context for these opportunistic infections and malignancies to take place and progress.

Overt manifestations of AIDS should be differentiated into mild and severe forms. The milder or *prodromal* (early warning) form afflicts a large portion of high-risk groups. While this form is usually not fatal, scientists estimate that approximately 10 percent of infected people will go on to develop the severe form. The severe form is very serious, however, and over half of those infected die within two years.

The mild form, also known as *AIDS-related complex* or ARC, generally lasts for at least three months or longer. This form may be a precursor to full-blown AIDS. Alternatively, it may never progress beyond the range of symptoms listed below:

- Swollen lymph nodes in several areas
- Fever and night sweats
- Chronic diarrhea

• Weight loss and gradual emaciation

The more severe form of AIDS may manifest as any combination of a variety of opportunistic infections. Two of the most prominent conditions are *Pneumocystis carinii* pneumonia (PCP) and *Kaposi's sarcoma* (*KS*). Besides PCP, other opportunistic infections may contribute as well, albeit less extensively. Some of the more common are as follows:

• *Pneumocystis carinii* pneumonia is a severe parasitic infection of the lungs. It is the most common life-threatening opportunistic infection in AIDS, accounting for half of all diagnosed cases. The PCP protozoan parasite is found widely in the environment and in the lungs of humans. Since exposure to the organism has no adverse consequences for healthy individuals with normal immunity, PCP is rare in the United States. In children with AIDS, lymphoid interstitial pneumonitis can also destroy lung tissue.

This opportunistic infection is of particular interest because of its relatively recent emergence in the West outside of AIDS: It has been noted in severely malnourished infants, adults with leukemias and *lymphomas* (cancers of the lymph nodes), patients receiving chemotherapy, and organ-transplant patients treated with immunosuppressive drugs.[55]

• *Candidiasis*, a fungal condition that commonly affects the mouth and esophagus in many AIDS patients. As will be discussed, this infection can damage the nervous system, create nutritional deficiencies, and further impair immunity. It is of interest that this infection also appears to be afflicting large numbers of women in the United States.

• *Cytomegalovirus*, (*CMV*), an infection which may lead to meningitis and colitis. While the virus appears to be inactive in many AIDS patients, it is usually detectable in the patient's blood. Some research suggests that this virus may serve as an important co-factor in the development of AIDS.

• *Atypical microbacterial infections*, which are normally extremely rare or harmless, and can crop up anywhere in the body of a person with AIDS. One of the more frequently seen types, *M. avium*, attacks bone marrow and the liver. This microbacteria is so ubiquitous that it is found in high concentrations in much of our country's water supply.

● *Chronic herpes simplex*, a virus that can cause ulcerating anal and oral herpes. It is interesting to note that herpes (as well as candidiasis) has been increasing at an alarming rate in the young heterosexual population of the Western world.

● *Cryptosporidiosis*, a microbe that instigates prolonged diarrhea and may thus indirectly interfere with adequate absorption of foodstuffs.

● *Cryptococcosis*, a fungal infection that may lead to meningitis.

● *Toxoplasmosis*, due to the action of *Toxoplasma gondii*, a protozoa that infects the brain and lungs. It is interesting that *Toxoplasmosis* (and CMV) have been observed as a complication *in utero* (hence present at birth) as well as among immunocompromised infants (being transmitted through the milk from a carrier mother).

● Other microbial infections such as tuberculosis, salmonella, amebiasis, and so on.

Another associated phenomenon in AIDS is the concommitant presence of malignancies. The most common of these is Kaposi's sarcoma. Other less common cancers are central nervous system lymphomas, undifferentiated non-Hodgkins lymphoma, and undifferentiated Burkitt's-type lymphoma. It is felt that the spectrum of these malignancies will broaden over time.

● *Kaposi's sarcoma*, or KS, is a form of skin cancer which manifests primarily as diffuse brown or purple spots on the skin, normally confined to the legs. It may or may not be accompanied by grossly swollen lymph nodes in the neck. It may or may not develop in the internal organs of the body. Until recently, KS was a rare malignant skin tumor that mainly affected elderly men of Mediterranean descent. It was limited to the skin, rarely affected other organs, and responded well to treatment; patients often recovered and went on to live productive lives.

Early in the evolution of AIDS in the Western world, clinicians were attracted to the presence of KS in a group of young homosexual men in the United States, as it was not a previously known condition. It was also observed to be an unusually aggressive variety of KS, which was not previously part of the clinical picture. Other researchers then became aware of this more aggressive variety of KS in the equatorial regions of Africa.

Recently this type of KS has been observed in organ-transplant recipients as well as in cancer patients undergoing chemotherapy.[56] This implies that KS primarily affects those patients with compromised immune systems. It has also been observed that KS patients without the complications of opportunistic diseases tend to have a better prognosis and exhibit a more stable clinical picture. In some AIDS patients, this malignancy has taken a less aggressive form, implying some residual integrity in their immune systems.

Other manifestations of AIDS involve neurological complications, including dysfunction of the central nervous system, cranial nerves and peripheral nervous system. This apparently involves both viral and nonviral infections, tumors, and miscellaneous diagnoses. Subacute encephalitis, atypical aseptic meningitis, viral myelitis, Cryptococcosis, Candida Albicans, *Treponema pallidum*, atypical mycobacterium, CMV, toxoplasmosis, *Herpes simplex* and *Herpes zoster* encephalitis, has been implicated in the neurological complications of AIDS patients.[57]

Now let us briefly consider AIDS at the microscopic level. Here several observations seem consistent with a diagnosis of advanced AIDS. A prominent feature is an abnormal ratio of T-helper to T-suppressor cells, generally due to a deficit in the former. In healthy persons, the ratio of helpers (T_4) to suppressors (T_8) is about 2: 1, but in AIDS this ratio is reversed, with three suppressors to every one helper. Not only are the numbers of cells imbalanced, but the helper cells themselves often demonstrate abnormal functioning. Furthermore, B-cells appear to be functioning abnormally by producing excessive quantitites of antibodies which appear ineffective against the AIDS virus and other opportunistic infections. Elevations of both IgE and IgD have been observed in immunodeficiency disorders, including AIDS. Low levels of IgE, the antibody implicated in allergy, are associated with an improved prognosis for AIDS patients.[58]

It is worth noting that some of these microscopic observations are also shared by other infectious states. What is peculiar to AIDS, however, is the fact that HIV appears to focus on the T-helper cell so that the immune system loses its ability to repel usually harmless infectious agents. Under such circumstances even the common cold may seriously jeopardize the condition of a person with AIDS. By contrast, the person who does not have AIDS, or who has the milder form (ARC), usually can overcome these infections, sometimes with the help of powerful antibiotics. This suggests that antibiotics are ineffective unless the immune system itself retains at least some capability to neutralize potential disease entities. In other words, the body must ultimately have the natural reserves to maintain and rejuvenate itself.

If, indeed, HIV is the primary disease entity involved in the severe form of AIDS, it presents a formidable challenge to the sophisticated high-tech approach of modern medicine. The virus is capable of changing its genetic structure, which, in turn changes the very proteins (many times per minute) in the envelope that would be targeted by a vaccine. For this reason effective vaccines are an unlikely possibility. Antibiotics are used to treat the opportunistic bacterial infections as they arise, but they have not had any effect on the virus. Anticancer drugs are used to treat the Kaposi's sarcoma, but they cannot change the overall course of the disease. *More importantly, however, these drugs further suppress the immune system, thus rendering the individual more susceptible to opportunistic infections.* None of the many anti-viral drugs have been capable of stopping the virus from destroying T-helper cells and nerve cells, and medicine has only begun to explore possibilities for reconstituting the ravaged immune system once the virus has been eradicated.

If HIV exposure alone is "sufficient" cause, and if the mean incubation is at least five years, then the epidemic could soon become as virulent as the famous Black Plague, which wiped out more than a quarter of London in 1665.[59] However, in spite of the fact that this has been touted as one of the worst plagues of all time, let us maintain a perspective and recall that London was also "plagued" with unsanitary conditions, overcrowding, and poverty. Let us not forget that, even without antibiotics, the majority survived! This again underscores the relative importance of the basic constitution and condition of the host when confronted with a virulent agent.

Given the increasing threat which AIDS presents, we may benefit by reflecting on some of the conditions which have favored the appearance of this immunologic anomaly at this time in human history. Let us leave the mechanisms of T-cell action and viral transmission to consider some of the environmental factors which may weaken our immunocompetence. By doing so we may gain valuable insights into ways to prevent and relieve this dread phenomenon.

[1] Edelson, R. L. and F. M. Fink, "The Immunologic Functions of Skin," *Scientific American* (1984), 252(6): 46–53.

[2] Golub, E. S., "The Nature of Immune Reactions," in *The Cellular Basis of the Immune Response* (Sunderland, Mass.: Sinauer Associates, Inc., 1981), pp. 306–7.

[3] Johnston, R. B. and R. M. Stroud, "Complement and Host Defense against Infection," *J. Pediatrics* (1977), 90: 169.

[4] Schottelius, M., "Die Bedeutung der Darmbakterien fur die Ernahrung," *Arch Hyg* (1902), 42: 48–70.

[5] Mackowiak, P. A., "The Normal Microbial Flora," *N. Eng J Med* (1982), 307(2): 83–87.

[6] Ibid.

[7] Sprunt, K. and W. Redman, "Evidence Suggesting Important Role of Interbacterial Inhibition in Maintaining Balance of Normal Flora," *Ann Intern Med* (1968), 68: 579–90.

[8] Allison, M. J. et al., "Inactivation of *Clostridium Botridium* Toxin by Ruminal Microbes from Cattle and Sheep," *Appl Environ Microbiol* (1976), 32: 685–8.

[9] Gordon, H. A. and Pesti, "The Gnotobiotic Animal as a Tool in the Study of Host Microbal Relationships, "*Bacteriol Rev* (1971), 35: 390–429.

[10] Shedlofsky, S. and R. Freter, "Synergism between Ecologic and Immunologic Control Mechanisms of Intestinal Flora," *J Infect Dis* (1974), 129:296–303.

[11] Flesher, A. R. et al., "*Legionella Pneumonophila*: Growth inhibition by human pharyngeal flora," *J Infect Dis* (1980), 142: 313–7.

[12] Collins, F. M. and P. B. Carter, "Growth of *Salmonellae* in Orally Infected Germ-free Mice," *Infect Immun* (1978), 13: 172–9.

[13] Mackowiak, P. A., Op. cit. (1982), p. 89.

[14] Mandel, I. D., "The Functions of Saliva" (New York: School of Dental and Oral Surgery, Columbia University, in press, 1986), p. 11.

[15] Pollock, J. J. et al., "Fungistatic and Fungicidal Activity of the Human Parotid Salivary Histidine-rich Polypeptides on Candida Albicans," *Infect Immunol* (1984), 44: 702.

[16] Heneman, H. S. and M. S. Greenberg, "Cell-protective Effect of Human Saliva Specific for Herpes Simplex Virus," *Arch Oral Biol* (1980), 25: 257.

[17] Tenovuo, J. et al., "Interaction of Specific and Innate Factors of Immunity: IgA enhances the antimicrobal effect of the lactoperoxidase system against Streptococcus mutans," *J Immunol* (1982), 128: 726.

[18] Mandel, I. D., "Immunologic Properties of Saliva and the Prevention of Oral Disease," Columbia University College of Physicians and Surgeons, Symposium: Nutrition and the Immune System (1987).

[19] Ibid.

[20] Ibid.

[21] Nishioka, H. et al., "Human Saliva Inactivates Mutagenicity of Carcinogens," *Mutation Res* (1981), 85: 323.

[22] Isemura, S. et al., "Cystatin S, a Cysteine Proteinase Inhibitor of Human Saliva," *J Biochem* (Tokyo, 1984), 96: 1311.

[23] Stainer, R. Y. et al., "Effect of the Environment on Microbial Growth," in *The Microbial World*, 5th edition (Englewood Cliffs, N.J.: Prentice-Hall, 1986), p. 210.

[24] Ibid., p. 205.

[25] Hamburger, R. N., "Of Many Things," *Ann Allergy* (1978), 40: 374.

[26] Wendler, I. et al., "Neutralizing Antibodies and the Course of HIV-induced Disease," *AIDS Research and Human Retroviruses* (1987), 3(2): 157.

[27] Burger, H. et al., "Transient Antibody to HIV and T-lymphocyte Abnormali-

ties in the Wife of a Man Who Developed AIDS," *Amer Coll Phys* (1985), 103: 545.

28 Walker, C. M. et al., "CD8+Lymphocytes Can Control HIV Infection in Vitro by Suppressing Virus Replication," *Science* (1986), 234 (4783): 1563.

29 Klurfield, D. M. et al., "Alterations of Host Defenses Paralleling Cholesterol-induced Atherogenesis," *J Med* (1974), 10: 49.

30 Buttke, T. M., "Inhibition of Lymphocyte Proliferation by Free Fatty Acids. I. Differential Effects on Mouse B and T Lymphocytes," *Immunology* (1984), 53: 235.

31 Buttke, T. M. and M. A. Cuchens, "Inhibition of Lymphocyte Proleiferation by Free Fatty Acids. II. Toxicity of Stearic Acid toward Phytohemagglutinin-activated T Cells," *Immunology* (1984), 53: 507.

32 Pourbihloul, S. et al., "Inhibition of Lymphocyte Proliferation by Free Fatty Acids," *Immunology* (1985), 56: 659.

33 Bumet, S. M. and D. O. White, "Viruses," in *Natural History of Infectious Disease*, 4th edition (New York: Cambridge University Press, 1979), p. 66.

34 Ibid., p. 67.

35 Hardy, W. D., "The Virology, Immunology, and Epidemiology of the Feline Leukemia Virus," in *Feline Leukemia Virus*, ed. Hardy W. D. et al. (New York: Elsevier North Holland, 1980), pp. 33–78.

36 Burger, H. et al., "Transient Antibody to HIV and T-cell Abnormalities in the Wife of a Man Who Developed AIDS," *Ann Intern Med* (1985), 103: 545.

37 Findlay, S., "AIDS Is Rising among Heterosexuals," *USA Today*, 20 July 1987.

38 Altman, L. K. "Inherited Factor May Play a Role in Risk of AIDS," *New York Times* (1987), 5 Oct. 1987.

39 Folks, T. et al., "Induction of HIV Infection from a Nonvirus-producing T-cell Line: Implications for latency," *Science* (1986), 231: 600.

40 Dunnett, B., "Drugs That Suppress Immunity: Drug users have a new reason to kick the habit," *American Health* (1986), 5(9): 43.

41 Marshall, E., "Immune System Theories on Trial," *Science* (1986), 234 (4783): 1490.

42 Taylor, R. E. and B. Meier, "Consumers and States Force Food Industry to Question the Use of Suspect Chemicals," *Wall Street Journal*, 20 Nov. 1986, p. 37.

43 Sperling, D., "Sidney Wolfe: 'The Ralph Nader of medicine' is tough on bad doctors and dangerous drugs," *USA Today*, 19 Mar. 1986, sec. 4D.

44 Weiner, M., "What Makes Immunity Fail?" in *Maximum Immunity* (Boston, Mass.: Houghton Mifflin Co., 1986), pp. 140–64.

45 Burnet and White, "Viruses," p. 61.

46 Tizard, I. R., "The Fate of Neutrophils," in *Immunology. An Introduction* (Philadelphia, Pa.: Saunders College Publishing, 1984), p. 49.

47 Ibid., p. 50.

48 Virgin, H. W. and E. R. Unanue, "Supression of the Immune Response to

Listeria Monocytogenes. I. Immune Complexes Inhibit Resistance," *J Immunol* (1984), 133: 104.

[49] Badgley, L., "Immune System: Nature's intelligence confronts modern technology," *Intern J Hol Health Med* (1985), 3(4): 26.

[50] Silberner, J., "Networking AIDS," study by S. Muller et al., reported at the Sixth International Congress on Immunology, Toronto, Canada, *Science News* (1986), 130(4): 58.

[51] Cherubin, C. E., "Infectious Disease Problems of Narcotic Addicts," *Arch Intern Med* (1971), 128: 309.

[52] Mol, B. et al., "Inverted Ratio of Inducer to Suppressor T-lymphocyte Subsets in Drug Abusers with Opportunistic Infections," *Clin Immunol Immunopathol* (1982), 25: 417.

[53] *Nutrition Research* (1984), vol. 4, pp. 537–43.

[54] See Ted Kaptchuk's authoritative book, *The Web That Has No Weaver* (New York: Congdon & Weed, Inc., 1983).

[55] Gong, V., "AIDS—Defining the Syndrome," in *Understanding AIDS* (New Brunswick, N.J.: Rutgers University Press, 1985), p. 6.

[56] Ibid., p. 6.

[57] *Medical News*, "Neurological Complications Appear in AIDS," *JAMA* (1985), 253 (23): 3379.

[58] Report "Immunoglobulins in AIDS," *Oncology Times*, Aug. 1986.

[59] Castleman, M., "AIDS Goes Hetero," *Medical SelfCare* (1985), 30: 18–20.

2. Nutrition for Immunity: The Scientific Perspective

The Health-promoting Value of Diet

Ever since the birth of the pharmaceutical industry in the 1920s, the medical view of health and disease has become increasingly divorced from respect for the body's self-regulating and self-regenerative capacities. With the explosive popularity of "wonder drugs," the appeal of corrective medicine almost instantly eclipsed preventive medicine as a scientifically valid approach to health care. The mechanistic paradigm of Western medicine drew the emphasis of treatment away from root causes to address symptoms, mechanisms, and the final pathological states themselves. As the seemingly miraculous power of drugs began to captivate America's health-care consumers, the traditional emphasis on self-care and preventive medicine faded into obscurity. This opened the doors for the elusive microbial diseases that have infiltrated our society today: herpes, candidiasis, salmonella, and AIDS, to name a few. We have lost sight of the fact that when our immune systems are weak or somehow compromised, these conditions will wreak havoc on our population.

Anyone with a sincere interest in understanding AIDS or any other infectious disease must be willing to grapple with the basic question of *disease resistance*, which refers to the host's (the individual's) biological strategies of protection against potential disease-causing entities. With AIDS, medical science has established several causes of lowered resistance or depressed immunity. These include anticancer treatments (radiation and chemotherapy), routine use of immunosuppressive drugs in transplant patients, excessive use of heroin and other illicit drugs, and recurrent or persistent viral and parasitic infections. Malnutrition, too, has recently been recognized as an immunodepressive factor. This recent acknowledgment has brought much needed attention to the possibility that nutritional excesses, as well as deficiencies, may play an important role in compromising the immune system. In other words, one need not be a starving Ethiopian to be at greater risk for contracting AIDS.

The raw materials constituting the human body consist of proteins, carbohydrates, fats, vitamins, minerals and water. Some of these constituents are stored and synthesized by the body itself, but all are ultimately obtained from our daily diet. The ongoing regeneration of our many trillions of cells and sub-cellular components depends entirely upon the food we eat. But more importantly, optimal functioning of these cells and tissues is largely a function of proper nutritional balance. Even subtle imbalances in nutritional status could alter cellular functioning in important ways. These changes may either manifest directly as disease or may predispose the body to physiological and psychological stresses, eventually resulting in disease.

Nutrition is, like immunology, genetics, and molecular biology, a relatively young scientific discipline. Even so, much information has already been obtained to provide a reasonable understanding of the synergism between nutritional factors and immunocompetence. As the authors of the landmark book, *Nutrition and Immunity*, point out, ". . . the interaction [between nutrition and immunity] is profound because it is bidirectional: nutritional status influences host immunological function and the response to pathogenic challenge; conversely, infectious disease, whether acute or chronic, has a detrimental influence on the nutritional state."[1]

Broadly speaking, the relationship between nutrition and immunity entails a dual source of environmental stress: an ecological milieu characterized by: (a) frequent contact with a wealth of foreign substances (antigens) and microbes, and (b) inappropriate dietary and life-style patterns. Although both areas are controllable to some degree, with few exceptions (b) is usually far more controllable than (a). Antigens and microbes are everywhere, and obviously we cannot confine ourselves to a sterile "bubble-boy" environment. On the other hand, dietary habits and other life-style practices (such as exercise, which may in turn influence our nutritional status) are the most practical aspects of maintaining sound immunity.

Nutritional support for immunity includes a wide variety of components, all varying according to biochemical individuality, age, activity levels, and other factors. Nutritional factors antagonistic to sound immunity includes those recognized by the National Cancer Institute and other prestigious organizations as detrimental to overall health: foods that are heavily processed, high in cholesterol, fat, protein, simple sugars, and chemical additives. Simple avoidance of such foods is a powerful first step toward strong disease resistance. Conversely, some dietary factors—namely complex carbohydrates, fiber, vitamin C and B-complex, potassium, magnesium and other minerals—can enhance immune responsiveness by eliminating toxins and regenerating the lymphoid and lymphatic tissues, cells, and other components. This of course provides an added edge of protection and enhances the possibility of recuperation from disease.

Millions of Americans expose themselves daily to factors which are likely to weaken the immune system over time: white sugar, fatty junk foods, food additives, agricultural chemical residues, alcoholic beverages, recreational drugs and prescription medications. Many Americans probably have sufficient genetic strength to sustain a modicum of resistance toward the numerous opportunistic microbes and chemical toxins in the environment. Thus, whereas the immunodepression of AIDS is persistent and progressive, most of these "average Americans" are struck with only temporary periods of depressed immunity, during which they may "catch" colds or get "struck" by the flu. But even these transient spells of weakened immunity could be sufficient to allow a virus like HIV or herpes to establish a foothold in the body. Furthermore, given the rate and magnitude of technological change today, it may be just a matter of time before many Americans compromise their immune systems and become vulnerable to otherwise harmless viruses and microbes.

It is therefore imperative that the connection between nutrition and immunity is clearly mapped out and scientifically substantiated, and this is the purpose of this chapter. In recent years, largely due to improvements in biological research technologies, scientists have made many important discoveries on the relationships between nutrition and immunity. A number of recently published books offer comprehensive scientific documentation on these relationships, including: *Nutrition and Immunity* (Gershwin *et al.*, eds.); *Immunology of Nutritional Disorders* (R. K. Chandra, M. D.); *Malnutrition and the Immune Response* (R. M. Suskind, M.D., ed.) and *Nutrition, Disease Resistance, and Immune Function* (R. R. Watson, M.D., ed.). Medical review articles listed in the appendix provide additional support for the nutrition-immunity link.

Let us now consider these relationships in more detail.

(1) Excessive dietary fats. Since the sixties, when the relationship between heart disease and dietary fat first made headlines across the country, many of us have grown increasingly conscious of the various disease-promoting effects of fatty, oily foods. Indeed, fats are by far the most often incriminated of our modern dietary menaces. In particular, four basic effects of dietary fats may be cited.

 a. Altered lymphocyte receptor binding. As discussed in the last chapter, the receptors located in the membranes of lymphocytes (T-cells and B-cells) play an essential role in the recognition of foreign and potentially disease-causing entities. These receptors are composed of glycoproteins (complexes of glucose and protein) and are constantly influenced by the cell membrane in which they are embedded. High levels of saturated fat in the cell membrane produces a reduced fluidity in the membrane, while unsaturated fats increase the fluidity. A less saturated membrane allows receptors to move in and out of the membrane more smoothly in order to be regenerated. Furthermore, a high saturated-fat content in the membrane may adversely alter the physical structure and electrical affinity of the receptors, resulting in abnormal recognition of viruses, bacteria, or other antigens.[2]

b. Oxygen deprivation. Following ingestion of milk, butter, cheese, cream or other fatty foods, red blood cells (RBCs) tend to cluster together inside of blood vessels. As RBCs are essential carriers of oxygen for tissues throughout the body, the clumping effect leads to a reduced capacity to carry oxygen. A lack of oxygen may jeopardize normal metabolism in these tissues, as well as favoring undesirable bacterial colonization and proliferation of malignant cancer cells. Some doctors have proposed that RBC clumping could cause strokes or a reduced mentality in the elderly.

c. Poor blood circulation. The slowing of blood circulation may be caused by cholesterol buildup along the walls of blood vessels, leading to narrowing and occasional blockage of these vessels. Any interference with blood flow can negatively affect the body as a whole, as the blood provides essential nutrients, oxygen, and other substances to all tissues and organs, and various immune components are carried along the myriad circulatory and lymphatic channels to perform important immune functions. Poor circulation is further encouraged by a lack of physical activity; sludge or fat droplets can form in the large lymph channels in the chest and abdomen and float to blood vessels where they may cause some degree of interference with blood flow.

d. Free radicals/oxidized fats. Free radicals are natural molecules formed in the body by the metabolization of fats, by radiation, and even by physical and emotional stress. A free radical possesses an unpaired electron in its outer orbit which renders it highly reactive and unstable. Paired electrons usually spin around molecules, giving molecules electrical balance and stability. If they lose one of these electrons, however, they become highly reactive and are capable of *oxidizing* (plucking electrons from other molecules) and thereby damaging cells and tissues throughout the body. If excessive free-radical activities occur in our bodies, we end up having more cells destroyed than we can create. The result is degeneration, plain and simple.

White blood cells are richly endowed with unsaturated fats, which are highly vulnerable to free-radical damage. Thus anything which promotes free-radical production can seriously weaken the immune system as well as other body systems. The main dietary culprits are fatty, oily, and highly refined foods and particularly foods that have been cooked with high temperatures (fried or deep-fried).

While the immune system's functioning is impaired by free radicals, it also naturally generates its own free radicals in the process of eliminating harmful microbes and viruses. Indeed, any time inflammation occurs, there is an excess of free-radical activity. Any time the body is called upon to step up its metabolic rate (i.e., under "stress" conditions), free radicals are formed as waste from the cell's energy production. Under normal conditions, these same free radicals are removed by the antioxidant enzyme *superoxide dismutase* (SOD) as well as by a system of other enzymes and nutrients.

Certain kinds of animal fats have unique detrimental effects. The fat in cheese, for example, is hydrolyzed to irritating fatty acids, including butyric, caproic, caprylic and longer carbon chain fatty acids. It seems that some of the changes that occur in fats and cholesterol through the aging of cheese may adversely affect health.[3] Several forms of oxidized cholesterol that occur with aging or with overcooking of food can cause rapid damage to artery walls.

While saturated fats are often incriminated, it is important to realize that *any excess* of dietary fats, whether saturated or unsaturated, can have undesirable consequences. Even excesses of linoleic acid (an essential fatty acid) can weaken the immune system, probably by free-radical damage.[4] Overcooking of unsaturated fats (vegetable oils) produces free radicals which damage cells and tissues throughout the body, promoting a host of degenerative disorders. This includes altered functioning of antibodies and macrophages, as well as T-cells and B-cells. Hence everything in moderation—including the essentials!

(2) Excessive sugar. Observations of diabetics suggest that a high concentration of sugar in the blood lends itself to a greater susceptibility to infection. Uncontrollable infection leading to gangrene is five times more common in diabetics, and infection of the feet is seventy times more common. Other types of infection to which diabetics seem more prone include skin abscesses, meningitis and ear infections. Vaginal yeast infections and recurrent skin problems are often the first presenting symptoms of diabetes. The exact causal relationship between high blood sugar or altered sugar metabolism and reduced immune function is unknown. But if we regard diabetics as the upper limit of the blood-sugar spectrum within the general population, then "normal" people who subject themselves to an abundance of refined carbohydrate foods— hence repeated albeit temporary highs in blood sugar levels—may also show some degree of altered immunity.

Another interesting fact is that various immune-related disorders appear to be closely associated with altered sugar metabolism. *Rheumatoid arthritis* (an autoimmune disease) is often accompanied by hyperinsulinism and hypoglycemia, both of which have been associated with excess consumption of sugary foods, including white sugar, honey, white flour, fruits and fruit juices, and so on. Other conditions of altered immunity which may be linked with consumption of refined or simple carbohydrates are various allergies, abnormal skin conditions, polio, and rheumatic fever.[5]

Some research shows that sugary foods may directly inhibit immune function. For instance, overconsumption (100 grams) of simple carbohydrate from glucose, fructose, or sucrose (white sugar) can significantly decrease neutrophil phagocytic activity for up to five hours and longer, and can also decrease lymphocyte transformation.[6,7,8] These findings have important implications in light of the fact that the average American consumes more than 100 pounds of white sugar per year, not to mention simple sugars coming from fruits, fruit juices, ice cream, pastries, and other sources.

(3) Low dietary fiber. Fiber plays a versatile role in maintaining health, and there is no substitute for a whole-grain-based diet, which is the best way to obtain fiber. Fiber assists in the crucial elimination of fecal matter from the intestines. By doing so it supports removal of toxic matter, including carcinogens, and helps maintain the health of the intestines, blood and body as a whole. Fecal accumulation in the intestines may entail a potentially lethal mixture of intestinal flora, endotoxins, exotoxins, and blood-derived products, which may then enter the circulation via the intestinal lymphatics or by absorption from the peritoneal cavity.[9] The result is "septic shock" and probably a tendency toward antigen overload and various immune-related problems.

Except for cancer of the lung, colon cancer kills more people than any other—about 50,900 deaths a year—and it is the most frequent cancer killer of all for those who do not smoke. Colon cancer is accompanied by high levels of bile acids in the colon, which appear to result from high-fat diets. The feces of people on a typical high-fat American diet contain more bile acids than those of Japanese, Chinese, or U.S. Seventh Day Adventists, all of whom eat less fat and substantial amounts of fiber, and have lower rates of colon cancer than average Americans.[10] Futhermore, there is a high degree of intestinal bowel obstruction associated with a known diagnosis of advanced cancer originating in the pelvis.[11] Because of these and related findings, both the American Cancer Society and the National Cancer Institute have begun recommending an increase in America's consumption of fiber-rich whole grains and vegetables.

Besides maintaining normal bowel functions, diets high in fiber are associated with better weight control, as fiber helps displace nutrients and prevents a high absorption of energy-rich foodstuffs. (Refined-carbohydrate foods have the exact opposite effect.) This is important because obese people tend to have more infectious diseases than people of normal weight, and their mortality rate from infections is higher.[12] High-fiber diets are also linked with a lower incidence of appendicitis, Crohn's disease, various cancers, diabetes, hypoglycemia, and various gastrointestinal disorders.[13]

(4) Excessive animal protein. Protein-rich diets are typically high in animal products, including red meat, poultry, eggs, fish and all dairy products. Excess protein is broken down in the liver and excreted through the kidneys as urea, or blood urea nitrogen. Due to its diuretic action, urea causes the kidneys to work harder and excrete more water, and valuable minerals such as calcium, potassium, and magnesium are lost in this process. Studies have shown that young men consuming diets containing more than 95 grams of protein daily develop a negative calcium balance, even with very high calcium intakes.[14] It is interesting to note that the incidence of osteoporosis is significantly higher among societies with high protein intakes than among those with low protein intakes. Eskimos, for example, who consume extremely large amounts of protein *and* calcium have the highest incidence of osteoporosis in the world. By contrast, for many African peoples subsisting on low-protein, low-calcium diets osteoporosis is extremely rare or utterly absent.

Ever since saturated fat was recognized as a major risk factor for both heart disease and cancer, the dairy industry has been promoting low-fat dairy products. (Not surprisingly, when calcium was recently found to be helpful in the prevention of colon cancer, the number of T.V. commericals and magazine ads for milk increased dramatically.) Unfortunately, the issue of fat reduction completely ignores the protein aspect. In fact, when fat is removed from whole milk to produce skim milk, the relative protein content doubles. Therefore low-fat milk may be even less appropriate as a calcium source than regular milk. But the most healthful sources are dark leafy green vegetables, sea vegetables, whole grains, beans, seeds and nuts. In addition, sunlight (stimulating vitamin-D synthesis) and moderate exercise are very important in helping one maintain normal calcium levels.

While most people think of calcium as a bone-fortifying nutrient, calcium plays an even more critical role in neuromuscular excitability, cellular adhesiveness, transmission of nerve impulses, normal myocardial function, and activation of enzymes and hormones. It mediates immune functions via the nervous and circulatory systems as well as through several key enzymes in which it functions as a co-factor. Hence when calcium levels are lowered as a result of dietary imbalances (e.g., high protein intakes), or lack of sunshine and exercise, many undesirable conditions may arise, including chronic fatigue, hypertension, multiple sclerosis, osteoporosis, cancer and various immune and endocrine disorders.

(5) Synthetic drugs and chemical additives. Often called the "biochemical mastermind" of the body, the liver serves as the central clearing-house for all unassimilated nutrients and toxins, and the mastermind of many thousands of biochemical processes, including immune functions. Blood flows from the intestines through the liver before entering a major vein, the *vena cava*, and then moving on to the heart and general circulation. The liver filters out most of the carbohydrates, proteins, and fats which have been absorbed by the gastrointestinal tract, and enables their proper usage or storage. Carbohydrates, for example, are stored in the liver as *glycogen*, which gradually releases the sugar for energy needs between meals. But excessive sugar consumption and overeating in general could overload the liver's nutrient-processing capacity, perhaps causing a tendency toward abnormal blood sugar levels, overweight, and impaired immunity.

The liver is also responsible for cleansing the blood by removing any wastes, contaminants, or toxins which might damage cells throughout the body or interfere with healthy functioning. These potentially hazardous substances include pesticides, herbicides, preservatives, artificial colorings and other additives, which might be absorbed along with food, as well as many metabolites which are created within the body itself. With repeated exposure to those poisons, and with a lack of minerals, vitamins, and other nutritive substances which support proper processing, the liver cells may eventually become overburdened and begin to break down. The undetoxified chemicals, as well as unprocessed sugars and amino acids, may then enter the general circulation, posing a heavy stress on the immune system and body as a whole.

(6) **Heavy metals.** The principal toxic minerals, also known as *heavy metals*, are aluminum, arsenic, cadmium, lead and mercury. Our food, water and air have become increasingly contaminated with cadmium, mercury, and lead. These metals suppress all aspects of immune functioning, depressing phagocyte responses, reducing cell-mediated and humoral immunity, and increasing susceptibility to infection.[15] Even very low, theoretically safe levels of these metals may incur serious damage on the nervous system, particularly in growing children.[16] Various free radicals such as the hydroxyls and lipid peroxides are formed in the presence of some heavy metals.

Substantial concentrations of cadmium are found in agricultural fertilizers which readily pass up the food chain, from soil to plants to animals. Cigarette smoke and the electroplating and battery industries are additional sources of cadmium. In homes there are several sources of this toxic metal, including cadmium-plated trays and vessels, and soft water that remains in contact with galvanized or black polyethylene pipes. In an August 15, 1987 article "High-Cadmium Diet: Recipe for Stress?", *Science News* reported on studies showing that cadmium increased anxiety and decreased stress-coping ability in rats. Elevated cadmium levels have been observed to impair host resistance, B- and T-cell response, antibody response, and phagocyte response.[17] Cadmium may also threaten our vitality by lowering the availability of zinc, which is essential to immunocompetence; signs of zinc deficiency may indicate high cadmium levels.

Increasing concentrations of mercury are being detected in many freshwater fish and shellfish, and this seems primarily due to industrial pollution of freshwater rivers and lakes. More within the realm of control, mercury exists in the silver amalgams used widely by dentists. Most dentists will tell you that *they* are more at toxic risk than yourself, since they have to handle it often and ostensibly the mercury is not in direct contact with the blood capillaries. However, this line of reasoning is inconsistent with recent data indicating that mercury may leach from silver fillings into the bloodstream to cause immune suppression and other toxic effects. For example, one dentist removed amalgam fillings from three patients and observed a proportionate increase in T-cells. When the amalgam was restored, the T-cell levels dropped again. This suggests that amalgam fillings chronically depress this vital cell population.[18] Alloys of nickel, which is also used in dental work, may have a similar effect on immune function.[19] These effects of dentistry warrant serious attention, especially for those suffering from AIDS or those concerned about preventing AIDS.

Aluminum may present a problem for those using aluminum cookware; it has been linked with neurological disorders, reduced bone density, and poor absorption of the minerals selenium and phosphorus. Lead is another common culprit. Many people today have a lead level five hundred times greater than our ancestors had, probably due to automobile exhaust and other air pollution, lead-containing paints, and the presence of lead in the typical American diet and public water supply.[20] Lead toxicity is associated with brain damage, neuritis and kidney cancer.[21]

(7) Food and chemical antigens. Antigens, foreign substances, enter the body through the air we breathe, the water we drink, and the food we eat. As said before, the immune system is designed to neutralize antigens and eventually remove them through the body's various excretory channels. The liver is an extension of the immune system; it may become weakened by: (a) daily overload of food additives, agricultural chemicals, and the toxic by-products of a high-protein, high-fat diet, as well as by (b) a lack of important nutrients such as trace minerals, vitamins, and complex carbohydrates. This undesirable combination works in a similar way to bring about a weakening of the immune system.

Under healthy circumstances, any substance which the immune system recognizes as foreign to the body is eventually rendered harmless by antibody activity and various other immune mechanisms. For example, cow's milk, which has a high antigen content, elicits the production of antibodies when its proteins are incompletely digested in the stomach. Improper food combinations, such as cornflakes, milk, and orange juice for breakfast, or the popular fast-food meal of cheeseburger, French fries, and milk shake or coke may enhance this possibility. In light of our present knowledge of nutrition, this constitutes a lethal combination.

The lymphoid tissues can be both antigenically overstimulated and malnourished, resulting in a depletion in their immunologic reserves—the phenomenon of *antigen overload* due to excessive exposure to foreign proteins, bacteria, viruses, and artificial chemicals. Overtaxed and weakened in this way, the immune system may be incapable of countering an elusive disease entity such as the AIDS virus (HIV).

Lastly, some people demonstrate an allergic reactivity to food and chemical antigens, and various sources are known to contribute more than others. Dairy products, eggs, citrus fruits, tomatoes, yeasted wheat bread, and numerous artificial chemicals are among the most allergenic sources for susceptible individuals. For such cases consumption of these substances may further stress immunity and contribute to antigen overload. Many of the reactions arising from food and chemical hypersensitivity may be delayed, variable, and seemingly unrelated. It is imperative that people be aware of these potential problems and investigate various modes of diagnosis.[22]

(8) Antibiotic residues in animal foods. The use of antibiotics has skyrocketed since their inception several decades ago. Whether this is due to increasing incidence in infectious disease, or to changes in diagnostic procedures, is unclear. The problem is further exacerbated by the heavy use of antibiotics for food-animals on American farms. Modern society's escalating exposure to antibiotics through the medical and agricultural systems may have reached a dangerous level, creating both resistant microorganisms and deleterious effects on the human immune system.

Animals on modern farms are raised on unhealthy diets under poor living conditions—over-crowding and low physical activity—making them susceptible to infectious diseases. In order to keep such animals from falling ill, antibiotics are constantly added to their feed.[23] In 1970 approximately 1,300 tons of antibiotics were fed to animals on U.S. farms. While the precise effects of antibiotic residues in the meat supply are unknown, a Federal task force concluded in 1972 that there is "an imminent harzard" to human health posed by the low-level feed use of antibiotics in cattle, hogs, and chicken. (Also, nearly 500 million dollars worth of antibiotics are added to cows' feed annually, and these antibiotics are passed on to humans in the dairy products made from the milk of these cows.) Common sense tells us that animals raised in this manner are unhealthy; in fact, many develop malignant tumors which are removed in the slaughterhouse before the meat is marketed![24]

A central problem with the trace quantities of antibiotics found in many commercial animal products is that these substances may actually *promote* the generation of harmful microflora in the human gut. Organisms that are resistant to the specific antibiotics used can multiply when competing or regulating microorganisms are removed. These antibiotic-resistant bacteria may be associated with conditions of depressed immunity. For example, such bacterial imbalances have been linked to a common yeast infection called candidiasis.

Candida albicans is a yeast which naturally inhabits the intestines and is kept in check through intimate interactions with "normal" intestinal microflora. When this important balance is upset, the yeast begins to multiply and becomes pathological. According to Dr. Iwata of the University of Tokyo, it begins to secrete *neurotropic* (nerve-associated) and *mutagenic* (genetic mutation-causing) toxins, which can harm the nervous system and other systems throughout the body. Infection commonly takes place in the skin, nails, mouth, vagina, bronchi, or lungs, as well as the bloodstream.[25] Moreover, deficiencies of magnesium, zinc, and essential fatty acids are commonly caused by pronounced Candida infection.[26] Each deficiency in turn creates its own concomitant problems, such as various trace-mineral imbalances. The combined effect of these nutritional imbalances and neurotoxic and mutagenic effects could be substantial immunodepression.[27]

Candida albicans also evidently has a sweet tooth: like many other microorganisms it loves simple carbohydrates. Unlike other microbes, however, it tends to cause extreme cravings for simple-sugar food. It also appears to thrive on other dietary yeasts and inorganic substances (artificial food additives, medications, etc.). A diet containing high levels of refined carbohydrate, yeasted or fermented foods, chemical additives and trace amounts of antibiotics, will tend to promote the development of Candidiasis. In the coming years this problem may become a national crisis of the same magnitude as AIDS and cancer.

(9) Emotional stress. The immune and nervous systems are inextricably linked, both directly and indirectly, anatomically as well as chemically. These connections serve to integrate their activities so that the functions of one can influence those of the other. The nervous system's regulatory influence on T-cells is further brought out by the fact that nerves generally end in regions rich in T-cells and avoid the areas that contain the developing B-cells.[28] Although much remains to be learned about the complex mutual interactions of the immune and nervous systems, extensive documentation has established the effect of psychological factors or stress on susceptibility to infectious disease.[29] This relationship is further complicated by the integral connection between nutrition and stress-coping ability (see Appendix E, Relationship between Nutrition and Stress).

Numerous studies have linked distressing life events to depressed immune function. Early studies indicated that separated and divorced women have increased mortality rates for some disease. Recently researchers found that separated and divorced women showed lower immune responses than married women. Within the former group, those with a continued feeling of attachment to the husband or ex-husband whether persistent resentment or longing—reported greater feelings of depression and showed diminished immunocompetence.[30] Other examples of how life's stresses may influence the immune system are presented in the chapter 4, "Lessons from the New York Study."

The Essential Macronutrients

Considerable nutritional information suggests that the diet most appropriate for healthy immune functioning fulfills these four criteria: (1) high in complex carbohydrate and fiber; (2) low in protein; (3) low in fat; and (4) low in additives and synthetic chemicals. Nutritionally speaking, this translates into a diet of whole grains and grain products, beans and bean products, land and sea vegetables, and supplemental portions of seeds, nuts, fish, and fruits. Also, because additives and agricultural chemicals are preferably avoided, one is advised to buy organically grown whole grains and vegetables whenever possible. This also means avoiding many so-called "health foods" or those labelled "100 percent natural," as these are often vitamin-fortified, heavily processed, or contain flavorings, emulsifiers, or other kinds of additives. Our modern food system has yet to arrive at satisfactory definitions for the terms "natural" and "organic."

Each of the four primary dietary requirements is discussed below.

(1) *A Diet High in Complex Carbohydrate and Fiber.* The human body needs energy at all times, and especially in times of persistent physical demand and psychological stress. Of all the nutrients, carbohydrates provide the most efficient and most readily available source of energy for bodily functions. The brain and other neural tissues can utilize only carbohydrates for energy.[31] Depending on the workload, the immune system must derive enough energy to adequately perform its protective functions when provoked by food and chemical antigens, viruses, bacteria, and toxins. If these immunologic challenges are strong and persistent, the immune system can derive adequate energy from carbohydrates in order to carry the extra burden.

Some of this energy is held in reserve in the liver and muscles as glycogen. When the blood sugar is low, these stores are called upon to meet additional energy demands. In times of physical exertion, these stores of energy may make the difference between endurance and exhaustion. In times of repeated infectious challenges, these stores can make the difference between immunocompetence and immune breakdown. Protein and fat are far less efficient energy sources, and these are utilized for energy only when the carbohydrate supply is depleted (e.g., fasting conditions). When ample carbohydrate is available for energy, proteins can then participate in body functions specific only for proteins. For this reason carbohydrate-rich foods may be regarded as protein-sparing foods. A lack of these foods could contribute to imbalances or problems in protein-dependent processes, including enzyme and antibody production and immune responses in general.

Cereal grains offer the greatest concentration of complex carbohydrates and fiber. Because these foods take longer for our bodies to digest and absorb, they tend to provide energy in a more gradual and sustained way, thus ensuring that energy is more or less consistently available over the long term. It is primarily the fiber content which determines the relative speed of sugar release: the higher fiber content leads to slower absorption and more sustained energy levels. Furthermore, the physical consistency of a plant food may determine how the carbohydrate is utilized by the body. For example, the grinding of brown rice into rice flour changes the body's response to the food.[32] The ground form yields sugar (and energy) more rapidly than does the unground form. Similarly, apples taken in the form of apple purée or apple juice provide more rapid release of sugar than in the unprocessed form.[33] By breaking down some of the plant cell walls, cooking has the effect of making the complex sugars of grains and vegetables more available for digestion.

Carbohydrates combine with other nutrients to form important compounds called *glycosaminoglycans* which perform the vital function of detoxifying harmful substances that are manufactured by or taken into our bodies. They also combine with proteins to form large glycoprotein molecules that may surround viral entities and prevent them from reaching a target cell and causing infestation.[34]

Avoidance of foods high in simple sugars makes sense for a number of reasons. The "empty calories" of a high-sugar diet may lead to a number of problems, including overweight, dental carries, mineral deficits, and even psychological problems such as hyperactivity and depression. High sugar consumption has also been associated with the elevation of *serum triglycerides* (blood fats) in some people.[35] High levels of these fats may aggravate heart disease and problems associated with poor circulation.[36] Refined grains, fruits and fruit juices, alcohol, caffeine, and dietary fats in general tend to raise the triglyceride levels; other evidence suggests that cholesterol levels are increased slightly by replacing complex carbohydrates with simple sugars.[37]

One of the widely recognized benefits of a balanced, grain-based diet is its fiber content. In terms of immunity, fiber's role is primarily to dilute, bind, inactivate, and remove carcinogens, cholesterol, bile acids, and various toxic substances found in our food supply.[38,39] Fiber enhances the movement of waste materials through the intestinal tract and increases the amount of feces passed. The relatively smooth and rapid movement of fecal material prevents harmful substances from prolonged contact with the intestinal mucosa, thus minimizing absorption and possible toxicity. This may explain why high-fiber diets prevent colon cancer as well as various other cancers.[40,41] Another effect is to reduce some of the nutrient absorption and to induce satiety, thereby supporting better weight control. This too could benefit people susceptible to immunologic disorders, since overweight has often been associated with lower immunocompetence.

Balanced consideration of energy needs should reflect an appreciation of the overall nutritional advantages and appropriateness of food sources. Organically grown whole cereal grains, legumes and vegetables provide a superb supply of fiber, proteins, essential fatty acids, vitamins and minerals. In addition, this combination is naturally low in sodium and fat. Thus they offer tremendous food value over the empty calories of refined carbohydrate foods such as white bread, pastries, candies, and plain white sugar. Blood sugar imbalances such as diabetes or hypoglycemia are partly associated with excessive consumption of simple sugars in the form of refined grain products, candy, soft drinks, ice cream, and fruit juices.[42,43] Furthermore, refined-cabohydrate foods in the Western diet tend to contain higher quantities of saturated fats and contaminants due to more extensive processing.

Cereal grains have served as the nutritional mainstay for human societies throughout history: whole barley, rye and wheat breads, and oatmeal for European; corn and wild rice for American Indians; millet and other grains for African and South American peoples; wheat, rye and buckwheat for citizens of the Soviet Union; and rice and millet for most of Asia. Among those populations with the highest longevity in the world, the diet is predominantly grain-based. This makes sense from the viewpoint of one's ability to cope with stress: when our energy and total nutritional needs are properly met, we can live each day more fully and deal more effectively with everyday issues and conflicts. Our quality of life improves along with the quality of our diet. Regular consumption of whole cereal grains is an integral step toward a better quality of life.

(2) *A Diet Moderately Supplied with Protein.* In addition to its well-known role in promoting growth and physical stature, proteins are necessary for the formation of essential body compounds, including enzymes, hormones, sperm, antibodies, and many other components. The plasma proteins help regulate the distribution of fluids both inside and outside of cells, as well as the acid/alkaline balance of the blood. All of these protein-dependent phenomena, as well as the availability and assimilation of protein itself, may have considerable impact on immune responsiveness. Lymphoid functions rely on a constant and balanced source of protein to regenerate phagocytic cells, lymphocytes, and antibodies.

Fortunately there are many healthful sources of protein available to us. Contrary to popular belief, however, the most appropriate source of protein is not animal but vegetable. Although it is true that animal products provide a quick and easy source of protein, the biological costs may be quite high. Most red meats, for example, contain 50 percent fat (mostly saturated), and substantial amounts of cholesterol and sodium as well. Dairy products contain highly antigenic proteins which may overstimulate antibody production and eventually overburden the immune system. In addition, ice cream, butter, cheeses and eggs tend to contain excessive quantities of saturated fats and cholesterol, and synthetic hormones, antibiotics, and preservatives persist in higher concentration in these foods as well. To say that the protein found in animal sources is the "highest quality" reflects very limited thinking. In nutritional science one needs to consider the whole food, not just one small aspect.

Due to their excessive protein content, meats, dairy foods and eggs produce toxic by-products in the body. These foods are generally high in *purines*, which are the primary building blocks of our DNA and RNA. Excessive amounts of purines break down in the body to form uric acid, which then collects in the joints and may precipitate attacks of gout in susceptible individuals.[44] High uric-acid levels are associated with uric-acid kidney stone formation, arthritis, gout, triglyceridemia, and type IV hyperlipoproteinemia, which itself may be a risk factor for cardiovascular disease.[45] In addition, by virtue of protein's high nitrogen content, protein-rich meals may lead to the production of ammonia in the intestines, and this can be highly toxic to intestinal lymphoid tissues, and weakening to the body as a whole. It could also set the stage for propagation of undesirable pathogens along the intestinal tract.

Another problem with high dietary protein, as mentioned earlier, is its relationship with calcium metabolism, as protein may directly upset our body's calcium balance. When the protein content is high, acids are produced and released into the blood. A homeostatic mechanism causes some of the calcium stored in the bones and other areas to be used as a buffer in the blood. High levels of calcium are then passed on to the kidneys to be excreted. This, in turn, contributes to the tendency to form painful calcium kidney stones.[46] Since the Western diet is extremely high in protein, it is not surprising that calcium kidney stones are the most common type of stone found among people living in affluent countries. Consumption of low-protein foods would therefore help prevent the formation of such stones and would be of particular benefit to those who suffer from recurring stones.[47]

The integrity of the kidney (renal) system bears an essential relationship to the health of the immune system. The kidneys help filter the blood and thus serve a complementary function to the lymphatic system. Furthermore, by maintaining a proper acid-base balance in the blood, the kidneys enable the biochemical reactions of immunity to proceed smoothly. Excess dietary protein causes destruction of kidney tissue and progressive deterioration of kidney function.[48] People in industrial societies commonly lose 75 percent of their kidney function by the time they reach eighty years of age.[49] This may mean that there has been gradual weakening of the kidneys for some time, perhaps even since ones' early adult years. Because the kidneys have such a tremendous extra capacity, such losses may not manifest overtly. However, when one takes in extra protein or toxic substances, the kidney may not be capable of handling these stresses optimally, and this would subsequently place a toxic burden on the rest of the body. Fortunately, people with partial damage to their kidneys, when placed on a low-protein diet, are able to preserve much of their remaining kidney function.[50]

Under normal conditions, protein is broken down in the liver, and the waste products are excreted through the kidneys. Failure of either of these organs to function normally results in a buildup of toxic protein-digestion by-products. Accumulation of such toxic substances, in addition to a general imbalance in nutritional status, is likely to promote the development of immune-related disorders.[51] Diets which are low in protein enable people with kidney or liver failure to recover dramatically.[52,53] Excessive protein consumption may thus have a direct weakening effect on the liver (any food in excess would), and this could also influence the condition of the immune system because of the liver's important role in many detoxification and lymphoid processes.

There is no reason to consider either meat or dairy products as essential to health. Thousands of years of grain-based dietary practices, many still observable in parts of the world today, are sound testimony that vegetable foods can provide more *appropriate* proportions of protein and other nutrients while avoiding or minimizing possible toxic effects. The relatively long intestinal tract and lack of canine teeth (proportional to molars and incisors) suggests that the human body is not evolutionarily designed for the concentrated protein content of animal foods. Moreover, modern sources of animal protein lack any semblance to that eaten in small quantity by our ancestors. In addition to their generally high saturated-fat content, most of today's meat and dairy products are loaded with antibiotics and hormones, both of which may contribute to a wide variety of modern health problems.

Unlike the average American diet, the macrobiotic diet emphasizes foods that are naturally low in protein. With the exception of the legumes, all vegetable products tend to be lower in protein content than animal products. Legumes such as soybeans, chick-peas, and lentils can yield too much protein; if consumed in excessive amounts they too may contribute to protein overload and further promote immunolgic deterioration, especially in the presence of an overburdened renal system. For this reason macrobiotic dietary guidelines suggest small amounts of beans, seeds, and nuts, and relatively larger amounts of grains and vegetables. Sea vegetables are cooked with the beans because they provide minerals which enhance amino-acid absorption. Fish of the non-fatty, white-meat variety is reserved for occasional use, or for individuals who are more physically active.

Another aspect of "quality" concerns the capacity of proteins to stimulate the immune system. If a food protein enters the body in whole or undigested form, then that protein can stimulate the production of antibodies. Sometimes this produces an inflammatory reaction (allergy); other times it leads to a benign antibody response. In either case, however, the immune system is compelled to react. The ideal diet would include proteins that are easily digested. Most cow's-milk proteins are not easily broken down and are the most antigenic substances in the modern diet. By contrast, the predominant proteins in typical macrobiotic foods are of very low antigenicity (rice, millet and rye being amoung the most neutral). A mildly antigenic diet is less burdensome to the immune system and enables it to deal more effectively with other sources of stimulation, such as toxins, microbes, and cancer cells.

Although a single plant food may not provide all the essential amino acids, different plant foods taken together can easily fill the protein bill. In her book *Diet for a Small Planet*, Francis Moore Lappe tells how to obtain sufficient protein by incorporating a variety of vegetable sources, including whole cereal grains, beans, and leafy vegetables. Lappe also explains that individuals adhering to the standard meat-centered American diet are inadvertently substituting 16 pounds of edible grain for one pound of meat each time they sit down to dinner. Thus, meat-eating is an extremely wasteful practice that may eventually have serious consequences for our global food system. For the sake of future generations and long-term agricultural prosperity, we would do well to shift away from reliance on animal foods for protein. As Buckminster Fuller once said, "Think globally, act locally."

(3) *A Diet Low in Fat.* Everyone needs some amount of body fat to ensure that various biological processes are adequately fulfilled. For women, the minimum amount is 13 to 15 percent of total body mass; for men it is only 3 to 5 percent. We use fat to ensure hormone production, vitamin transport (A, D, E and K), normal body temperature, and energy reserves. As integral constituents of cell membranes, fats mediate the flow of nutrients, ions, hormones, and other organic substances between every cell's internal and external environments. Despite the importance of these functions, our dietary fat requirements are relatively small. Living in a temperate climate, we can fully satisfy our daily nutritional requirement for fat by consuming a large handful of sunflower seeds, or the equivalent of one tablespoon of vegetable oil.

There are basically two kinds of dietary fat: saturated and unsaturated. Much of the fat in red meat, lard, butter, whole milk, hard cheeses, and poultry is saturated. Simply speaking, saturated means the fat is chemically dense and compact, in general, the more dense or solid a fat is, the more saturated it is. The denser fats are more difficult for the body to emulsify (liquefy) and assimilate, and are invariably accompanied by cholesterol. By contrast, the fats in grains, vegetables, and fruits, are *unsaturated*—they have a more dispersed structure. With the exception of palm and coconut oil, these fats are easier to emulsify and assimilate. Polyunsaturated fat, the least dense form of unsaturated fat, is also the easiest to assimilate and has a cholesterol-lowering effect. In chemical terms, a fat molecule is termed "saturated" when all of its available carbon bonds are occupied by hydrogen atoms; unsaturated fats have more carbon bonds left free.

Diets high in saturated fats have been implicated as a risk factor in heart disease and various cancers (breast, pancreatic, prostatic, colon, ovarian), as well as in diabetes, high blood pressure, liver disease, rheumatoid arthritis, and other immune-related diseases. Fats place an unnecessary burden on the body by slowing the blood flow, blocking blood flow, and thereby inhibiting essential nutrients and oxygen from getting to cells and tissues. By severely reducing the blood flow to specific areas of the body, fat produces a tendency toward angina, atherosclerosis, inner ear problems, reduced lung function, and stroke. It is interesting to note that obesity, a problem linked with excessive saturated-fat intake, is also associated with a greater susceptibility toward infections and lack of specific antibody responses. Under fasting conditions, however, antibody specificity is one of the last immunological attributes to be maintained, sometimes even until death.[54]

The irony of dietary fats is that while one type may help avert the ill effects of another (e.g., unsaturated fats counter the cholesterol-raising effects of saturated fats), too much of *any* type of fat can contribute to poor immune responsiveness and degeneration. When taken in excess, for example, polyunsaturated fats may undergo excessive oxidation in the body, a process which releases highly unstable and reactive molecules (free radicals) that cause tissue damage and malignant conditions. Excessive intakes of vegetable oils can profoundly jeopardize numerous aspects of the immune response.[55]

On the other hand, polyunsaturated fats (PUFAs) serve many important functions in overall health, including the following:

—Diets deficient in PUFAs inhibit the production of antibodies, probably by first affecting the T-helper cell.[56,57]

—Diets rich in PUFAs demonstrate a beneficial effect in preventing deterioration of kidney function in people with chronic renal disease.[58]

—Essential fatty acids have antibacterial, antifungal, and antiviral action, primarily by promoting T-cell activity and the production of certain hormone-like substances (prostaglandins).[59]

Since the diet must contain *some* unsaturated fatty acid for immune protection, the key is to provide moderate amounts of linoleic acid, the essential polyunsaturated fat obtained only from plant sources, including whole grains, legumes, nuts and seeds. Cold-pressed vegetable oils, such as sesame and corn oils, are good sources when used sparingly on an occasional basis. Occasional consumption of salmon, bluefish, whitefish, mackerel, and other types of coldwater fish will provide a beneficial fatty acid called *omega-3* (*eicosapentanoic acid*), which is also found in most sea vegetables and some northern land plants.

For the maintenance of good health, fatty foods such as hamburgers, roast beef, butter, cheese, creamy desserts, and others should be minimized, especially during the hotter months of the year. Shifting to a natural diet based on whole grain and vegetables automatically lowers fat intake and reduces the risk posed by the fat-soluble toxic chemicals usually found concentrated in fatty meats and dairy products, free-radical release, and overall stagnation of blood and organ functioning.

(4) *A Diet Free of Additives.* The typical American diet is replete with artificial substances which may collectively fall into the category of "additives." These include thousands of preservatives, flavorings, emulsifiers, texturizers, colorings, and other modifiers that have entered the commercial food market. These substances enable long-distance food transportation, longer shelf-life, and various sensorial qualities to compensate for otherwise tasteless or textureless refined foods. Additives also include agricultural chemicals such as antibiotics in animal feed, as well as fertilizers, pesticides, and herbicides used on our modern food crops. The increasing consumption of hot dogs, hamburgers, French fries, and various junk foods (candy bars, soft drinks, etc.) has, over the last forty years, exposed the human body to a barrage of strange chemical compounds for which there is no known biological value whatsoever.

Some three thousand artifical and "natural" additives are now circulating throughout the American food supply. According to Samuel Epstein, M.D., in *The Politics of Cancer*, conservative estimates place the number of chemical additives consumed annually—including preservatives, flavoring agents, stabilizers, and artificial colors—at about *nine pounds per year.* Therefore, over several decades of consuming the average American diet, the individual will have received *several hundred pounds of food additives.* Since many of these chemicals were introduced only recently, we may not even have begun to see the possible repercussions on our biological integrity. In a very real sense, those of us who continue to consume such chemical-laden foods have unwittingly become participants in a potentially catastrophic experiment, and we can only speculate on what the cumulative, long-term results might be.

The biological effects of most additives on the body are either unknown, unclear, or unproven by strict scientific standards. Research on food additives has often been marred by technical limitations and inadequate protocol designs. For example, most experimentation involves short-term animal studies, and results may differ greatly between species as well as within the species tested, varying according to age, sex, diet and other factors. More important, substances that appear harmless to one species may actually be dangerous to human beings. This may have to do with biochemical differences in excretory or detoxification mechanisms between species, or it may involve the way these substances interact with elements in our food and water supply. Finally, what may seem to be a safe level of carcinogen by one experimental design may be found to cause cancer by another. This discrepancy may depend on dosage concentration, frequency of dosage, and other variables.

Perhaps the most important point about food additives is again simply that our bodies have no evolutionary precedent for dealing with these artificial compounds. This raises some fundamental questions. For instance, what happens to these artificial substances if they enter our cells and collect in our tissues? What happens to our immune system's clean-up artists, the macrophages, when they come across an additive, consume it, and attempt to break it down? How much of these insults can the liver and immune system handle before they begin to break down? Unfortunately, science may be a long way off from answering such questions. In light of our own limitations in studying this problem, it would be wise to avoid these substances as much as possible. In doing so we may not only preserve the life of our soils (and their mineral balance in particular), we may also save ourselves from serious degenerative disease ten years down the road.

What follows is a list of some of the documented relationships between food additives and physiological responses:

• Sulfiting agents (sulfur dioxide, sodium metabisulfate, and potassium metabisulfite) are commonly used in restaurant salads, dried fruits, supermarket vegetables, avocado dips, wines, and shrimp to prevent spoilage. Severe chemical reactions with these substances can take place and may result in asthma attacks accompanied by weakness, cyanosis, chest tightness, shock and coma.[60]

• Monosodium glutamate (MSG) is a flavor enhancer often used in Chinese restaurants, as well as in a large variety of common commercial foods. Reactions provoked by this substance include nausea, headache, chest tightness, facial pressure, weak limbs, a burning sensation, and psychiatric problems.[61,62] One of the serious long-term effects of ingesting MSG may involve substantial brain damage.[63]

• Nitrites and nitrates, preservatives often used in packaged meats and various other foods, are converted in the body to nitrosamines, which appear to be strongly associated with stomach and gastrointestinal cancers.[64]

• Tartrazine, or FDC Yellow No. 5, is a yellow coloring agent added to common processed foods, including orange drinks, imitation lemonades, ice creams, instant puddings, pie fillings, Italian dressings, cake mixes, imitation butter flavoring, imitation fruit extracts, packaged frozen dinners, various types of candies and other products. Many over-the-counter drugs also carry tartrazine. Reactions include itching, hives, runny nose, and asthma; and occasional rash, fast heartbeat, shortness of breath, and chest pain have been observed in sensitive people.[65]

• Azo dyes, benzoates, annatto, BHT, BHA, and various meta-bisulfites have been implicated in immediate reactions (hives, edema, runny nose, etc.), as well as, less commonly, hyperactivity, irritability, contact dermatitis, and other skin problems.[66]

The actual dangers of long-term ingestion of many common additives have yet to show themselves. A few studies, however, have found long-term manifestations of damage to organs, birth defects, and malignant cancers.[67] That such drastic results had to be born out of long-term trials is unfortunate, but it should also prompt us to think and choose more wisely. Fortunately human beings do not have to be guinea pigs, but have the power to discriminate and make appropriate decisions. In spite of all our gaps in quantitative knowledge, at least we know that additives are not essential nutrients, not designed in any way to support human life.

Food additives are only a problem insofar as we fall into the trap of basing our choices on sensory gratification and forgetting the essentials of life. Whole grains, vegetables, and fruits, organically grown if possible, are free of all but unavoidable environmental contaminants. They are the only safe and sensible way to maintain our biological health.

The Effects of Dairy Foods

Mothers play an important role in determining the future health of their children. When mothers eat sugary, fatty, or adulterated foods during pregnancy, or feed their infants cow's milk or formula milk instead of breast milk, they are promoting the development of weak constitutions in their infants. Our country's obsession with dairy foods may play a very insidious role in the immunological problems of today's young and old alike. Just as human milk is ideally designed for human development, cow's milk is biologically designed for cows. Perhaps one of the gravest mistakes in human history was the introduction of cow's milk into the human diet. In their provocative book, *The Animal Connection*, medical doctors Agatha and Calvin Thrash state:

Considering its widespread use, even to the point of force-feeding, how strange that very little investigation has been done along the lines of establishing with certainty that milk satisfies all the expectations of the consumer and claims of the producer. Many problems have been identified even with the small amount of research that has been done. Milk may contribute to the formation of kidney stones, may cause intestinal malabsorption and diarrhea, and may even *cause* malnourishment of the older infants, especially leading to iron deficiency anemia.[68] Good evidence has been presented that milk products are associated with the development of cancer, skin lesions, musculoskeletal abnormalities, pulmonary obstruction, immunological disorders, and liver function abnormalities.[69]

John A. McDougall, M.D., author and nutrition expert, points out that dairy products are the leading cause of food allergies and have been linked with no less than forty-five diseases (see "Dairy Products and Eggs are Avoided on a Health-supporting Diet," *The McDougall Plan*, 1983, New Century Publishers, Inc., Piscataway, N.J.). Among the few other medical authorities to turn thumbs down toward the consumption of dairy foods is Frank Oski, M.D., author of *Don't Drink Your Milk* (1983, Mollica Press, Syracuse, N.Y.). In Oski's well-informed opinion, there are sufficient grounds to place cow's milk on the official hazardous food list.

Let us now consider more specifically the possible immune-related problems associated with milk products and their consumption. Though the list is by no means extensive, it does point out some important yet often overlooked areas of concern.

(1) *High antigen (foreign protein) content.* Whenever the immune system is posed with a substantial load of foreign substances or antigens, a general state of antigen overload (also called immune overload) may result, whereby the immune system becomes overstressed and simply cannot adequately respond to various foreign stimuli. Approximately 25 different antigens (foreign proteins, which trigger an immune response) have been identified in milk; the most antigenic of milk proteins are those which are not easily digested, namely casein and lactalbumin. Antigen overload may contribute to the development of immune-deficiency disorders such as AIDS;[70] and, regular consumption of dairy products has been implicated in certain cancers of the immune system, such as Hodgkin's disease.[71] Other antigenic substances such as various antibiotics and steroids are often found in commercial cow's milk and

may further contribute to antigen overload. Finally, most of the milk's protein content is in the form of the highly antigenic casein, of which about 40 percent is indigestible and may contribute to allergic reactions —another form of physiological stress on the immune system.

(2) *Contamination with disease-causing bacteria and viruses.* In recent years Americans have seen a rise in salmonella and other food-borne infectious diseases. Eggs and dairy products are among the primary sources of salmonella and other contaminants such as staphylococci, E. coli, and viruses linked with leukemia. Veterinarians have found leukemia viruses (which bear some semblance to the AIDS virus) in more than 20 percent of dairy cows; goats, sheep, and chimpanzees fed cow's milk may go on to develop leukemia.[72] There is some speculation that the original AIDS virus may have been a mutation of a cow's leukemia virus, which was then passed on to humans via dairy products. "Raw" dairy products carry the greatest risk for bacterial contamination. Staphylococcal food poisoning is most often associated with nonfat dry milk, cheese and butter. Whether or not an *overt* infection develops, the presence of these bacteria and viruses in milk may constitute a *covert* source of antigenic stimulation, hence an added stress to the immune system.

(3) *Excess protein, producing transient acidosis and calcium excretion.* The immune system and other bodily systems function best when the blood is slightly alkaline (about 7.2 pH). But dairy products and other foods high in protein tend to cause a transient rise in blood acidity, which elicits calcium release from the bones and hence a net *excretion* of dietary calcium. A 1985 study by the National Dairy Council found no significant change in calcium balance when the diets of postmenopausal women were supplemented with three 8-ounce glasses of milk (1500 mg of calcium, or nearly twice the RDA) for one year; the researchers attributed this obvious failure to improve calcium balance to "the average 30 percent increase in protein intake during milk supplementation."[73] Thus even though milk is high in calcium, much of the mineral may be lost indirectly in the homeostatic response to its high-protein content. The nitrogenous compounds which result from the digestion and metabolism of protein can place a heavy load on the kidneys, further affecting the condition of the blood. High protein consumption yields the highly toxic nitrogenous compound, ammonia, which may increase the risk of carcinogenesis in intestinal tissues. (It is interesting to note that a high-calcium diet has recently been associated with a decreased risk of developing colon cancer.)

(4) *Toxigenic bacterial colonization of the upper small intestine.* Cow's milk is designed for calves; human milk for humans infants. Cow's milk induces generation of bacteria designed to metabolize a calf's diet and to promote other species-specific intestinal functions. Ingestion of milk supports generation of many kinds of bacteria in the human small intestine that are found in calves.[74] To propagate most effectively, these bacteria probably utilize some of the foodstuffs intended for human digestion. Such bacteria may weaken our immunity by constant secretion of toxins and by upsetting the balance of healthy bacteria throughout the gastrointestinal tract. Many beneficial intestinal bacteria thrive in a symbiotic way with lymphoid tissues of the intestines and therefore may serve as important immunological co-factors. There is some evidence that elimination of milk products from the diet improves the prognosis for candidiasis, the yeast infection stemming from an imbalance of intestinal bacteria.

(5) *Improper calcium to phosphorous ratio.* Calcium is generally best assimilated and utilized in the body when ingested in an approximately 2: 1 ratio with phosphorous. Phosphorous can combine with calcium in the intestinal tract and interfere with calcium absorption. Dairy products tend to be very high in phosphorous (often in a 1.2: 1 ratio), so much of the calcium may not be absorbed. Many nutritionists believe that only foods which have a calcium-to-phosphorous ratio of 2: 1 should be used as the main source of calcium. Foods such as processed meats, fabricated potato chips, canned fruit desserts, and carbonated beverages are also high in phosphorous. Some medical scientists suggest that excessive phosphates may be associated with osteoporosis (bone loss) in the course of aging, though the data is conflicting.[75]

(6) *Increased vitamin and mineral requirements.* Doctors Calvin Thrash and Agatha Thrash contend that habitual consumption of cow's milk and cow's-milk products may increase the need for vitamin A and zinc, and probably also for iron, calcium, and vitamin B_{12}.[76] All of these nutrients, but especially vitamin A and zinc, are now recognized as key micronutrients for maintaining sound immunocompetence. There are probably a variety of reasons for an increased risk of certain nutritional deficiencies; these may include the following: (a) the high-protein content of milk may deplete potassium, magnesium, B-vitamins, and bone calcium; (b) bacterial growth associated with certain nutrient deficiencies (e.g., iron and zinc), as certain bacteria will interfere with intestinal absorption (point number 4) and usurp the available nutrient supply; and (3) since dairy products are high on the food chain, they may contain

unsafe levels of environmental contaminants such as pesticides and herbicides, which increase the demand for certain nutrients to help eliminate these toxic substances.

(7) *Toxicity due to improper breakdown of lactose. Lactose* is a prominent carbohydrate found in all dairy products, as well as in mother's milk. During infancy, the body normally produces several kinds of *lactase*, an enzyme which breaks down the sugar. In many Asians and Africans, however, lactase deficiency develops between infancy and adult life, leaving these people unable to digest the sugar properly after their early growing years. But the problem may be even more widespread than previously thought. Because lactase production declines substantially after the early years of life, there is reason to believe that even Caucasions develop some degree of lactase deficiency by 13 or 14 years of age. Lactose is converted to lactic acid by putrification and fermentation; most of the products of this process are toxic and irritating, including esters, the acids, and certain of the *amines*, such as tyramine and nitrosamine.[77] The general acidic effect of improper lactose utilization is reflected by increased hydrogen in the breath of individuals with reduced lactase activity.[78] It is interesting to note that neither milk fat nor lactose itself has been shown to be allergenic. It seems, however, that the allergenicity of cow's-milk protein is synergistically enhanced by reaction with lactose. In milk-hypersensitive individuals, the skin reactivity to *beta-lactoglobulin* (milk protein) was increased one hundred-fold by prior reacting with lactose.[79]

(8) *Toxicity due to excessive intakes of vitamin D.* Vitamin D's chief function is to enhance absorption of calcium in the intestines, though recent research also indicates that it supports important functions of the immune system.[80] (This may explain, in part, the seemingly therapeutic effect of sunlight for tuberculosis patients.) Nicknamed the "sunshine vitamin," vitamin D is synthesized by the activating effects of the sun's rays on a form of cholesterol present in the skin called *provitamin D*. It is also supplied by oily fish such as cod, tuna, and salmon. Both sources supply the inactive form, which must then be converted by the liver and kidneys to the active form, vitamin D_3. High intakes of calcium (e.g., from dairy products) appear to have a "down-regulating" effect on calcium-binding protein, which then causes a diminished ability to absorb calcium.[81] Moreover, regular use of D-fortified milk may carry toxic effects. Noted vitamin D authorities, Jim Moon, Ph. D, of the British Columbia Cancer Research Center and Dr. Mildred Seelig,

president of the American College of Clinical Nutrition, have linked pathological calcification (accumulation of calcium in the joints and soft tissues) with consumption of the synthetic vitamin D_2 (now banned) and D_3 (still added to dairy foods to prevent rickets). Vitamin D_3 may be toxic when consumed in excess in the form of either fortified milk or fish oils. In sum, the sun seems to be the best and safest source—fifteen minutes daily and without a sunscreen, which prevents vitamin-D synthesis.[82]

Taken together, these eight points strongly suggest that regular consumption of dairy foods—even low-fat milk—is not as healthy as flamboyant magazine ads and beguiling television commercials (all sponsored by the dairy industry) would lead us to believe. To the contrary, as a consequence of their high consumption in America, cow's-milk products may constitute one of the most serious unrecognized insults to our biological integrity. Indeed, it seems quite possible that the unprecedented dairy consumption of the past few generations has done more harm than good to our human *genome* (collective genetic make-up) and immunological integrity in general.

One of the most unique and important nutritional aspects of the macrobiotic approach to AIDS is elimination of cow's milk from the diet. Two of the main problems with dairy products with respect to immunity include: first, the antigenic quality of cow's-milk proteins; and second, the naturally declining ability to break down the simple sugar, lactose. Here we are concerned primarily with the former problem, although lactose intolerance (which appears to occur, at least marginally, in all people after infancy) as well as other problems mentioned previously, play basic supportive roles in immune dysfunction. The serious magnitude of immunosuppressive effects of cow's-milk proteins was recently stated by Dr. Charlotte Cunningham-Rundles, at a 1986 symposium called "Nutrition, Infection, and the Immune System," sponsored by the Institute of Human Nutrition, Columbia University's College of Physicians and Surgeons.[83]

According to Cunningham-Rundles, who has carried out extensive research in the area of dietary antigens and immunosuppression, the gastrointestinal tract serves the essential role of preventing absorption of antigens (all foreign substances) into the bloodstream. This occurs primarily through the local distribution of the unique antibody called IgA, which is secreted throughout the gut, lungs, and any other area lined with mucosal tissues. Tremendous amounts of IgA are constantly used up and recycled in proportion to exposure to foreign particles (antigens) in our air, food, and water. This process demands a considerable supply of dietary amino acids, minerals, vitamins, and other supportive nutrients. The absorptive surface of the gastrointestinal tract is extensive —by far our largest body of tissue interfacing with the outer world— and covered with the secretory IgA molecules. If IgA is lacking, the highly antigenic cow's-milk proteins such as casein enter the blood circulation in original whole form and stimulate the immune system to produce antibodies and other components that dispose of the antigens.

Two of the twenty-five antigenic cow's-milk proteins, casein and bovine gammaglobulin, are highly *immunogenic*, which means they pose a heavy demand on the immune system to produce large amounts of antibodies and complement. Under ideal circumstances, undigested or unbroken-down cow's-milk protein and other food antigens are retained in the gut and excreted along with other fecal matter. In some instances, however, as in the case of IgA deficiency, food proteins such as the highly indigestible casein are absorbed into the bloodstream in whole, undigested form and contribute to the development of a variety of auto-immune-related diseases, including rheumatoid arthritis, lupus erythematosus, Hodgkins' disease, brain tumors and various other cancers.[84]

It now appears that lack of IgA is one of the most common yet undiagnosed immune deficiencies. This condition exists naturally in prenatal development and in newborn infants due to immaturity of the immune system during early life. Mother's milk provides the necessary IgA to fulfill development and functional integrity of the developing infant's intestinal and respiratory tracts, while cow's-milk formula is totally devoid of this essential antibody. It is interesting to note that of sixty AIDS patients interviewed, all had been formula-fed with the exception of one, who had been breast-fed for less than three months.[85]

Furthermore, in adult individuals, pronounced IgA deficiency is far more common than previously realized. In 1985, at Memorial Sloane-Kettering Hospital in New York, of all patients seen, about half had *hypogammaglobulinemia*, or depleted levels of various antibodies—that is, combined deficits of IgG, IgA, and IgM, or lack of IgA alone. By some estimates, measurable IgA deficiency exists in about 1 in 700 in the United States and to a lesser extent in other countries. In the average hospital visit by patients and their asymptomatic family members, the condition is as common as 1 in every 300 individuals.[86] This high incidence is particularly alarming because IgA deficiency is a sub-clinical entity; it is not overtly manifested or readily diagnosed by outward appearances. Moreover the possibility of widespread *marginal* deficiency in modern societies cannot be ruled out.

As said before, the normal immune response to entry of antigen involves formation of antigen-antibody complexes. These immune complexes are ordinarily engulfed and dissolved by the natural complement compounds described earlier in this chapter. Individuals with this condition show low levels of complement within 30 to 60 minutes of drinking only 100 milliters (about 3.4 ounces) of milk, the amount commonly used in one bowl of cereal.[87] This implies that the very high levels of complexes rapidly use up the body's reserves of complement. As complement levels drop, the high levels of antibody-antigen complexes continue to circulate throughout the body without being broken down and excreted. These immune complexes result in various problems. For example, as stated at the 1986 Columbia symposium on nutrition and immunity, the kidneys become infiltrated and choked with the complexes, promoting development of nephritis, arthritis, vasculitis and abnormalities in brain function.[88]

(This last manifestation prompts the question: Could there be some relationship between the three generations of infants receiving cow's-milk formula in lieu of breast-feeding and subsequent heavy dairy consumption, one on hand, and the increasing prevalence of learning disabilities among young Americans on the other? The La Leche League, the major educational organization in support of breast-feeding, has determined from large cross-sectional studies that children who had been breastfed have higher average IQ's compared to children who had received formula feeding.)

In sum, with continual intestinal absorption and chronic exposure to cow's-milk proteins and other food and chemical antigens, the immune system cannot sustain normal levels of complement and dispose of these and other immune complexes. The result of this antigen overload is depressed immunity, whereby the immune system is overstressed and unable to appropriately host effective immune responses to other potentially harmful influences—viruses, bacteria, toxins, and so forth. It is worth recalling reports of the abnormally high levels of circulating casein-antibody complexes among persons with either AIDS or ARC. Notably, the immune complexes found in *both* healthy homosexual men and in AIDS patients are unusually low in complement proteins, which logically represents the results of repeated exposure to multiple antigens.[89] In other words, even healthy gay men appear to have highly stressed immune systems *prior* to contracting AIDS.

It is worth noting that immune deficiency is commonly acquired as a result of radiotherapy, chemotherapy, and surgery on the colon. These applications appear to upset the immunologic integrity of the gastrointestinal tract, making it quite permeable to antigens and resulting in much higher levels of circulating immune complexes. It is therefore imperative that people receiving such treatments avoid all dairy products, even though such foods may appear appealing due to their easy palatibility. Soft-cooked grains and vegetables would be a far more judicious dietary choice for preserving one's immune competence.

The concern most Westerners, particularly lacto-vegetarians, have about milk stems from concern about calcium. Because Americans generally get their calcium from dairy products, many are unaware that this essential micronutrient may be readily obtained from sea vegetables, leafy green vegetables, beans, seeds and nuts. For example, one cup of kale yields 206 milligrams (mg); collards, 280 mg; mustard greens, 310 mg; turnip greens, 267 mg; and broccoli gives nearly 200 mg in a one-cup serving. These are all quite close to the amount supplied by milk—about 300 mg in a half liter (approximately eight ounces). One of the richest sources of calcium among the land vegetables is lambsquarters (*Chenopodium album*), a delicious, leafy green "weed" which flourishes throughout Europe, America, and many other areas of the globe. In cooked form it supplies 400 mg per cup—more than is required in one day. Sea vegetables tend to provide even more calcium. By dry weight, 100 grams of hijiki sea vegetable (*Hizikia fusiforme*) provides 1,400 mg; wakame (*Undaria pinnatifida*), 1,300 mg; and arame (*Eisenia bicyclis*) yields 1,170 mg.[90] These delicious vegetables from the sea are regularly consumed in macrobiotic diets. Meeting our calcium needs is therefore mainly a matter of reeducating ourselves in the ways of proper food selection.

Another example of the confusion over dairy as a source of calcium involves its presumed role in preventing and treating colon cancer. In November, 1985, the *New England Journal of Medicine* reported that calcium supplements were effective in reversing the growth of cancer cells in colon-cancer patients. This evoked an emphatic response by the press in favor of dairy foods and seeded the fallacious notion that milk was a way to prevent colon cancer. Curiously enough, however, other studies suggest that diets high in animal protein and fat tend to *encourage* the development of colon cancer![91,92] Furthermore, diet-and-disease studies have suggested a link between high dairy consumption and some common illnesses, including heart disease,[93] breast cancer,[94] ulcerative colitis,[95] and Hodgkin's disease,[96] a cancer of the immune system. The development of Hodgkin's disease may involve continuous overstimulation of the immune system by dairy proteins, eventually leading to the breakdown of the immune system and manifesting in this form of cancer.[97] This line of thinking corresponds with these authors' contention that antigen overload through repeated consumption of dairy products and adulterated foods contributes to the development of AIDS.

The Marvelous Micronutrients ━━━━━━━━━━━━━━━━━━━━

Vitamins and minerals are integral components of a great many chemical processes in the body, from the fundamental activity of enzymes to the metabolism of macronutrients and the synthesis of immune components, hormones, and even DNA, our genetic material. Many holistically minded physicians believe the ideal proportions of these micronutrients may be the key to strong immunity. They observe that nutrient deficiencies often accompany illnesses associated with depressed immunity. Indeed some surgeons have actually proposed *inducing* nutritional deficiencies to promote immunosuppressive drug treatment for patients receiving organ transplants.[98]

If poor nutrition supports depressed immunity, then providing nutrients in the proper quality and balance can bring about the opposite: an immune-enhanced condition. This relationship may have far more validity than most medical scientists presently realize. But, there is still considerable misunderstanding about the way micronutrients are utilized and how to supply them appropriately. Many people believe that vitamin and mineral imbalances result simply from a lack of a specific nutrient in the diet, but this implies an oversimplied view of nutrition. Of course, one's habitual diet may not contain enough of these micronutrients. In the case of vitamins, the diet may contain an excess of refined and adulterated foods and a lack of whole, unprocessed, and organically grown vegetable foods. In the case of minerals, the soil in which the food was grown may be depleted of minerals, perhaps as a result of modern agricultural methods, cattle raising, and acid rain.

But this is only part of the story of micronutrient deficiency. The diet may not consist of enough *variety* to provide the proper proportions of micronutrients. Eating too many high-protein foods may lead to a loss of calcium, potassium, magnesium, and vitamin B_6. Consuming too many animal products in general and not enough vegetable-quality foods may produce deficiencies in vitamins C and B-complex, beta-carotene, potassium, magnesium, and the essential fatty acid called linoleic acid. In addition, white sugar, white flour products, junk foods, artificial sweeteners, and highly refined table salt are not only devoid of balanced nutrition but also tend to upset body chemistry.

Other less obvious factors involved in micronutrient deficiencies include the following:

1. **Lack of water, regular exercise, or glandular function** can prevent the manufacture and replacement of new cells, and may diminish the body's detoxification potential, making it more vulnerable to toxic chemicals in our food, air, and water. The body's response to rising toxicity involves accelerated glandular functions, which in turn increases the utilization—and hence depletion—of essential nutrients. Our body needs enough water during times of physical exertion or blood toxicity to aid in the excretion of acids and toxins. Physical movement or exercise promotes the functioning of the lymphatic system (which is also glandular) and thereby boosts this system's blood-cleansing abilities.

2. **Emotional stress** tends to rob the body of valuable nutrients through a variety of direct and indirect mechanisms. The body's digestive capacities are compromised during periods of intense stress, so nutrient absorption and utilization may be limited. Excretion of minerals tends to accompany anxiety or "fight or flight" responses. Stress frequently brings on self-destructive behaviors characterized by poor eating habits and abuse of alcohol, tobacco, caffeine and drugs. Bingeing on sweets or sugary foods is a common method of "coping" in modern society; in certain individuals, sugar increases anti-anxiety substances in the brain called *endorphins*.[99] However, this only accentuates the problem by promoting hypoglycemic tendencies and depletion of minerals. Lastly, eating fatty foods as a coping method increases the need for antioxidants such as vitamins A, C, and E, as well as zinc, copper, and selenium. In addition to health-promoting diet and lifestyle habits, we must all learn to relax and adopt an attitude of compassion and forgiveness toward ourselves and others.

3. **Physical strain**, either from working long hours with little rest and recreation, or from exerting oneself excessively through vigorous aerobic activities, heavy construction work, and so on, may also bring on micronutrient imbalances. Excessive physical activity releases lactic acid in the blood, which tends to elicit the uptake of certain minerals. In addition, as discussed previously, the process of aging carries with it an increased demand for certain vitamins and minerals which may in turn slow the rate of aging. Getting enough sleep every night is an important aspect of preventing physical strain or trauma for people of all ages.

4. **Medications and common medical procedures** can deplete the body of some micronutrients, both vitamins and minerals. Medications may

interfere with nutrient metabolism (and vice versa) or may produce toxic side effects which increase the need for certain nutrients, notably the antioxidants mentioned above. Some medications lead to increased excretion of valuable vitamins and minerals. Surgery or radiation treatments can adversely affect organs involved in nutrient digestion and metabolism, especially the liver and intestines.

5. **Excessive amounts of toxic trace minerals** (aluminum, calcium, lead, mercury, etc.) can be absorbed into food and water from the use of copper or aluminum cookware, copper or lead plumbing, chemical fertilizers and pesticides, car exhaust fumes and cigarette smoke. In many parts of America, the soil contains toxic heavy metals which are then passed onto the plants, and then to the animals or humans eating these plant foods. In general, toxic chemical substances tend to be more concentrated in fatty animal products such as hamburgers, roast beef, butter, cheese, or ice cream. These substances will either be stored in fatty tissues or pose an increased demand on the liver, the organ primarily responsible for detoxification processes and nutrient metabolism.

6. **A weak digestive system** may be unable to absorb and utilize much of the food consumed. People who engage in a predominantly sedentary life-style or who have consumed excessive amounts of sugar and fatty foods tend to have more sluggish digestive tracts and may be unable to properly utilize whole, unrefined foods. Some people lack enough gastric or pancreatic juices to aid in the proper breakdown of proteins and carbohydrates, which in turn may alter the metabolism of micronutrients. For whatever reason, a weak digestive system will be unable to extract and assimilate sufficient amounts of micronutrients.

Over the past two decades growing interest has centered on the possible role of vitamins and minerals for the prevention and treatment of disease. Until recently, however, studies have focused primarily on single-nutrient deficiencies rather than on combinations of these micronutrients and their dynamic interrelationships. It is now recognized that, under normal physiologic conditions, micronutrients can and do interact with one another in complex ways. The enormous amount of interplay occurring simultaneously among vitamins, minerals, and hormones involves a diverse array of biochemical antagonisms and synergisms. This picture of mutual interdependence is the key to determining the optimal set of levels for each micronutrient, and it is critical to an accurate understanding of their essential modes of action. For example, iron absorption can either be inhibited or enhanced by various nutritional factors. Vitamin C, lactose, fructose, sucrose, and alcohol are synergistic or supportive, while egg proteins, certain fatty acids, zinc, calcium, and magnesium are antagonistic or inhibitory toward iron.[100]

The following information on micronutrients and their influences on immunity was extracted primarily from three sources. First, drawing from several of Dr. William Beisel's review articles: the 1980 Federal Proceedings (Volume 39), the 1981 *Journal of the American Medical Association* (Volume 245), and the 1982 *American Journal of Clinical Nutrition* (Volume 35). Among the several authoritative textbooks used, we highly recommend *Nutrition and Immunity* (1985, Academic Press, Inc.) by M. Eric Gershwin, Richard S. Beach, and Lucille S. Hurley, research scientists of the University of California's Division of Clinical Immunology and Departments of Nutrition and Internal Medicine in Davis, California. This text provides an excellent synthesis of the medical literature concerning the relationship between nutrition and immunocompetence. It should be mandatory reading for all medical students.

Vitamins

With all the media coverage of nutrition in recent years, no other group of nutrients has received more attention than vitamins. They have emerged in the public limelight as modern elixirs, at once beautifying and energizing. Now they are also being recognized as possible keys to the prevention and treatment of cancer, heart disease, AIDS, allergies, arthritis, and many other modern diseases. Our perspective in this section, as in the rest of this book, is holistic and integrative, focusing on the major vitamins involved in strong immunity. Vitamins are indeed important to health, but they are simply one integral part of our total biological needs.

Vitamins are classified into two general categories: *fat-soluble* and *water-soluble*. The four fat-soluble vitamins, which include vitamins A, D, E, and K, are biochemically related because all are synthesized with the help of cholesterol, and all require fat or bile for absorption. The nine water-soluble vitamins include the vitamin B-complex (B_1, B_2, B_6, B_{12}, folic acid, pantothenic acid, nicotinic acid, biotin) and vitamin C (ascorbic acid or ascorbate). This group is excreted more rapidly than the fat-soluble vitamins, which are stored to various extents in fatty tissues. Plants are the primary source of all vitamins except B_{12}, which is produced by microorganisms. The typical American diet tends to be deficient in B_1, B_2, B_6, folic acid, C, and E, probably due to its heavy reliance on meat, dairy, and highly processed and adulterated food products.

Vitamins play a key role in many aspects of control or regulatory mechanisms, including those of the immune system and of interactive systems. Many vitamins seem to mimic the actions of hormones, some being so similar to hormones that only small differences exist. For instance, vitamin D acts with hormone-like properties on the DNA in the cell's nucleus, and this is as would be expected, since vitamin D is chemically a *sterol*, similar in structure to the steroid hormones. Many of the B vitamins act as *co-enzymes* and can therefore mediate many fundamental biochemical processes throughout the body, including those involved in the immune response. Largely because of their role in enzyme reactions, vitamins and vitality go hand in hand.

Dietary recommendations should include awareness of both the protective effects of a food and the way it complements other foods in the diet to promote the balanced biochemistry essential to health. In this regard, a basic awareness of the complex web of micronutrient interrelationships is helpful, because it suggests the use of whole natural foods as an excellent way to provide micronutrients in safe, appropriate proportions. Over millions of years of evolution our metabolic capacities have been fine-tuned to satisfy our nutritional needs. The recent introduction of isolated nutrients (vitamin and mineral supplements) represents a deviation from our evolution, one which may carry harmful repercussions. Does excessive use of supplements compromise our ability to assimilate vitamins from natural sources? Could supplements upset the balance of other nutrients in the body, possibly with long-term or virtually imperceptible repercussions? A growing body of research suggests the answer is "yes" to both questions.

Besides being designed by nature to utilize nutrients in the collective form of whole foods, we may also consider the principle of biochemical individuality: that everyone's needs are unique and changing.[101] *Recommended Daily Allowances* (RDAs) are best viewed as average figures or "ball-park" approximations. Among people matched for sex and age, variations of twenty-fold or more in individual requirements may be found. Nutritional scientists attribute these variations primarily to genetic and physiologic differences between individuals.

The principle of biochemical individuality also relates to the possibility of subclinical vitamin deficiencies, or so-called *marginal deficiencies*. Some people will need more, while others need less. For those individuals with extreme deficiencies, large doses of vitamins could be helpful as a temporary measure. The same may apply to those persons who have difficulty absorbing, processing, or storing vitamins. However, the "megavitamin" approach carries many risks and must be followed with extreme caution. Results from several studies indicate that abnormally high dosages of vitamins C, B₆, A, and others can have toxic side effects.[102]

Another important point concerns the way nature designed the body to recognize and assimilate vitamins and minerals. In natural foods, most vitamins and minerals are bound to protein molecules. When these protein-bound (*chelated*) micronutrients enter the body, the protein portion enables the micronutrients to be carried and utilized far more efficiently than if they had been presented in isolated form (as in vitamin supplementation). For example, vitamin A and its metabolites are bound to various retinoid-binding proteins in plasma and tissues which facilitate absorption, transport, and the mediation of their biological activity.[103] Vitamin B₆, another immune-enhancing vitamin, depends on a variety of protein complexes for its proper transfer and utilization within the body.[104]

Taken together, these points highlight the importance of procuring vitamins and minerals in the form of an unrefined, whole-foods diet. The differences in the physiological and biochemical effects of consuming supplements versus whole foods are considerable. For this reason the National Academy of Sciences, in their 1982 landmark publication, *Diet, Nutrition and Cancer*, stated that nutrition from whole foods was far superior to vitamin and mineral supplements. In 1986, several major nutritional organizations including the American Institute of Nutrition and the American Society for Clinical Nutrition issued guidelines for increasing whole-food consumption while minimizing intakes of vitamin and mineral supplements. Alice Smitherman, president of the American Dietetic Association (ADA), said, "Most Americans can and should get all the nutrients they need to be healthy from food rather than supplements." Both the ADA and AMA released guidelines questioning the use of supplements.

With these points in mind, we now present some of the evidence for the immune-enhancing benefits of single nutrients. All nutrients are dynamically interwoven as integral parts of the whole food.

(1) *Vitamin A*. Otherwise referred to as *retinol* or *beta-carotene*, vitamin A has for many years been recognized for its potential role in preventing cancer and infectious diseases. In fact, the discovery that vitamin A might play an important role in immune processes was made over 50 years ago.[105] At the same time, relatively little is known about

vitamin A's contribution to other body functions, with the notable exceptions of the eye and mucous membranes. In the eye it serves as a key constituent of the pigment systems necessary for peripheral and color vision. Night blindness is a typical sign of major deficiency.

Vitamin A's best known protective function is to support *nonspecific* resistance to infectious disease by maintaining the integrity of skin and mucous membranes. Since vitamin A is essential to the maintenance of normal epithelial tissues, a deficiency may allow entry of bacteria or other pathogens that would ordinarily be excluded from intact mucosal surfaces (i.e., opportunistic microbes).[106] It is also needed for the production of antibacterial enzymes in tears, saliva, and sweat.[107] Modest increases in dietary vitamin A enhance resistance to infection in animals and humans, and boost various kinds of immune responses. The incidence of spontaneous infections was observed to increase in vitamin-A deficient humans.[108]

In addition to general immune mechanisms, vitamin A, particularly in the form of beta-carotene, has a powerful effect on *specific* immunity, stimulating both cell-mediated and humoral responses. Beta-carotene is a plant-derived provitamin form of vitamin A; after absorption in the intestine, it is converted to two molecules of retinol in the intestinal mucosal cells. According to researchers at the National Cancer Institute and at John Hopkins School of Hygiene and Public Health, beta-carotene is the most promising micronutrient to aid in cancer prevention. They have found that people with low levels of beta-carotene may be four times more likely to develop lung cancer than those with normal levels of the nutrient. The researchers asserted that the low vitamin levels were precursors to, and not effects of, the cancer. They also admitted, that other nutrients (vitamins E, B_6, zinc, fiber, etc.) could be responsible for the observed relationship, and encouraged more whole-food consumption as opposed to vitamin supplementation.[109]

In other studies of human blood samples, various forms of vitamin A seemed to inhibit the conversion of chemically altered body cells into cancerous cells.[110] The vitamin was observed to afford direct protection against tumors induced by chemical carcinogens.[111] The functioning of T-helper cells is also enhanced by vitamin-A levels, and this may constitute an important aspect of the anticancer action of retinoids.[112] Vitamin A also works as an antioxidant to protect the integrity of cells against harmful elements in the environment (radiation, additives, fats, drugs, etc.), and this is thought to play a key role in protection against cancer.

Studies of the immune system suggest that vitamin A is essential for normal antibody production in response to a specific antigen, and under many circumstances may act to enhance antibody production if supplemented at higher than normal levels. Diets deficient in beta carotene or vitamin A resulted in significantly depressed immune responsiveness based on several standard measures. Vitamin A has been shown to enhance the activity of human natural-killer (NK) cells and to potentiate the cytotoxic effect of T-cells against tumor cells. At higher concentrations, however, vitamin A actually suppressed this latter effect, suggesting that its influence on cytotoxicity is dose-dependent and most effective within a moderate range. (This supports the case against megavitamin therapy.)

As mentioned above, vitamin A is best consumed in the form of its provitamin, beta carotene, which forms part of the pigments of many green and yellow vegetables. Excellent sources include: carrots, collard greens, kohlrabi, kale, broccoli, parsley, turnip greens, dandelion greens, mustard greens, watercress, leek greens, endive, chicory, pumpkin, and squash (acorn, butternut, and hubbard). Sea vegetables and most forms of freshwater algae are very high in beta carotene. Since vitamin A is stable at rather high temperatures, very little is destroyed in the process of cooking.

It is interesting to note that vitamin-A deficiency is a major nutritional problem throughout the world, second only in incidence and prevalence to protein-calorie malnutrition. Although the problem seems more widespread in tropical and subtropical regions of the globe (southeast Asia, Africa, India, Brazil, and others), the Western world is clearly not exempt. In fact, several large surveys have reported that vitamin A, iron and calcium were the three essential nutrients most likely to be supplied in marginal amounts in most American diets, and Black and Hispanic groups were most frequently implicated as vitamin-A deficient. A 1987 study reported in *Toxicology and Applied Pharmacology* (vol. 85, No. 3) found that certain common industrial pollutants (PCPs, PBBs, and dioxins), can reduce the concentration of vitamin A circulating in the blood and stored in the liver.

(2) *B-complex.* The B-complex is comprised of various vitamins that are usually found grouped together in nature. Among the more prominent of the B-complex vitamins are thiamin, riboflavin, niacin, pyridoxine, folic acid and pantothenic acid. Within the body there are many interrelationships among the B-vitamins, and the functions of different members of the group overlap to some extent because of their common involvement in enzyme systems. Anemia, nervousness, in-

somnia, lack of appetite, weakness in the legs, lethargy, and burning sensations in the feet are all common symptoms of B-complex deficiency. In recent years science has found that the immune and nervous systems are intimately dependent upon adequate supply of the B-complex vitamins. Indeed, without a proper supply and balance of B-vitamins, our immune system and our health would suffer tremendously.

Vitamin B_6, or *pyridoxine*, is one of the best studied of the B-vitamins and plays a fundamental role in supporting strong immunocompetence. This vitamin participates crucially in the direct line of protein, carbohydrate and lipid metabolism, and acts as a co-enzyme in amino-acid metabolism and in red blood cell formation. Due to its central location in the metabolism of major nutrients and its integral role in both the immune and nervous systems, considerable attention should be given to providing vitamin B_6 through appropriate dietary practice.

Vitamin-B_6 deficiency depresses both cellular and humoral immunity. Effects of the deficiency include atrophy of lymphoid tissues, absence of delayed skin hypersensitivity reactions, and inhibition of the expected rejection of skin transplants. Diminished antibody production is observed following antigen challenge, and both B-cells and T-cells exhibit abnormal proliferation when stimulated by antigens. The activity of thymic hormone (*thymosin*) is diminished during B_6 deficiency. In addition, pyridoxine deficiency is accompanied by decreases in serum levels of essential antibodies (IgA), total numbers of T- and B-cells in the blood, T- to B-cell ratio, spleen cell numbers, and thymus size and weight; it has also demonstrated the ability to inhibit tumor growth. In short, vitamin B_6 appears to contribute in numerous ways to strong immunocompetence.

Vitamin B_6 requirements are proportional to the protein content of food because protein metabolism places a heavy demand on B_6 supply. For persons following the standard American diet of high-protein and refined-carbohydrate foods, vitamin B_6 deficiency may be a major problem. The most concentrated and appropriate dietary sources of B_6, in descending order, include: brown rice, barley, oats, rye, corn, whole wheat, peanuts, walnuts, cabbage, kale, peas, turnips, Brussels sprouts, cauliflower, soybeans and soybean products (miso, *tempeh*, *tamari* soy sauce, and *tofu*), yams, and various species of white-meat fish (cod, flounder, etc.). Vitamin B_6 is lost through the refining of grains, as in the production of white flour.

Other members of the B-vitamin family—pantothenic acid, folic acid, biotin, thiamin, and riboflavin—influence various aspects of immunity. Deficiency of either pantothenic acid and folic acid is associated with decreases in spleen size and functioning, T- to B-cell ratio, serum antibody levels and functioning, and overall host resistance to infection, as well as inhibition of tumor growth. Pantothenic-acid deficiency appears to inhibit the stimulation of antibody-producing cells and their ability to produce new antibodies. Thiamine (B_1) and riboflavin (B_2) are mild immune-system promoters which, under deficiency conditions, are associated with most of the effects listed above, and play key roles in the maintenance of mucosal membranes, formation of red blood cells, and metabolism of carbohydrates.

Preferable dietary sources for these vitamins include brown rice, wheat, barley, oats, corn, rye, soybean and soy products, kidney and other beans, broccoli, Brussels sprouts, kale, kohlrabi, endive, parsley, parsnips, dandelion greens, watercress, cauliflower, lentils, leeks, almonds, peanuts and chicory. If possible, the cereal grains should usually be consumed in unground form.

Vitamin B_{12} (*cobalamin*) deserves special consideration because of the common notion that strict vegetarian diets are inadequate sources of the vitamin. In addition to its well-known role in maintaining health of the nervous system, vitamin B_{12} has demonstrated critical importance in the integrity of immune function, exerting a profound regulatory influence on both T-helper and T-suppressor cells. Deficiency leads to decreased T- and B-cell proliferative responses, white blood cell phagocytosis and ability to eliminate bacteria, and an increase in blocking antibodies. Vitamin B_{12} participates along with folic acid in the synthesis of the hemoglobin in red blood cells, and contributes to cell longevity, DNA and RNA synthesis, white blood cell longevity, health of the central nervous system, synthesis of proteins and fats, and in the breakdown (*catabolism*) of carbohydrates.

In contrast to the other B vitamins, B_{12} is required in extremely small amounts—less than one millionth of a gram (1 mcg). Healthy people receive some B_{12} from the millions of beneficial bacteria found in their intestinal tracts. For people consuming the typical American diet, vitamin B_{12} stores in the body tend to exceed the daily requirement by 1000-fold.

Vitamin B_{12} can be obtained in sufficient quantity from macrobiotic diets if one gives proper attention to food selection and preparation, to the way of eating, and to other aspects of life-style such as physical activity. Among strict vegetarians, B_{12} deficiency seems to occur primarily only in the presence of a gastrointestinal upset, and may be due to unrecognized diseases of the stomach and small intestine. Vitamin B_{12} problems among strict vegetarians may also be attributed to an imbalanced or overly narrow diet, lack of chewing, overeating, and lack of exercise. Excessive use of fruits, soy products, concentrated sweeteners, cigarette tobacco, antibiotics, and vitamin C and B_{12} oral supplements, may also increase the rise of B_{12} deficiency.

A critical review of the thirty or so B_{12} deficiency cases reported among vegetarians in the medical literature revealed no solid scientific basis to indicate that dietary B_{12} deficiency was the cause.[113] It should be noted, however, that B_{12} deficiency has also been observed among non-vegetarians consuming diets concentrated in refined flour products, white and artificial sugar, heavily processed foods, canned and conventionally grown vegetables, alcohol, and dairy products—though of course medical journals rarely report these cases.

Foods providing trace amounts of B_{12} in the standard macrobiotic diet are unpasteurized miso, tempeh, *natto*, tamari soy sauce, sea vegetables, pickles, fish and some organically grown vegetables. During a therapeutic regime, it is especially important to carefully monitor the diet to include the various vegetable-quality sources listed here. One should guard against overcooking and excessive washing of organic produce, since these practices tend to eliminate B_{12}-producing bacteria harbored in these foods. In degenerative states such as cancer and AIDS, use of fish or any animal product should be limited, due to toxic by-products; however, this is generally only a temporary measure, and such adjustments are made according to individual condition.

Vitamin pills are an inappropriate source of B_{12} since these pills tend to contain breakdown products of B_{12} which have an antagonistic effect that can promote subsequent B_{12} deficiency, even when adequately supplied by the diet.[114] In the case of a pronounced B_{12} deficiency, injections of the vitamin may bring about a quick replenishment of body stores; however, medical doctors recommend this course only in acute deficiency states, since B_{12} urinary excretion is high following injection.[115] Due to the malabsorption states that often accompany AIDS, a 1,000 microgram injection with hydroxycobalamin may be advised.

It is important to emphasize that the average American diet may tend to lack balanced proportions of B-complex vitamins. This is largely a result of heavy reliance on refined cereal grain products, sugary foods and adulterated or highly processed foods in general. Excessive caloric intakes (overeating) may also contribute by upsetting the digestive system; in addition, metabolism of carbohydrates and proteins, when consumed in excess, requires a larger supply of various B vitamins, including B_{12}. Many of these vitamins have an integral relationship with bacterial colonization in the large intestine, and this may have some bearing on antibiotics' capacity to alter the balance of B-complex vitamins in the body.[116] This illustrates how some of the finer biologic interrelationships of the body may indirectly influence immunocompetence.

(3) *Vitamin C.* Otherwise known as *ascorbic acid* or *ascorbate*, this vitamin is primarily a product of the plant kingdom. While most mammals produce their own vitamin C, humans, monkeys, and guinea pigs must obtain this vitamin from plant sources. The natural ascorbate-synthesizing ability of most four-legged animals probably affords them a relatively high resistance to infections and the ability to heal wounds rapidly. The fact that humans and other primates have lost the ability to produce vitamin C may be one reason for our greater susceptibility to infections and allergies. It is well-established that in cases of acute *scurvy* (resulting from vitamin-C deficiency), many infections become chronic, wounds heal less easily, and other complications frequently result.[117]

Although early research by acclaimed chemist and Nobel Prize laureate Linus Pauling suggested that vitamin-C supplementation alone could improve immune function in individuals with various cancers and the common cold, to date there are no convincing data to support his conclusions.[118] One reason for this failure may be that other aspects of life-style—in particular, the subjects' dietary practices—were not controlled. In addition, according to Pauling and other scientists, later studies may have failed to produce positive results because the supplementation levels were too low. When the body is in a diseased state, extra vitamin C is needed to counteract harmful biochemical reactions involving free radicals.

As discussed before, free radicals are unstable molecules which lead to destruction of cells and tissues in the body and are generated in excess following consumption of fatty, oily, adulterated foods, as well as by too much smoking, alcohol consumption, or drug use. Free radicals are also produced as natural by-products of the immune response to infections. Vitamin C works as an important *antioxidant* and free-radical scavenger. When too many free radicals are being generated, vitamin C helps minimize the potential destruction of cells, tissues, and organs.

Vitamin-C deficiency causes a depression of the immune response toward cancers, viruses, fungi, and other pathogens. Vitamin C supports white blood cell mobility and "cell-eating" functions, as well as the healing of wounds.[119] The vitamin-C content of WBCs tends to decrease during viral infections, pregnancy and in elderly persons.[120] Animals and humans fed deficient diets are more susceptible to infectious diseases than controls fed diets adequate in vitamin C, and show reduced antibody production and T-cell responses.[121] Vitamin C may also influence immunity indirectly by enhancing one's ability to deal with stress: it counteracts the immune-suppressive effects of *corticosteroids* (natural stress-related hormones), yet simultaneously assists in the anti-inflammatory function of these steroids.[122]

Since vitamin C also acts as an antioxidant, it may also protect against cancer by preventing the formation of carcinogens and tumors in the body. Vitamin C inhibits the formation of nitrosamines by reacting with nitrite before the nitrite can combine with amines in the diet to form carcinogenic compounds.[123] (Nitrites and amines are the metabolic breakdown by-products of red meat.) In addition, vitamin C acts as an antioxidant by preventing lipid (fat) peroxidation, thus preventing formation of dangerous free radicals.[124] For these reasons, frequent consumption of animal products and fried foods may greatly increase the body's need for vitamin C.

It is interesting to note vitamin C's interrelationships with other nutrients. The vitamin has a synergistic effect when taken with other antioxidants; for example, the more vitamin C one takes, the less vitamin E one needs, and vice versa.[125] It aids in the metabolism of the amino acids (phenylalanine and tyrosine), converts the inactive form of folic acid to the active form (folinic acid), and may have a role in calcium metabolism.[126] It also protects thiamine, riboflavin, folic acid, pantothenic acid, and vitamins A and E against oxidation, as well as the brain and spinal cord from destruction by free radicals.[127] Lastly, intestinal absorption of iron is greatly increased by adequate levels of vitamin C. It is therefore yet another of nature's masterful touches to have included abundant amounts of both vitamin C and iron in most varieties of dark leafy greens.

We are very encouraged by the extensive case studies by Dr. Robert Cathcart of California, who has investigated the relationship between vitamin C and immune-related disease. In many cases, the toxicity of AIDS induces an acute scurvy and creates the need to bring large amounts of vitamin C into the body tissues.[128] Since early 1983, Dr. Cathcart has treated more than 200 individuals diagnosed with either AIDS or ARC. His treatments emphasize large doses of vitamin C (ascorbate) along with a wholesome diet excluding all junk foods. On the average, this approach has consistently doubled the life expectancy of AIDS patients and considerably reduced major symptoms, resulting in less disability before death.

Dr. Cathcart's findings indicate that vitamin-C supplementation, in the context of a balanced nutritional program, may enhance recovery from acute viral diseases such as the common cold, influenza, hepatitis, mononucleosis (EBV infection), viral pneumonia; and from persistent viral infections such as herpes, chronic hepatitis, and AIDS.[129,130] Clinical research by Russell Jaffe, M.D., Ph. D., of Vienna, Virginia, lends support to many of Dr. Cathcart's observations of AIDS patients.[131] Dr. Jaffe's eclectic protocol for AIDS lays special emphasis on attitudinal changes, allergy testing, and balanced nutrition.

Although more time may be needed to assess the overall efficacy of these approaches, it does appear that large doses of vitamin C, combined with a balanced diet, positive attitude, and regular exercise, can protect and support the immune system of a person with AIDS. The effects have been especially impressive in AIDS cases involving pneumocystis carinii pneumonia (PCP) and during the use of antibiotics for opportunistic bacterial infections. In addition to its role as a free-radical scavenger, vitamin C counteracts the allergic reactions to antibiotics that are commonly seen in people with AIDS.[132]

These pioneering studies indicate that AIDS patients should avoid all oily foods, fatty dairy products, red meats, drugs, and other free-radical-producing substances. Instead they should consume plenty of dark or bright green vegetables, which are by far the richest sources of vitamin C. These include broccoli, Brussels sprouts, collards, kale, parsley, turnip greens, carrot tops, sprouts, cabbage, cauliflower, kohlrabi, mustard greens, watercress, and many others. Compared to green vegetables, citrus fruits contain less vitamin C per gram and are too concentrated in simple sugars; their intake should be limited. Since vigorous cooking may easily cause a loss of this vitamin, gentle steaming is preferable to boiling or heavy steaming. As a general rule, steam until the color of the vegetable is slightly enhanced, or until it begins to lose its crispiness.

As regards supplementation, we do not advocate the administration of massive doses of vitamin C for AIDS or related conditions, except perhaps as a temporary measure in advanced PCP or during the antibiotic therapy for other opportunistic infections. As Dr. Cathcart himself acknowledges, megadoses of vitamin C in AIDS patients usually lead to a lifelong dependency; if vitamin-C supplementation is withdrawn from patients following a prolonged period of massive doses, sudden death results.[133] While it is probably true that additional vitamin C is necessary in toxic or diseased conditions, the nutrient can be adequately supplied by regularly consuming the vegetable-quality foods listed above and maintaining a health-promoting mode of living. Try wild strawberries in the summertime.

(4) *Vitamin D.* Otherwise known as the "sunshine vitamin," vitamin D is the only vitamin that we are able to manufacture ourselves—with a little help from the sun, that is. The sun's ultraviolet rays are necessary for activating a form of cholesterol, which is present in the skin, and converting it to vitamin D. Provitamin D is found in both plant and animal tissues, such as in fish-liver oils. Vitamin D enables proper absorption of calcium from the intestinal tract, and the breakdown and assimilation of phosphorus, which is required in bone formation. It also aids in the synthesis of those enzymes in the mucous membranes which are involved in active transport of available calcium.

Too much vitamin D can easily suppress the immune system. The vitamin has been shown to suppress the production of interleukin-2 by human WBCs, which would in turn put a damper on proliferation of T-helper and T-suppressor cells and antibodies.[134] Perhaps vitamin D functions to prevent excessive lymphocyte and antibody proliferation; on the other hand, perhaps too much vitamin D could be dangerous because of its immunosuppressive effects. The above study suggests that for people already in an immunodepressed condition (e.g., AIDS), it would be unwise to take vitamin-D supplements or to drink vitamin D-fortified milk. Infants occasionally hyperreact to the amounts of vitamin D found in fortified milk, often resulting in further medical complications. Also, "hypervitaminosis D" causes high levels of calcium and phosphorus in the blood and excessive urinary excretion of calcium, leading to calcification of soft tissues and of the walls of the blood vessels and kidney tubules—a condition known as *hypercalcemia*.[135]

This should not in any way detract from the importance of vitamin D in establishing immunocompetence. As long as the vitamin is supplied adequately through getting out in the sun regularly, such problems become nonexistent. Vitamin-D deficiency has been found to decrease phagocytic ability.[136] Vitamin D-deficienct rickets is often accompanied by infections. While children with rickets were found to have normal bactericidal capacity of WBCs to E. coli, all had impaired phagocytosis.[137] This suggests that vitamin D exerts a supportive influence primarily on the nonspecific immune functions.

Vitamin D is best obtained by getting out in the sun for 15 minutes daily. Its effects on calcium utilization may be enhanced by regular physical activity. Dietary sources, which may be desired especially during the winter months, include various fish oils (bonito, tuna, lingcod, sea bass, swordfish, halibut, herring, cod, and soupfin shark), tuna, halibut, shrimp, and, to a limited extent, grain and vegetable oils. Cortisone, a drug commonly used in the treatment of allergies, arthritis and other inflammatory conditions, is an antagonist and may depress vitamin-D levels in the body.[138]

(5) *Vitamin E.* Recent research suggests that vitamin E (*tocopherol*), like its fat-soluble cousin vitamin A, may be useful in preventing various kinds of cancer. This vitamin aids in the formation of red blood cells (RBCs), and helps maintain the integrity of the vascular and central nervous systems, as well as the kidney tubules, lungs, genitals, liver, and RBC membranes. There is a high concentration of vitamin E at sites of cortisone synthesis in the adrenal glands. The adrenals pump out cortisone during stress or the "fight or flight" response, and this brings on an increased requirement for vitamin E.[139] This vitamin plugs into many important functions throughout the body, both directly and indirectly. In particular the immune system appears to be highly sensitive to even small drops in vitamin-E levels.[140]

The most impressive studies to date on vitamin E have focused on its interactions with beta-carotene and selenium. All three micronutrients function synergistically in the prevention of lung cancer.[141] Other research has found an antioxidant role of vitamin E in the prevention of breast disease and cancers associated with nitrosamines, the carcinogens found in most barbecued or heavily fried meats. The cooperative action of selenium and vitamin E preserves cell membranes from destruction by oxidation products and retards the breakdown of red blood cells.[142] Vitamin E protects the lungs from air-pollution damage, and interacts with selenium to protect various white blood cells from damage by bactericidal free radicals.[143,144]

Earlier we mentioned that free radicals play a role in radiation- and chemical-induced transformation of various types of cells, including immune cells. Depending on nutritional supply, some cells are far more vulnerable than others. A 1986 study found that selenium and vitamin E function synergistically as radiation-protecting and toxicity-preventing agents.[145] The substances appear to work in a complementary yet opposite fashion, altogether supporting the body's natural modes of protection against harmful radiation, toxic chemical exposure, and other forms of free-radical-related damage.

In animal studies, diets supplemented with vitamin E led to enhanced antibody production when challenged by bacteria and other infectious organisms.[146] Again, this humoral response is further enhanced by the synergistic effect of selenium. Moderately elevated vitamin-E levels in the blood, in addition to raising the antibody response, have been observed to improve white-blood cell bactericidal activity and phagocytosis.[147] A deficiency in vitamin E has been shown to result in decreased lymphatic organ size, T- and B-cell proliferation, white-blood cell function, inflammatory response, and host resistance to infection.[148] There is some evidence that vitamin E exerts an influence on the maturation of T-cells, as well as enhancing T-helper cell activity.[149,150] In the presence of thymus-derived factors, vitamin E enhances the immune responsiveness of B-cells.[151]

Some scientists believe that vitamin E stimulates the immune system primarily by reducing the production of *prostaglandins* (PGs). This class of natural, hormone-like chemicals have been called "the yin and yang of the inflammation cycle of the body" because they turn inflammation on and off.[152] Three kinds of prostaglandins are synthesized from the three essential fatty acids in our diet: (1) linoleic acid from plants; (2) eicosapentenoic acid from cold-water fish and cold-weather vegetables; and (3) *arachadonic acid* from meats such as beef, pork, poultry, and other warm-blooded animals, including ourselves—we can synthesize this EFA from linoleic acid. The first two types of PGs, derived from the EFAs of plants and fish, tend to inhibit the inflammatory process. The third type, derived from the EFAs of meat, tends to promote inflammation. Vitamin E is thought to inhibit the third type of prostaglandin, thus preventing excessive inflammation from taking place.[153] It also appears that this particular "meat-derived" prostaglandin suppresses T-cell activity.[154] Thus vitamin E may indirectly support immune response by lessening the amount of inflammation and boosting T-cell function.

Modern nutritional science has only begun to grasp the power of food because only recently have such fine and integral relationships been revealed. The synergistic interactions of vitamins E, beta-carotene, and selenium are testimony to the body's natural metabolic integrity. When science attempts to view only one of these nutrients in, say, the prevention of lung cancer, the results are inconsistent or insignificant. But when all three are viewed collectively, a much more positive picture emerges. Balance is of the essence: *a lack* of vitamin E depresses many essential aspects of the immune response, while *excess* of this vitamin has a similar effect on immunity. The principle of balance (or excess) applies to vitamin B_6, vitamin A, and probably all other essential micronutrients as well.

Vitamin E is most abundant in plant foods, while extremely low in animal products. The best dietary sources for this vitamin are the following: whole wheat berries, barley, brown rice, oats, rye, corn and sesame oils, miso, tofu, tempeh, natto, sesame and alfalfa seeds, dark leafy greens, and lightly roasted nuts such as walnuts, almonds, and peanuts. Note that the average American diet is likely to be deficient in vitamin E due to its easy removal or inactivation during food processing (e.g., refining of grains and vegetable oils) together with its fairly rapid excretion from the body.[155] The need for this vitamin goes up during pregnancy and newborn infancy, during heavy or frequent exposure to air pollution, and following consumption of highly processed and oily foods.

Minerals and Trace Elements ───────────────────

The Lord God formed man of the dust of the ground, and breathed into his nostrils the breath of life; ... for dust you are, and to dust you will return.

Genesis 2: 7; 3: 19

The elements in our physical body are also in our earth and sea. As fundamental to life as the air we breathe, mineral elements are found in the tissues and fluids of all living things—humans, plants, and animals —and play a role in every biochemical process within our bodies. Any cell that lacks proper mineral balance will fail to perform at its optimum level. Today, as scientists continue to discover new facts about the nature of human nutrition, there is a growing consensus that many of today's health problems, from general fatigue to the common cold to cancer, may be related to mineral deficiencies or imbalances. Indeed, the potential effects attributed to mineral imbalance are so wide-ranging as to possibly encompass birth defects, mental illness, and even accident injuries.

Like the vitamins, minerals are generally consumed in minute amounts, but are important regulators of all body processes. They are somewhat arbitrarily divided into two broad categories. First there are the bulk or *major minerals*, so-called because they are present in relatively high amounts in body tissues. These include calcium, phosphorous, iodine, sulfur, magnesium, sodium, chlorine, and potassium. All other minerals are called *trace elements* because they are found in tiny yet specific amounts. These include cadmium, chromium, cobalt, copper, germanium, iodine, iron, lead, lithium, manganese, molybdenum, nickel, selenium, silicon, titanium, vanadium, and zinc. Some of these may be toxic to the body if present in quantities which, although seemingly insignificant, are nonetheless still too high for the body to handle.

The list of mineral-dependent functions is extensive, since every biologic process in the body requires minerals of varying kinds and proportions. They are known to function in the following important mechanisms: as co-factors in metabolic reactions (e.g., magnesium is required for all macronutrient metabolism); as components of organic compounds such as enzymes, hormones, and others; as ions affecting muscle contractility and acid/alkaline balance; as major constituents of bone structure; and as co-factors in digestion and elimination, in detoxification processes, and in the transport of oxygen from the lungs to the cells. The human body can survive longer without all the essential vitamins than it can without the essential minerals. Indeed, we could not begin to utilize vitamins from food were it not for minerals.

Optimum concentrations of some trace elements are very low (measured in parts per million, or micrograms per gram, mcg). However, the toxic limits of some are quite close to the recommended intakes. This means that a highly delicate balance exists for many trace elements between toxicity, vitality, and deficiency. According to Dr. Roman Kutsky, expert in mineral biochemistry, this balance could easily be upset by improper mineral supplementation, due to excessive trace amounts of precipitating ions.[156] These precipitates could form in sensitive tissues such as kidney, heart, and brain, with possibly fatal consequences; in addition, certain imbalances of ions could disturb intracellular enzyme reactions and pH, or affect the irritability of muscle or nerve.[157]

Most of the minerals, especially the trace elements, are highly toxic to the body when present in excess. One example is iron, which is most concentrated in red meats, but also exists in more balanced proportions in dark leafy greens and sea vegetables. Excessive iron levels are associated with increased risk of both cancer and infectious disease.[158] In the presence of either microbial infection or cancerous tumor, the body attempts to withhold iron by storing it in the liver and spleen. As cancer spreads, the iron content of the plasma decreases proportionately.[159] This seems to be a healthy response on the part of the host, because the low plasma levels of iron make it more difficult for cancer cells and infectious organisms to thrive. On the other hand, if too much iron is stored in the liver for an extended period of time, the hepatic tissues begin to deteriorate, possibly promoting cirrhosis, diabetes, and other problems, including depressed immunity and greater susceptibility to infection.[160]

The problem of iron imbalance becomes magnified when there is too much iron being supplied to the body from iron-rich foods (primarily red meats). An excess of vitamin C, which enhances iron absorption, might further contribute to iron overload. In the case of either cancer or microbial infection, the iron-rich diet may promote a condition of iron excess which supports the disease state. This effect would be amplified by the fact that iron overload suppresses T-cell functions, T- and B-cell mobility, and may even distort the normal structure and functioning of DNA.[161,162,163] Finally, modern diets which include substantial amounts of red meats or iron supplements tend to deplete the body's zinc levels, since iron is biochemically antagonistic to zinc.[164] Such dietary patterns would therefore tend to promote a lowering of the T-cell response, which is directly dependent on proper zinc balance.[165]

Some of the minerals in our environment are overtly toxic. In a large retrospective 1986 study of 2,000 lead-poisoning cases, researchers at the Tennessee Technological University found a relationship between high levels of lead and learning disabilites. Many cases of lead poisoning involve children biting on pencils or ingesting old paint, but others may result from overexposure to automobile exhaust fumes, pesticides, tobacco smoke, coal burning, ink, plastics, hair dyes and some cosmetics. Cadmium is found in refined white flour, white rice, sugar, coffee, tea, tobacco, and probably most foods grown with phosphate-based fertilizers. Excess cadmium can interfere with the balancing of other minerals and nutrients, possibly leading to hypertension, heart disease, and abnormal functioning of the liver and kidneys. It is of interest to note that excessively *low* levels of certain toxic trace elements can also be harmful. Recent research has found that when the trace mineral lithium is too low, approximately 80 percent of patients have manic-depressive tendencies.

Other common sources of toxic metals include the aluminum in cooking utensils and coffee pots, lead and copper plumbing, and the mercury and nickel alloys used in dental fillings. The relatively high levels of chlorine, lead, and aluminum found in our modern water supply probably play an important role in the poor health of millions of Americans. These potential sources of toxicity are difficult to study because their effects are cumulative and extremely gradual. At the present time, until long-term studies are conducted, we can only logically assume that our drinking water harms the immune system. Drinking water should be filtered or obtained from uncontaminated wells and springs.

Since there is insufficient space to discuss all the beneficial minerals, we shall only focus on a few of those known to be essential to sound immunity. These are the trace elements zinc, manganese, and copper. We must emphasize, however, that there is considerable evidence for the immune-enhancing effects of other mineral elements, notably magnesium, calcium, germanium, and selenium.[166,167] Interested readers are referred to the extensive documentation and superb discussion presented by medical scientists in *Nutrition and Immunity* (see bibliography), and to recent issues of *Nutrition Update*, a comprehensive research journal devoted to holistic health and nutrition.

As with the vitamins, the key to nutritional success is in providing minerals in sufficient quantity and balanced proportions. No nutrient acts independently of other nutrients, and trace elements have highly specific relationshps to many key body functions. The safest way to accurately satisfy our mineral requirements is by adhering to a wholesome vegetable-quality diet. This point cannot be overemphasized. The food sources listed in the discussion on trace elements are derived from Dr. Roman Kutsky's *Handbook of Vitamins, Minerals and Hormones* (1981) and from Kirschmann and Dunne's *Nutrition Almanac* (1984).

(1) *Zinc.* Zinc has received a lot of good press lately, and for good reason: it is required for normal growth and development and plays an integral part in many metabolic and immunologic processes. For example, it is needed for carbon dioxide metabolism, and serves as a co-factor for enzymes involved in protein and carbohydrate metabolism. It is required for production of some eighty enzymes in humans, as well as for the synthesis of RNA and protein. The trace element is also necessary for fertility, sexual development, prostate functioning, and adrenal steroid and growth-hormone secretion.

Zinc is a necessary ingredient in T-cell immunity. A deficiency can produce atrophy of the thymus gland and a reduction in the number of mature T-cells. As a result, many cell-mediated immune functions are impaired, including T- and B-cell bactericidal activity, natural-killer cell activity, and other immune responses.[168] Low levels of zinc have been associated with reduced antibody response, abnormal proportions of antibiodies, and defective cell-mediated immunity.[169]

In addition, patients with immunodeficiency diseases, in addition to the typical array of depressed immune responses, frequently exhibit low levels of serum zinc; and zinc repletion is associated with the restoration of many of these immune functions.[170] It is also interesting that a hallmark of the physiological response to invasion by pathogenic microorganisms or their toxins is a transient decline in serum zinc, with a concomitant sequestering of zinc from the liver.[171] These observations suggest the possibility of an integral interplay between zinc and the immune response. Perhaps one effect of the repeated infections seen among most of the high-risk groups for AIDS is an upset of this essential balance, thus contributing to the pathogenesis of the syndrome.

Supplementation with zinc is somewhat arbitrary since no one really knows how much intake is appropriate. While zinc's importance in immunity is incontestable, supplementation could actually have a deleterious effect. Certain immune cells (macrophages and neutrophils) are depleted as a result of high zinc intakes, and this could be undesirable if there is a danger of bacterial infection, or when infection is already present.[172] High zinc intakes might inadvertently promote candida fungal infections as well.[173] Lastly, too much zinc leads to a depletion of copper.

Given these drawbacks of zinc supplementation, whole foods are clearly the best alternative. Prominent dietary sources for zinc include whole wheat, brown rice, rye, barley, oats, buckwheat, oysters, tuna, shrimp, crab, sunflower and pumpkin seeds, various sea vegetables (kombu, wakame, etc.), corn, lentils, peas, watercress, parsley, okra, and carrots.

(2) *Manganese.* Manganese appears to be important in the maintenance of structural integrity of heart and kidney cell membranes, tissue oxygen uptake, food absorption, neurotransmitter synthesis, fertility, insulin synthesis, and fat and carbohydrate metabolism, and homeostatic blood-clotting mechanisms.[174] It is a component of the body's primary antioxidant, superoxide dismutase, and there is some evidence that it may help to counteract the immunosuppressive effects of corticosteroids.[175]

Although much is known about the immunosuppressive effects of excess manganese, relatively little is known about its specific positive effects on the immune system. The most likely effects would be on the plasma membranes of important cell types employed in the immune response, since changes in membrane structure or fluidity could in turn influence the binding affinity for antibodies and other lymphocytes.[176] Manganese may also act as a co-factor in an enzyme associated with stimulation of macrophages. Finally, there may also be an interaction between manganese and calcium, which is specifically involved in lymphocyte activation by mitogens.[177] At this point it seems likely that manganese mediates immunocompetence predominantly by indirect means, that is, as a key component of carbohydrate and lipid metabolism, as an antioxidant, and as a co-factor in various enzyme systems.

The most abundant and balanced sources of manganese are the following: brown rice, barley, oats, buckwheat, rye, whole wheat, kelp, wakame, kombu, dulse, sunflower seeds, almonds, walnuts, parsley, celery, Brussels sprouts, broccoli, watercress, kale and other dark leafy greens.

(3) *Copper.* Copper plays an essential role in respiration, and functions as a co-factor for many important enzymes, called *cuproenzymes,* which catalyze oxidation reactions. Among these enzymes is *tyrosinase,* which enables the conversion of tyrosine to melanin, which determines skin pigmentation and influences neuroendocrine processes involving the pineal gland. It is intimately involved in body healing processes, bone formation, hair (and skin) color, purine excretion, connective tissue maintenance, and red blood cell and hemoglobin formation. By and large, however, copper's most significant role is as an integral structural feature of many enzymes in metabolic processes.

Copper has also been recognized for some time as a protective factor against infection. Deficiency of this element has been linked to lowered resistance to infectious challenge, greatly increased mortality following infection, and shortened lifespan.[178,179] By virtue of its divalent action in copper sulfate, copper appears to be essential to proper functioning of virtually all of the immune system's cell types.[180] Both dietary excess and deficiency can adversely affect immunity. The trace element also seems to be involved in the inflammatory process, at certain times potentiating and at certain times inhibiting it.[181] Finally, copper is intimately involved in the three-dimensional structure of antibodies.[182]

Zinc and copper have a delicate inverse interrelationship in the body and tend to interact antagonistically to one another. Because of the extremely narrow range of our copper needs, zinc supplementation may elicit copper deficiency, and too much copper may upset the zinc balance. Also, excessive copper is linked with a wide range of psychiatric disorders, while copper deficiencies are associated with degeneration of heart tissue and blood vessels, such as may occur in some strokes and heart attacks.[183,184]

For the reasons stated above, supplementation with copper could be dangerous and should only be done under expert medical supervision. A far safer way to satisfy copper needs is by consuming whole, natural foods. Among the most favorable sources of dietary copper are whole wheat, barley, oats, rye, rice, almonds, walnuts, sunflower and sesame seeds, miso, tofu, tempeh, natto, kale, onions, leeks, okra, sea vegetables, and various species of non-fatty, white-meat fish.

The Mineral Crisis

More serious than our gargantuan Federal deficits here in the U.S.A. are the deficits in topsoil minerals around the world. These minerals are the basic food of soil microorganisms, which in turn provide their protoplasm as nourishment for plants. Over the past 10,000 years, these minerals have gradually been used up by natural "weathering" processes and as part of the natural soil cycle. But as they go, so also does the vitality of the soil and the vegetation it produces. Consequently, plants and trees are increasingly vulnerable to infestation by insects and harmful microbes, as well as to damage by ozone pollution and acid rain. It may be more than casual imagery to say that our dying forests around the world are the "AIDS" of Earth's ecosystem. Just as we humans are losing our resistance to the omnipresent microbes, so also are the forests losing their biological foundation and succumbing to the disintegrative forces of mankind. And both phenomena are strongly rooted in the mineral-content of our soils.

The natural 10,000-year demineralization process has been greatly accelerated, however, by conventional agriculture. The use of soluble artificial fertilizers causes imbalances in the soil mineral composition, and trace elements are gradually washed away along with the soil's valuable humus content. Intensive cultivation and monoculture farming practices lead to soil erosion, and the loss of valuable topsoil causes enormous mineral losses. This explains why so many minerals are grossly deficient in the typical American diet.[185] Many of our food crops, for instance, are deficient in several vital minerals, including magnesium, iron, selenium, zinc, manganese, and copper.[186] For this reason, we must not only reorient our agricultural system—with massive rock-crushing programs to remineralize the dying soils from which all food is ultimately derived—but also regularly consume ample amounts of sea vegetables.

Mineral-deficient soils produce mineral deficiencies in plant foods and in the domesticated animals which subsist on these plants. Since minerals are integral to every enzyme system in the body, many body systems may be adversely affected by any pronounced mineral deficiency. In particular, our immune systems stand a risk of gradually becoming substantially compromised.

Another contributing factor to micronutrient imbalance is intensive food-processing. In particular, the milling of whole grains depletes most of the grain's vitamin B6 and vitamin E, as well as the essential minerals chromium, zinc, iron and manganese. While synthetic vitamins may be added to enriched breads (*fortification*), the natural balance among vitamins that exists in whole grains before milling is lost. Indeed, vitamin and mineral supplements only became necessary when we began refining whole cereal grains. The nutritional content of our food supply may also be lacking due to long-term storage, long-distance transportation, overcooking, and soil depletion due to modern agricultural techniques.

The story of one trace element, chromium, provides a fascinating example of how Western diet and life-style upset important nutrient balances. Chromium appears to play a role in preventing diabetes and heart disease. Americans generally have low levels of chromium when compared to individuals from around the world. In one study, Oriental peoples averaged 4.5 times as much and other nationalities also had markedly more chromium in the blood.[187] There may be a link between the lower chromium levels and the higher rates of diabetes and arteriosclerosis in America, as well as a relationship with lead poisoning in America. Chromium deficiency makes one more susceptible to lead poisoning and Americans have the highest lead levels in the world. Refined foods are extremely low in chromium. The trace element is contained in the outer bran portion of cereal grains, and much is lost in the production of white flour. There is also an additive effect since our body's chromium needs increase in proportion to blood carbohydrate levels; thus higher intakes of simple sugars per se tend to deplete the body of chromium.[188]

There has been some concern that mineral deficiencies may also result by consuming high-fiber vegetarian diets. Earlier laboratory studies found that fiber binds minerals in the intestine and could therefore inhibit their absorption. This theory has recently been contradicted by a recent investigation which found no evidence of mineral deficiency for people on long-term, high-fiber vegetarian diets.[189] Oxalic acid binds minerals such as zinc, copper, iron and calcium and can inhibit their absorption. Since this acid is found in certain vegetables, including green peppers, spinach, Swiss chard and tomatoes, it may be wise to avoid or minimize their use.

People in poor health need to exercise special care to ensure that their nutritional needs are adequately fulfilled. Cancer and infectious disease pose an increased demand on the body's immune and nutrient reserves. Many people with AIDS have extremely poor levels of nutrient absorption, which are associated with multiple infections along the intestinal tract. For such individuals, accurate adherence to macrobiotic guidelines is critical, especially with a strong emphasis on thorough chewing and proper food preparation. In some cases moderate use of chelated vitamin and mineral supplements may be used as a temporary measure. Megadoses of vitamin C have been recommended on the premise that the body's requirements are greatly increased during times of infection, but this strategy may weaken the kidneys and the long-term effects are still unknown. Extreme caution must be exercised whenever vitamins and trace elements known to be toxic at high doses are provided in the form of a supplement.

As documented earlier, trace elements influence physiological, genetic, and psychological aspects of development from prenatal life through the stages of growth, maintenance, and aging.[190] Trace-element deficiencies are not peculiar to malnourished children of underdeveloped countries, but also manifest to an unknown extent in postindustrial countries throughout the world. For example, some observations suggest that marginal copper deficiency may occur widely throughout the population of the United States.[191] In light of the many studies suggesting an integral relationship between trace-element balance and the health of the nervous system, the possibility of borderline deficiencies or imbalances supporting learning disabilities, abnormal behavior and other psychological problems, offers ground for concern.

Is it just a coincidence that the rates of learning disabilities and viral diseases in America have been increasing over the last few decades? Is it merely coincidence that lack of minerals in the modern food supply has arisen at a time in which 1 out of every 5 Americans is in need of psychiatric help, while 1 out of every 4 dies from cancer? Given the integral connection between the immune and nervous systems, we think not. Our review of the literature suggests that the typical American diet may be an underlying causal force in both trends. Regular intakes of animal products, refined sugars, and highly processed foods could promote micronutrient imbalances which, in turn, could alter the functional integrity of the immune and nervous systems.

To reverse the current trend of physical and mental degeneration, we need to emphasize foods that are as pure, whole, and unadulterated as possible. Sea vegetables, for example, provide a rich source of many trace elements currently missing from much of our land-grown food. It is our experience that people who begin to eat sea vegetables regularly tend to notice remarkable improvement from fatigue, colds, allergies, low blood pressure, constipation, rheumatism, arthritis, acne, splitting hair, brittle fingernails, insomnia, anxiety, depression, and poor memory. At the same time junk-food dietary patterns are bound to upset the balance of essential vitamins and trace elements. For healthy immunity and biological functioning as a whole, one would do well to avoid such dietary practices altogether.

The immune system's functioning is impaired by free radicals, yet, paradoxically, it generates free radicals in the process of eliminating harmful microbes and viruses. Since white blood cells are especially rich in unsaturated fats, which are highly vulnerable to free-radical damage, dietary practices which promote free-radical production can seriously weaken the immune system. The main foods which cause this are fatty, oily, and highly refined foods and particularly foods that have been cooked with high temperatures (fried or deep-fried). In a 1984 issue of the *Journal of Holistic Medicine*, Elmer M. Cranton, M.D., and James P. Frackelton, M.M., summarize the practical solution to the free-radical problem as follows:

> Consumption of fats and lipids that have been processed, extracted, exposed to air, heated, hydrogenated, or in any way altered or removed from the food in which they naturally occur should be reduced as much as practical. Consumption of carbohydrates that are depleted of trace elements (white flour, white rice, sugar) should be minimized. Total caloric intake should be moderated to maintain weight within 20 percent of ideal body weight. The use of table salt should be restricted. Diets should contain ample amounts of fiber-rich whole grains and fresh vegetables. Patients suffering with extensive free-radical diseases should be stricter with diet until improvement occurs.[192]

The two medical doctors go on to state that ample amounts of vitamins E, C, beta carotene and the B complex, and balanced proportions of the minerals magnesium, zinc, selenium, manganese, and chromium, should be part of one's regular antioxidant-dietary intake. (Actually, copper, zinc, manganese, and selenium are essential to certain key enzymes produced in the body that provide most of our protection against free radical damage.) These nutrients are optimally supplied by a vegetable-quality diet based on organically grown whole cereal grains, root and green leafy vegetables, sea vegetables, beans, nuts, seeds, fruits, and fish.

In some areas of the country, especially those that have been chemically farmed for several years or longer, the soil is almost totally depleted of these trace elements, so the food crops and animals raised there are likewise depleted. Magnesium and manganese are grossly deficient in the typical American diet.[193] For this reason, we must not only reorient our agricultural system—with massive rock-crushing programs to remineralize the dying soils from which all food is ultimately derived—but also regularly consume ample amounts of whole, unrefined land and sea vegetables. (Minerals are also integral to virtually every one of the body's thousands of essential enzyme systems.)

In this chapter we explored the immunocompetence-promoting value of consuming whole foods—whole cereal grains, whole beans, vegetables, nuts, seeds, and fruits—rather than supplements. Beyond personal health, there are many reasons for selecting whole, ecologically grown foods. When we choose to eat in this way, we are not only lowering our risk of developing cancer, but also are promoting a food system that provides more food value per acre to sustain our increasingly overpopulated world. In addition, we are minimizing the possibility of further contaminating our drinking-water supply with agricultural chemicals; we are reducing the "greenhouse" and ozone-destroying gases produced by artificial fertilizers; and we are helping replenish the topsoil's fertility, upon which our future food supply depends.

[1] Gershwin, M. E. et al., "The Potential Impact of Nutritional Factors on Immunological Responsiveness," in *Nutrition and Immunity* (Orlando, Fla.: 1984), p. 1.

[2] Gershwin, M. E. et al., "In Vivo Effects of Fatty Acids," in *Nutrition and Immunity* (1985), pp. 271–9.

[3] "Spontaneously Occurring Antitoxic Derivatives of Cholesterol," *Am J Clin Nutr* (1979), 32: 40–47.

[4] Beisel, W. R. et al., "Single-nutrient Effects on Immunologic Functions," *J Am Med Assoc* (1981), 245(1): 53–58.

[5] Abrahamson, E. M., M.D., "The Glandular Jazz Band," in *Body, Mind and Sugar* (Information obtained through Dr. Abrahamson's personal communications with Dr. Burbank.) (New York: Avon Books, 1977), p. 174.

[6] Sanchez, A. et al., "Role of Sugars in Human Neutrophilic Phagocytosis," *Am J Clin Nutr* (1973), 26: 1180.

[7] Ringsdorf, W. et al., "Sucrose, Neutrophil Phagocytosis and Resistance to Disease," *Dent Surv* (1976), 52: 46.

[8] Bernestein, J. et al., "Depression of Lymphocyte Transformation Following Oral Glucose Ingestion," *Am Clin Nutr* (1977), 30: 613.

[9] Mayer, D. K., "Diagnosis and Management of Intestinal Obstruction in Individuals with Cancer," *Nurse Practitioner* (1986), 11(2): 36–46.

[10] Liebman, B., "How Fiber Fights Cancer," *Nutrition Action* (1984) (June issue p. 6. Cites a 1973 study in the *Journal of the National Cancer Institute*), 55: 1093.

[11] Mayer (1986), Op. cit.

[12] Palmblad, J., "Lymphomas and Dietary Fat," *Lancet* (1977), 1: 142.

[13] McDougall, J. A. and M. A. McDougall, *The McDougall Plan* (Piscataway, N. J.: New Century Publishers, 1983), pp. 116–22.

[14] McCarron, D., "Calcium, Magnesium, and Phosphorus Balance in Human and Experimental Hypertension," *Hypertension* (1982), 4 (supp 3): 33–27.

[15] Gordon, G., "New Dimension in Calcium Metabolism," *Osteopathic Annals* (1983), 11: 38–59.

[16] Weiner, M. A., "Nutrition against Immunity," in *Maximum Immunity* (Boston, Mass.: Houghton-Mifflin Co., 1986), p. 75.

[17] Beisel, W. R., "Single Nutrients and Immunity," *American Journal of Clinical Nutrition* (1982), 35: 417–68.

[18] Eggleston, D. W., "Effect of Dental Amalgam and Nickel Alloys on T-lymphocytes: Preliminary report," *J Prosthetic Dentistry* (May 1984), pp. 617–21.

[19] Weiner (1985), Op. cit., p. 77.

[20] Ibid., p. 76.

[21] James, G. V., "Trace Substances in Foods and Their Effect on Health," in *Nutrition and Killer Diseases*, ed. Rose, J. (Park Ridge, N. J.: Noyes Publications, 1982).

[22] Kushi, Michio, *Macrobiotic Health Education Series: Allergies* (Tokyo and New York: Japan Publications, Inc., 1984).

[23] Hall, R., *Food for Naught* (New York: Vintage Books, 1976), pp. 89, 97.

[24] Hunter, B. T., *Consumer Beware!* (New York: Bantam Books, 1971), pp. 117–18.

[25] Weiner, *Maximum Immunity*, pp. 232–9 for discussion on Candida.

[26] Galland, L., "Nutrition and Candidiasis," *J Orth Mol Psych* (1983), 14(1)

[27] Witkin, S. F. et al., "Inhibition of Candida Albicans-induced Lymphocyte Proliferation by Lymphocyte and Sera from Women with Recurrent Vaginitis," *Am J Ob Gyn* (1983), 147(7)

[28] Marx, J. L., "The Immune System Belongs to the Body," *Science* (8 Mar. 1985), 277: 1190–2.

[29] Jemmott, J. B. III, and S. E. Locke, "Psychosocial Factors, Immunologic Mediation, and Human Susceptibility to Infectious Disease: How much do we know?" *Psych Bull* (1984), 95: 78–108.

[30] Kiecolt-Glaser, J. and R. Glaser, reported by J. A. Miller in "Immunity and Crises, Large and Small," *Science News* (1986), 129(22): 340.

[31] McDougall, Op. cit., p. 110.

[32] O'dea, K., "Physical Factors Influencing Postprandial Glucose and Insulin Response to Starch," *Am J Clin Nutr* (1980), 33: 760.

[33] Haber, G., "Depletion and Disruption of Dietary Fiber: Effects on satiety, plasma glucose, and serum insulin," *Lancet* (1977), 2: 679.

[34] Weiner, Op. cit., p. 143.

[35] Antones, A., "The Influence of Diet on Serum Triglycerides in Sought African White and Bantu Prisoners," *Lancet* (1961), 1: 3.

[36] Williams, A., "Increased Blood Cell Agglutination Following Ingestion of Fat: A factor contributing to cardiac ischemia, coronary insufficiency, andanginal plan," *Angiology* (1957), 8: 29.

[37] Grande, F., "Dietary Carbohydrates and Serum Cholesterol," *Am J Clin Nutr* (1967), 20: 176; see also McDougall (1983), Op. Cit., p. 115.

190

38 McDougall (1983), Op. cit., p. 120.

39 Kelsay, J., "A Review of Research on Effects of Fiber Intake in Man," *Am J Clin Nutr* (1978), 31: 142.

40 Wynder, E. L., "Dietary Habits and Cancer Epidemiology," *Cancer* (1979), (Suppl) 43(4): 1955.

41 Greenwald, T. and E. Lanza, "Dietary Fiber and Colon Cancer," *Contemporary Nutrition* (1986), 11(1).

42 Jenkins, D., "The Diabetic Diet, Dietary Carbohydrate and Differences in Digestibility," *Diabetologia* (1982), 23: 477.

43 Burkitt, D., "Some Diseases Characteristic of Modern Western Civilization," *Br Med J* (1973), 1: 274.

44 Davidon, S., et al., "Gout and Hyperuricemia," in *Human Nutrition and Dietetics* (London: Churchill Livingstone, 1979), pp. 366–8.

45 Ibid., p. 368.

46 *Nutrition Reviews*, "Urinary Calcium and Dietary Protein" (1980), 38: 9.

47 Ibid.

48 Brenner, B., "Dietary Protein Intake and the Progressive Nature of Kidney Disease: The role of hemodynamically-mediated glomerular injury in the pathogenesis of progressive glomerular sclerosis in aging, renal ablation, and intrinsic renal disease," *N Engl Med* (1982), 307: 652.

49 Ibid.

50 Ibid.

51 Gloassock, R. J., "Nutrition, Immunology, and Renal Disease," *Kidney International* (1983), 24(16): 194.

52 Greenberger, N., "Effect of Vegetable and Animal Protein Diets on Chronic Hepatic Encephalopathy," *Digestive Disease* (1977), 22: 945.

53 Walser, M., "Does Dietary Therapy Have a Role in the Predialysis Patient?" *Am J Clin Nutr* (1980), 13: 1629.

54 Gershwin et al. (1985), Op. cit.

55 Rosenbaum, M., "Nutrients and Immune System" (1984), cited by Michael Weiner in *Maximum Immunity*, p. 81.

56 Ibid.

57 Morrow, W. et al., "Dietary Fat and Immune Function," *J Immunol* (1985), 135(6): 3857.

58 Barcelli, U. et al., "Is There a Role for Polyunsaturated Fatty Acids in the Prevention of Renal Disease and Renal Failure," *Nephron* (1985), 41: 209.

59 Das, U. N., "Antibiotic-like Action of Essential Fatty Acids," *Can Med Assoc J* (1985), 132: 1350.

60 Stevenson, D., "Sensitivity to Ingested Meabisulfites in Asthmatic Subjects," *J Allergy Clin Immunol* (1981), 68: 26.

61 Colman, A., "Possible Psychiatric Reactions to Monosodium Glutamate," *N Engl Med* (1978), 299: 902.

62 Schaumburg, H., "Monosodium L-Glutamate: Its pharmacology and role in the Chinese Restaurant Syndrome," *Science* (1969), 163: 826.

63 Olney, J., "Status of MSG Revisited," *Am J Clin Nutr* (1973), 26: 683.

[64] Fairweather, F., "Food Additives and Cancer," *Proc Nutr Soc* (1981), 40:21.

[65] Settipane, G., "Aspirin Intolerance, Subtype, Familial Occurence, and Cross-reactivity with Tartrazine," *J Allergy Clin Immunol* (1975), 56: 215.

[66] Juhlin, L., "Indicence of Intolerance to Food Additives," *Int J Dermatol* (1980), 19: 548.

[67] Miller, S., "Additives in Our Food Supply," *Ann NY Acad Sci* (1977), 300: 397.

[68] Editorial, "Milk Has Something for Everybody?" *JAMA* (1975), 232(5): 539.

[69] Thrash, A. and C. Thrash, *The Animal Connection* (Seale, Ala: Yuchi Pines Institute, 1983), p. 69.

[70] Silberner, J., "Networking AIDS," *Science News* (1986), 130(4): 58.

[71] Cunningham, A., "Lymphomas and Animal Protein Consumption," *Lancet* (1976), 2: 1184.

[72] Ferrer, J., "Milk of Dairy Cows Frequently Contains a Leukemogenic Virus," *Science* (1981), 213: 1014; also see the 1974 editorial "Beware of the Cow," in the *Lancet*, 2: 30.

[73] Recker, R. R. and R. P. Heaney, "The Effect of Milk Supplements on Calcium Metabolism, Bone Metabolism, and Calcium Balance," *American Journal of Clinical Nutrition* (1985), 41: 254.

[74] Jackson, A. A. and M. H. Golden, "The Human Rumen," *Lancet* (7 Oct. 1978), p. 764.

[75] Thrash, A. and C. Thrash, "Foods to Use Instead of Milk and Eggs," in *The Animal Connection* (Seale, Ala.: Yuchi Pines Institute, 1983), p. 62.

[76] Ibid., p. 81.

[77] Ibid., p. 111.

[78] Davidson, S., R. Passmore, J. F. Brock, and Truswell, A. S., "Diseases of the Gastrointestinal Tract," in *Human Nutrition and Dietetics* (New York: Churchill Livingstone, 1979), p. 407.

[79] Bleumink, E. and E. Young, "Identification of the Atopic Allergen in Cow's Milk," *Intern Allergy* (1968), 34: 521–543.

[80] Rigby, W. F., "The Immunobiology of Vitamin D," *Immunology Today* (1988), 9(2): 54.

[81] Bronner, F., "Intestinal Calcium Absorption: Mechanisms and applications," *Journal of Nutrition* (1987), 112: 1353.

[82] Holik, M. F. et al., "Photosynthesis of Vitamin D in the Skin: Effect of environmental and lifestyle variables," *Federal Proceedings* (1987), 46(5): 1876.

[83] Cunningham-Rundles, C., "Failure of the G. I. Tract Barrier in Patients with a Suppressed Immune System" (1986) (Lecture given at the symposium sponsored by the Institute of Human Nutrition, College of Physicians and Surgeons, Columbia University, New York, 4 and 5 December).

[84] Ibid.

[85] Cottrell, M. C. Unpublished clinical observations of a large group of AIDS patients practicing macrobiotics in New York City (1986).

[86] Cunningham-Rundles (1986), Op. cit.

[87] Ibid.

192

[88] Ibid.

[89] Euler, H. H. et al., "Precipitable Immune Complexes in Healthy Homosexual Men, Acquired Immune Deficiency Syndrome, and Related Lymphadenopathy Syndrome," *Clin Exp Immunol* (1985), 59: 267.

[90] Arasaki, S. and T. Arasaki, "Dietary and Medical Applications: Minerals," from *Vegetables from the Sea* (Tokyo and New York: Japan Publications, Inc., 1983), p. 45.

[91] Gregor, O., "Gastrointestinal Cancer and Nutrition," *Gut* (1969), 10: 1031–4.

[92] Drasar, B. S. and D. Irving, "Environmental Factors and Cancer of the Colon and Breast," *Brit J Cancer* (1973), 27: 167–72.

[93] Ornish, D., "Effects of Stress Management Training and Dietary Changes in Treating Ischemia Heart Disease," *JAMA* (1983), 249 (1983): 54.

[94] Dresar and Irving, Op. cit.

[95] Addy, D., "Infant Feeding: A current view," *Br Med J* (1976), 1: 1268.

[96] Cunningham, A., "Lymphomas and Animal Protein Consumption," *Lancet* (1976), 2: 1184.

[97] McDougall, J. A. and M. A. McDougall, "Dairy Products and Eggs Are Avoided," from *The McDougall Plan* (Piscataway, N. J.: New Century Publishers, Inc., 1983), p. 51.

[98] Jeon, D., "The Malice of Malnutrition," *Boston Magazine* (Nov. 1982), p. 120.

[99] Fullerton, D. et al., "Sugar, Opiods, and Binge Eating," *Brain Res Bull* (1985), 14: 673.

[100] Kutsky, R. J., *Handbook of Vitamins, Minerals, and Hormones* (New York: Van Nostrand Reinhold Co., 1981), p. 79.

[101] Williams, R., *Biochemical Individuality* (Austin, Tex.: University of Texas, 1956).

[102] Herbert, V., "Megavitamin Therapy: Facts and fictions," in *Food and Nutrition News* (1976), 47: 3–4.

[103] Ong, D. D., "Vitamin A-binding Proteins," *Nutr Rev* (1985), 43: 225–32.

[104] Rechcigel, M. ed., *CRC Handbook in Nutrition and Food*, sec. E., vol. 1 (West Palm Beach, Fla.: CRC Press, 1978).

[105] Green, H. N. and E. Mellanby, "Carotene and Vitamin A: The anti-infective action of carotene," *Br J Exp Pathol* (1930), 11: 81.

[106] Hays (1971).

[107] Rosenbaum (1984), Op. cit., p. 98.

[108] Dreizen, S., "Nutrition and the Immune Response—A Review," *Int J Vitam Nutr Res* (1978), 49: 22–8.

[109] Weisenthal, D., "Vitamin Deficiency Linked to Lung Cancer," *Veg Times* (1987), 118: 7.

[110] Wener, M. A. and K. Goss, *Nutrition against Aging* (New York: Bantam Books, 1983).

[111] Chandra, R. K., "Nutritional Deficiency, Immune Responses, and Infectious Illness," in symposium, *Fed Proc* (1980), 39: 3086.

[112] Malkovsky, M. et al., "T-cell Mediated Enhancement of Host-versus-graft Reactivity in Mice Fed a Diet Enriched in Vitamin A Acetate," *Nature* (1983), 302: 338.

[113] Immerman, A., *World Review of Nutrition and Diet* (1981), 37: 38.

[114] McDougall (1985), Op. cit., p. 53.

[115] Berlin, R., "Vitamin B_{12} Injections," *Brit Med J* (1985), 291, 56.

[116] Kutsky (1981), Op. cit., pp. 216–220.

[117] Cathcart, R. F., *Press Conference Statement* (New York: The Betsy Nolan Group, Inc. Public Relations, 5 Dec. 1987).

[118] Gershwin et al., eds., Op. cit., p. 254.

[119] Thomas, W. R. and P. G. Holt, "Vitamin C and Immunity: An assessment of the evidence," *Clin Exp Immunol* (1978), 32: 370–9.

[120] Beisel et al. (1981), Op. cit.

[121] Gershwin et al. eds. (1985), Op. cit., p. 254.

[122] McCarty, M. E., "Nutritional Insurance Supplementation and Corticosteroid Toxicity," *Med Hypothesis* (1982), 9: 15–156.

[123] Newberne, P. M. and V. Suphakarn, "Nutrition and Cancer: A review, with emphasis on the role of vitamins C and E and selenium," *Nutrition and Cancer* (1983), 5: 107–18.

[124] Germann, D. R., *The Anti-Cancer Diet* (Ridgefield, Conn.: Wyden Books, 1977).

[125] Kutsky (1981), Op. cit., p. 253.

[126] Kirschmann, J. E., *Nutrition Almanac* (New York: Nutrition Search, Inc. McGraw-Hill Book Co., 1984), p. 44.

[127] Kirschmann (1984), Op. cit. p. 44.

[128] Fuerst, M. L., "AIDS Patients Turn to Unproven Therapies," *Medical World News* (28 Apr. 1986), pp. 62–4.

[129] Cathcart, R. F., "Vitamin C in the Treatment of AIDS," *Medical Hypotheses* (1984), 14: 423.

[130] Cathcart (1987), Op. cit.

[131] Ibid.

[132] Ibid.

[133] Ibid.

[134] Rosenbaum (1984), Op. cit.

[135] Kirschmann (1984), Op. cit., p. 50.

[136] Chandra (1980), Op. cit.

[137] Stroder, J. and P. Kasal, "Evaluation of Phagocytosis in Rickets," *Acta Paediats Scand* (1970), 59: 288

[138] Kutsky (1981), Op. cit., p. 192.

[139] Harris, R. S. and K. Thimann, eds., *Vitamins and Hormones*, vols. 25–34 (New York: Academic Press, 1967–1976).

[140] Bendich, A. et al., "Dietary Vitamin E Requirement for Optimum Immune Responses," *J Nutr* (1986), 116: 675.

[141] Menkes, M. et al., "Serum Beta-carotene, Vitamins A and E, Selenium,

and the Risk of Lung Cancer," *N Engl J Med* (1986), 315: 1250.

[142] Kutsky (1981), Op. cit., p. 199.

[143] Crary, E. J. et al., "Potential Applications for High-dose Nutritional Antioxidants," *Med Hypothesis* (1984), 13: 77–98.

[144] Chandra (1980), Op. cit.

[145] Borek, C. et al., "Selenium and Vitamin E Inhibit Radiogenic and Chemically Induced Information in Vitro Via Different Mechanisms," *Proc Natl Acad USA* (1986), 83: 1490.

[146] Gershwin et al. (1985), Op. cit., p. 244.

[147] Beisel et al. (1981), Op. cit.

[148] Ibid.

[149] Gershwin et al. (1985), Op. cit., p. 248.

[150] Tanaka, J. et al., "Enhancement of Helper T Cell Activity by Dietary Supplementation of Vitamin E in Mice," *Immunology* (1979), 38: 727.

[151] Corwin, L.M. and J. Scholess, "Influence of Vitamin E on the Mitogenic Response of Murine Lymphoid Cells," *J Nutr* (1980), 110: 916.

[152] Badgely, L., "Fats," in *Healing AIDS Naturally* (San Bruno, Calif.: Human Energy Press, 1986), p. 80.

[153] "Prostaglandin Metabolism as Related to Vitamin E and Zinc Status," *Nutrition Reviews* (1982), 40: 338.

[154] "The Effect of Vitamin E on Immune Responses," *Nutritional Reviews* (1987), 45(1): 27.

[155] Kutsky (1981), Op. cit., p. 200.

[156] Ibid., p. 2.

[157] Ibid.

[158] Wenburg, E. D., "Iron in Neoplastic Disease," *Nutrition and Cancer* (1983), 4 (3): 223.

[159] Miller, A. et al., "Studies of the Anemia and Iron Metabolism in Cancer," *J Clin Invest* (1956), 35: 1248.

[160] McDougall, J. A. and M. A. McDougall, "Help Prevent Cancer with a Health-supporting Diet," in *The McDougall Plan* (Piscataway, N. J.: New Centuries Publishers, 1983), p. 40.

[161] Matzner, Y. et al., "Suppressive Effect of Ferritin on In Vitro Lymphocyte Function," *Brit Hamatol* (1979), 42: 345.

[162] de Sousa, M., "Lymphoid Cell Positioning: A new proposal for the mechanism of control of lymphoid cell migration," *Symp Soc Exp Biol* (1978), 32: 393.

[163] Whiting, R. F. et al., "Enhancement of the Chromosome-damaging Activity of Ferritin and Its Reaction to Chelation and Reduction on Iron," *Cancer Res* (1981), 41: 1628.

[164] Solomons, N. W., "Competitive Interactions of Iron and Zinc in the Diet: Consequences for human nutrition," *J Nutr* (1986), 116: 927.

[165] Allen, J. I. et al., "Severe Zinc Deficiency in Humans: Association with a reversible T-lymphocyte dysfunction," *Annal Intern Med* (1981), 95: 154.

[166] Koller, L. et al., "Immune Responses in Rats Supplemented with Selenium," *Clin Exp Immunol* (1986), 63: 570.

[167] Milner, J., "Effect of Selenium on Virally Induced and Transplantable Tumor Models," *Fed Proc* (1985), 44: 2568.

[168] Beach, R. S. et al., "Zinc, Copper, and Manganese in Immune Function and Experimental Oncogenesis," *Nutrition and Cancer* (1982), 3: 172.

[169] Gershwin et al. (1985), Op. cit., p. 209.

[170] Chunningham-Rundles, C. et al., "Zinc-induced Activation of Human B Lymphocytes," *Clin Immunol Immunorathol* (1980), 16: 831.

[171] Beisel, W. R., "Trace Elements of Infectious Processes," *Med Clin North Am* (1976), 60: 851.

[172] Beisel (1981), Op. cit.

[173] Rosenbaum, M., "Nutrients and the Immune System," cited by M. Weiner in *Maximum Immunity* (Boston, Mass.: Houghton Mifflin Co., 1984).

[174] Kutsky (1981), Op. cit., p. 125.

[175] McCarty, M. F., "Nutritional Insurance Supplementation and Corticosteroid Toxicity," *Med Hyp* (1982), 9: 15.

[176] Gershwin et al. (1985), Op. cit., pp. 201–4.

[177] Ibid., p. 204.

[178] Beach et al. (1982), Op. cit.

[179] Chandra (1980), Op. cit.

[180] Gershwin et al. (1985), Op. cit., p. 222.

[181] Milanino, R. et al., "Concerning the Role of Endogenous Copper in the Acute Inflammatory Process," *Agent Actions* (1979), 9: 581.

[182] Baker, B. L. and D. E. Hultquist, "A Copper-binding Immunoglobulin from a Myeloma Patient. Studies in Copper-binding Site," *J Bio Chem* (1978), 253: 8444.

[183] Preiffer, C., *Mental and Elemental Nutrients* (New Canaan, Conn.: Keats Publ., 1975), pp. 167–398.

[184] Kelly, W. et al., "Myocardial Lesions in the Offspring of Female Rats Fed a Copper Deficient Diet," *Exp Molec Pathol* (1974), 20: 40–56.

[185] Kollman, D. "Biochemist and Nutritional Consultant," (personal communications) (Klamath Lake, Oreg.: Cell Tech, Inc., 1986).

[186] Passwater, R. A. and E. M. Cranton, *Trace Elements, Hair Analysis and Nutrition* (New Canaan, Conn.: Keats Publishing, Inc., 1983); see also the USDA's 1979 analyses based on the 1963 data of Firman Bear of Rutger's University.

[187] Schroeder, H., *The Positions around Us* (Bloomington, Ind.: University Press, 1974), p. 126.

[188] Underwood, E., *Trace Elements in Human and Animal Nutrition*, 4th ed. (New York: Academic Press, 1977), p. 267.

[189] Anderson, B., "The Iron and Zinc Status of Long-term Vegetarian Women," *Am J Clin Nutr* (1981), 34: 1042.

[190] Gershwin, M. et al., "Trace Metals, Aging, and Immunity," *J Am Geriatr*

196

Soc (1983), 31: 374.

[191] Klevay, L. et al., "Evidence of Dietary Copper and Zinc Deficiencies," *JAMA* (1979), 241: 1916.

[192] Cranton, E. M. and J. P. Frackelton, "Free Radical Pathology in Age-associated Diseases: Treatment with EDTA chelation, nutrition, and anti-oxidants," *J Holistic Medicine* (1984), 6(1): 6.

[193] Passwater and Cranton (1983), Op. cit.

3. The Profile of Susceptibility

> It is more important to know what kind of person
> has the disease, than what kind of disease the
> person has.
>
> —Hippocrates

The Multifactorial View of AIDS

Despite its extensive coverage in the press and in books, Human Immunodeficiency Virus (HIV) may not be the cause—or not the sole cause—of AIDS. Antibodies for the virus have been found in at least 80 percent of people with AIDS, indicating previous exposure. This alone, however, does not prove a definitive cause-and-effect relationship. Indeed, the only way to prove HIV as cause would be to inject the virus into a large number of people who have been antibody-negative for several years. If a large percentage of the group then contracted AIDS, then HIV could be legitimately incriminated. Such an experiment would be ethically unthinkable. Moreover, it would require a large group of subjects to be followed for three years or longer to determine the rate of infection and disease manifestation. Differences in life-style patterns and in family history might account for variations in susceptibility among individuals.

AIDS research has come a long way in understanding *how* the virus can cause such grievous harm among so many young people. However, with at least two million infected and only a small fraction showing signs of illness, scientists are beginning to focus on the other side of the coin: *Why* have some long-time infected people not become ill? *Why* have certain people, unwittingly exposed to the virus, not become infected? The situation bears similarities to influenza. Among people exposed to influenza each year, some show flu symptoms, others experience mild illness, some are bedridden for a week, and a small percentage actually die. The main difference is that, with AIDS, the mortality rate is higher once the disease process is set in motion. This means we are dealing with a particularly lethal virus, but not necessarily one that is impervious to the protective mechanisms of the immune system.

No consensus has been reached on what exactly triggers AIDS in susceptible individuals.[1] It has been generally overlooked that HIV may only be the precipitating agent, the catalyst, for a disease process which may actually begin *prior* to infection by HIV. Unfortunately, rather than consider the conditions conferring resistance to infection, medical research has focused almost exclusively on the events which follow the initial stage of disease. Rather than study the underlying biochemical conditions which determine the progression of AIDS, the emphasis has been on the drastic symptomology and process of dying from the "full-blown" syndrome. At best, prevention itself is viewed only in the superficial terms of transmitting the virus, as if the Human Immunodeficiency Virus itself represents the entire disease. Given our current knowledge, however, it is doubtful that HIV exposure alone, without other predisposing factors or co-factors, dooms anyone to AIDS. Susceptibility and resistance, albeit far more complex than transmissibility, are essential considerations in approaching any form of infectious disease.

The concept of co-factors, while new to modern medicine, has long been an intrinsic focus of traditional medical philosophy and ancient healing systems. For example, the ancient Greeks believed that a proper balance of air, water, food, and sunlight, were essential to health, while other aspects of the environment promoted disease. Traditional medicine as practiced in China, Tibet, and India, still considers each individual case of illness as produced by a unique pattern of factors pertaining to one's daily way of life. Life-style patterns may vary considerably among individuals within cultures and sometimes even within families. The various aspects of unhealthy life-style and malnutrition belonging to each pattern comprise a "profile of susceptibility" for those groups deemed at risk for contracting AIDS.

A *co-factor* is defined as some agent (virus, microbe, toxin, nutrient, hormone, allergen, ect.) which contributes to the disease process. Usually when we speak of co-factors, we are speaking of the macroscopic manifestation—heredity, diet, rest, exercise, stress "coping" ability, allergy, and others. By definition, co-factors cannot work alone, but interact with other factors to compromise health and enhance the disease process. This constitutes the *multifactorial theory* of disease, in contradistinction to the *single-agent theory* espoused by conventional medicine. Some co-factors are tangible and controllable, while others are relatively obscure and uncontrollable. Some co-factors play a more primary role in predisposing one to disease, whereas others operate in a secondary way by stressing the organism further.

The multifactorial view is making a comeback since HIV was discovered. One reason this theory is becoming so prominent with AIDS compared to other diseases is that physicians are contending with a system that is both directly influenced by the environment and protecting against potentially harmful environmental influences. Genes, nutrition, foreign substances and stress are interwoven in the fabric of immune-competence. In the case of full-blown AIDS, doctors can no longer rely on the immune system to perform the work essential to healing after drugs have been introduced. Attacking the AIDS virus with drugs is usually futile, since the body only continues to deteriorate without an intact immune system.

Co-factors involved in the genesis of AIDS may consist of a wide range of dynamic elements which interact with HIV and the immune system. Many AIDS researchers now believe that one or more as yet unrecognized co-factors are necessary to turn an HIV infection into an actual disease; these harmful co-factors may render one susceptible to infection and support the disease process as a whole. Other co-factors may instead help the immune system counteract the AIDS virus; these beneficial co-factors may prevent infection *and* promote recovery from AIDS.

Factors which have been linked with weakened immunity—antibiotics, alcohol, marijuana, morphine, steroids, emotional stress, and typical American diets—may all be providing a background of vulnerability to HIV. Consider that the majority of cases have occurred among homosexual men, many of whom frequently take "poppers" (nitrite inhalants which enhance sexual sensations) and other recreational drugs which cause depressed immunity; most of the remaining cases have occurred among injectors of heroin, which is highly immunosuppressive (see section: "The Risk to Recreational Drug Users").

The revolutionary idea of multiple causes operating in synchrony may eventually supersede the specialized, narrow view espoused by modern medicine. The conventional approach is rooted in two fundamental theories: (1) *the germ theory*, of one type of *germ* causing one disease, and (2) *the genetic theory*, of one *gene* linked to one disease. The latter has been the primary counterpoint to the germ theory for several decades. Now both theories may be seen as encompassed by a broader theory of disease which asserts that various agents *collectively* either promote or inhibit disease processes. For example, natural brain chemicals (*peptides*) can be mediated by diet, regulatory hormones can be mediated by behavior, and the immune system is weakened by synthetic chemicals introduced through our food, air, and water. All bodily systems are influenced by genes, which are in turn switched on and off by various environmental conditions. Finally, all systems—especially the brain and nervous system—influence the body's immune status in a collective or synergistic way.

The multifactorial theory also sheds new light on our personal responsibility in promoting health and preventing disease. Infectious disease can no longer be attributed to a single insidious germ such as the HIV, herpes simplex virus, or papilloma virus. Instead, a multitude of factors may be interwoven in the disease process, most of which arise from individual choices made in daily life. No longer is there a place for "evil" germs or "enemy" cancer cells. These entities persist only in the context of other co-factors which support them; they are harmful only when we neglect to maintain strong immunity and overall vitality. Whether we will "acquire" a disease is not determined simply through contact with some harmful external agent, but through a wide range of environmental factors over which we exert varying degrees of control in daily life. We must learn to evaluate our own mode of living and the behaviors which either enhance or diminish our health and well-being.

Using sophisticated computer systems, scientists can now discern some of the diverse interrelationships of nutrients, chemical toxins, and physiological factors contributing to the disease process. While there are still more assumptions than definitive answers, our extensive research on the profiles of high-risk groups leads us to propose that co-factors—most of which are as yet unrecognized by modern medicine—play an essential role in AIDS. *The multifactorial perspective, if correct, provides an understanding of the practical basis for susceptibility to AIDS.* Herein lies humanity's hope for fully eliminating AIDS and restoring the health of millions of people around the world.

Understanding Transmission and Contagion

How does one acquire HIV, the so-called AIDS virus? First of all, this is a very fragile virus. When exposed to the open air at room temperature, it becomes nonfunctional within several seconds. The AIDS virus, HIV, can only survive and thrive in body fluids, especially blood and semen, although it has also be found in tears, saliva, urine, and vaginal secretions. This is one reason why HIV is not easily transmitted from one person to another. Unlike the common cold, AIDS is not strongly contagious in that a carrier can cough in your face and pass on the virus, nor can you get infected by sharing food or culinary utensils with an afflicted person. The two most critical aspects of transmission are the relative concentration of virus present in one's body fluids and the way these contaminated fluids are exchanged.

A study reported in the *New England Journal of Medicine* provides conclusive evidence that the disease is not spread through casual personal contact.[2] Out of 101 people who had shared homes with AIDS patients, there was no substantial evidence of transmission among family members who kissed, shared toothbrushes, drinking glasses, beds, towels, and toilets. Some scientists caution, however, that sharing of razors and toothbrushes, both of which may come into contact with blood, may possibly transmit the AIDS virus.

Studies of health-care workers exposed to body fluids of AIDS patients—as by needle pricks while drawing blood—have also reported an absence of risk for transmitting the virus.[3,4] It appears that clinicians giving injections are at low risk for contracting AIDS when a small dosage of the virus is inadvertently transmitted. Recently, however, several health-care workers whose skin was exposed to blood became infected by the virus. Officials from the Centers for Disease Control suggested that the virus may have passed through chapped or inflamed areas of unprotected skin, or through the mucous membrane in the mouth of one worker whose face was splashed with blood when handling a storage container before screening for antibodies. They stress that there is "no direct evidence" for HIV transmission through intact skin or by casual contact. Alternatively, this statement could also read "no one knows for sure." Only time can tell.

Since the virus has been isolated in saliva, kissing may theoretically represent an additional risk. The concern derives from a report issued by Zaki Salahuddin, M.D., Jerome Groopman, M.D., and colleagues from Harvard University.[5] An elderly Bostonian in his seventies had become impotent due to a surgical procedure. During the surgery, which involved a blood transfusion, he acquired the AIDS virus and subsequently infected his wife. At the time of infection their sexual relationship was, of necessity, restricted to kissing and hugging. This case may be unique to older people, however, since immune responsiveness decreases with age, perhaps making them more susceptible to the trace amounts of HIV occasionally present in saliva. To date, all other documented forms of sexual transmission have involved other forms of sexual activity. There is no other documentation supporting saliva-associated transmission of AIDS, for example, through sneezing, coughing, spitting, or sharing of food.[6]

Furthermore, we should note that only a small percentage of those with AIDS actually show the presence of the HIV virus in their saliva, and even then, as alluded to above, it is found in very low concentrations.[7] Unless large quantities of saliva are exchanged—as in passionate French-kissing—saliva is probably not an adequate medium for transmission. It is also plausible, as discussed in the next chapter, that saliva contains certain immune factors which deter or eliminate the AIDS virus.[8] To be on the safe side, it is probably best that infected individuals refrain from prolonged and intimate kissing, as recommended by the National Academy of Sciences.

In addition to sexual activity, the AIDS virus can be transmitted through sharing of contaminated needles, through infected blood and blood products, and from mother to child during and after pregnancy. Apparently it is *not* transmitted by mosquitoes, even though such insects (as well as tsetse flies, cockroaches, and others) may carry AIDS-virus-like segments in their genetic material.[9] Of the four recognized risk categories for transmission, sexual intercourse clearly constitutes the biggest threat to the greatest number of people. Let us now delineate these categories as follows:

1. *Semen and vaginal secretions can carry the virus.* Frequent and intimate sexual contact with more than one partner, regardless of one's sexual orientation, seems to represent a greater risk of receiving the virus from an infected sexual partner. However, some research also indicates that a single sexual contact—either homosexual or heterosexual—is sufficient to transfer the virus from one person to another. This observation has aroused much fear and anxiety around sexual practices, even prompting some people toward total celibacy.

The *mode* of sexual intercourse seems to play a significant role in spreading AIDS. Any sexual act which might rub or abrade the thin tissue that lines the colorectal wall may enhance the likelihood of infection if the virus is present. Hence anal intercourse, whereby semen is ejaculated into another's rectum, is far more risky than normal vaginal intercourse, although transmission can occur through this mode as well. A woman's vagina is far less prone to abrasion and absorption because of its tougher physical consistency and relatively low permeability, respectively. Local immune mechanisms also prevent the sperm from entering through the vaginal tissues.

An Australian report suggests, however, that damage to the vaginal or rectal lining and direct access to the bloodstream is not an exclusive requirement.[10] Eight women were artificially inseminated with semen from a symptomless carrier—inadvertently of course. Although the previously frozen semen had been gently placed into the vagina, four of these eight women became infected. Since the procedure was carried out ostensibly without causing any abrasion, it seems that a direct portal to the bloodstream is not necessary for sexual transmission to occur. In this case, it may be that a concentrated dose of HIV-contaminated semen, together with possible weaknesses in immunity, may have predisposed certain of the women to infection by the virus.

According to leading AIDS researchers, semen is a particularly rich source of virus in those people with a past history of venereal disease.[11] The T4 lymphocyte (T helpers) tends to accumulate in the semen of such individuals. These cells are key targets of the AIDS virus and may serve as a very rich source in the carrier's semen. Presumably, the semen's high T4 levels result from previous exposures to sexually transmitted disease-causing organisms such as herpes virus, candida, chlamydia, and so on. Other research suggests that the AIDS virus can bind to a molecule on the surface of sperm, to be taken directly to where it is least accessible—inside the T4 lymphocytes of a sexual partner.[12] This would constitute a far more efficient way for HIV transmission to occur. The use of spermicides may be a way to block the HIV "hitchhikers" from entering a new host. *Vasectomy*, which keeps sperm out of semen, is being considered, although the operation may be dangerous for an infected man, and the possible long-term effects of this procedure are unknown.

2. *Contaminated hypodermic syringes can carry the virus.* The sharing of intravenous (IV) drugs, a common practice among low-income drug addicts, has been implicated in transmission of the AIDS virus. By some estimates, more than two-thirds of New York City IV drug users are infected. In most major cities of the United States and Western Europe, this high-risk group continues to expand at an alarming rate, with the number of new cases currently exceeding that of gay and bisexual men. Educational programs regarding transmission via unsterile needles have been largely unsuccessful, but they may have important public health implications in Third World countries such as Haiti and Africa, where many medical clinics lack adequate sterilizing facilities and needles are often in short supply. With regard to IV drug users, perhaps closer scrutiny should be given to the underlying reasons for addictive behaviors and reliance on opiate drugs, and how such behaviors can be more effectively changed.

3. *The blood products used in transfusions for various medical purposes can carry the virus.* People receiving blood transfusions prior to 1985,

when the Red Cross began testing all donated blood for AIDS, are more likely to have been infected than those after 1985. In developed countries such as the United States, antibody-screening programs have greatly reduced the potential hazards of this procedure, and it is unlikely that contaminated blood could now be used in a transfusion in this country. For African countries, however, adequate screening programs are virtually absent, much of the blood supply is tainted, and blood transfusions continue to be a kind of Russian roulette throughout the continent. In both the United States and Africa, a significant number of AIDS cases among children have been transmitted by blood transfusions. Recently two organ-transplant patients were infected by the AIDS virus from a donor who originally tested negative.[13] Unless testing becomes foolproof, blood transfusions will remain a potential risk for transmitting the virus. (It is interesting to note that one of the two organ-transplant patients received a kidney and the other a liver; both organs play key roles in immunocompetence and both surgical procedures necessitate the use of strong immunosuppressive drugs.)

4. *A pregnant woman carrying the virus may infect her child.* Prenatal infection by the AIDS virus has been documented. Throughout embryonic development, the fetus is constantly in intimate contact with the mother's bloodstream, receiving essential nutrition and immune support. The flipside to this is that the fetus may also receive harmful substances and infectious organisms circulating in the mother's bloodstream, including the AIDS virus. Unless the mother has acquired some form of strong immunity beforehand, the virus will probably pass through the placental barrier to cause prenatal infection. According to most reports, however, the risk of in utero transmission is somewhere between 30 and 50 percent. Why some mothers transmit the virus easier than others may have something to do with differences in immunocompetence and composition of the placenta.

The AIDS virus has also been isolated in breast milk, suggesting that the newborn may become infected while nursing from a carrier mother. So, far, however, this possibility has not been definitively demonstrated; the existing data is largely circumstantial. Most research on postnatal transmission has shown an association with blood transfusions but not with breastfeeding.[14] Still, the possibility exists and should be guarded against. This is a serious dilemma for nursing mothers who would like to nurse their infants because of the many immune-strengthening benefits of breast milk.

Throughout the world, HIV is transmitted primarily through sexual intercourse. Hence the use of condoms has been advocated as a key measure for preventing spread of the virus. The most recent research suggests, however, that while sheaths help prevent the spread of HIV, they are not entirely foolproof. Their theoretical failure rate for preventing pregnancy is 2 percent, but the actual rate is 10 percent of all sexual encounters. Surveys in the United States show that 9.6 percent of couples had an unplanned pregnancy during the first year that they used condoms.[15] This may indicate that, despite the use of condoms, potentially one in every ten infected individuals can pass on virus during sexual intercourse—either male to female or vice versa.

In addition, the use of condoms as a preventive measure is fraught with practical limitations. Condoms are difficult to obtain in most developing countries, such as Africa and the Caribbean, where AIDS is widespread. Even in postindustrial countries, relatively few couples favor condoms, sometimes on the grounds of cost, availability, and cultural or religious conviction.[16] Furthermore, young people are less likely to use contraceptives properly than older people. Many object to using a condom because it reduces the hedonistic appeal of sexual intercourse. Spermicides, some of which appear to destroy the AIDS virus, are often shunned on similar grounds as well as their known toxic side effects.

Like syphilis and gonorrhea, AIDS is being classified as a sexually transmitted disease (STD). But as with these other diseases, the mode of transmission is only one aspect of the problem. Of very real significance is our immune system's amazing capacity to protect us from potential disease entities. By closely examining the human role in health and disease, we may come to see that acquired illness is largely our own responsibility, based upon our patterns of daily living. The life-style of the STD-prone individual concerns not only sexual practices, but also activities which may weaken immunity and render one more vulnerable to potential disease influences. Through healthy life-style we can promote sound health and powerful immunity, while through unhealthy life-style we diminish health and weaken our resistance to disease.

More attention should be directed toward the integral connection between immune strength and resistance to the elusive AIDS virus that is, the *milieu intérieur* or internal conditions which either promote or prevent disease *after* exposure to the virus.[17] This is not to underrate the role of transmission. It is imperative, however, that in studying risk factors for AIDS we distinguish between *susceptibility* and *transmissibility*, as each has its own unique behavioral profile. The latter involves behaviors that expose one to the virus, while the former involves behaviors which influence immune competence both before and after viral infection takes place. Since transmission and immune competence are both essential ingredients of the development of AIDS, both are integral considerations of any prevention program. Once transmission has taken place, however, strong immunity is our best hope for maintaining order and harmony within.

Gauging the Multifactorial Theory ———————

Given the widely held assumption that Human Immunodeficiency Virus is the primary factor in the *etiology* (cause and development) of AIDS, the overall emphasis of treatment and research has been to eliminate the virus and its effects. This prevailing focus is consistent with modern medicine's devout adherence to the germ theory, which propounds that viruses, bacteria and other microbes enter the body and cause disease regardless of the conditions of the host. Although the AIDS virus is usually just one of many viruses involved in AIDS, its specific capacity for destroying white-blood cell has given it the medical limelight as a prime suspect in the etiology of AIDS.

There are arguments both for and against HIV as the primary causal agent, the so-called single-agent hypothesis. The following is a simplified summary of these two opposing sides:

Supportive Evidence:	*Conflicting Evidence:*
Isolation of HIV occurred at about the time the AIDS epidemic began.	HIV has not been isolated from all the patients with AIDS symptoms.[18,19]
Injection of a simian HIV-anaglogue into monkeys has produced AIDS-like symptoms in some species.	Injection of blood from people with AIDS into monkeys has not produced the syndrome in these creatures.
Cluster outbreaks of AIDS among *seropositive* (antibody-positive, previous HIV exposure) persons in major American cities.	A substantial proportion of seropositive mothers in Africa have given birth to seronegative infants, suggesting maternal immunity.[20]

Supportive Evidence:

Conflicting Evicence:

Epidemiologic studies show chains of sexual contact in AIDS patients greater than expected by chance, and HIV can easily be transmitted via semen and other bodily fluids.

Endemic populations within certain areas of Africa show seropositivity but do not manifest signs of AIDS.[21] Many of these people also seem to be HIV-negative upon later testing.

HIV targets the T-cell, leading to severely depressed immunity and greater susceptibility to infection by opportunistic microbes.

A variety of other factors, including poor nutrition & overstimulation of the immune system by foreign substances, can lower T-cell numbers.[22]

HIV-tainted syringes are considered a major mode of transmission among heterosexual IV drug users.

Most IV drugs can directly cause immunosuppression, affecting the same cell types depleted in AIDS.[23]

Blood samples carrying HIV can transmit the virus to blood transfusion recipients, who may then go on to contract AIDS.

The effects of blood transfusions and the circumstances requiring their use suggest that immunodepression may precede infection.

An alternative to the single-agent view, as introduced earlier, is the multifactorial view, by which the AIDS virus is only one of a variety of factors which may bring about pronounced immune deficiency. Environmental factors which weaken the immune system in a subtle, gradual way throughout the lifetime of the organism may either directly or indirectly diminish the immune system's initial reaction to the AIDS virus. Other factors may influence activation of the AIDS virus once exposure and infection have taken place.

If the multifactorial hypothesis proves correct, then the AIDS virus itself, once established in the host, is merely another opportunistic entity. With regard to transmission, the multifactorial view asserts that there must be a *context* for HIV to establish itself in the body to begin the chain of events known as AIDS. This context seems to involve a compromised immune system, which is then peculiarly vulnerable to the AIDS virus. The larger context may include any combination of various environmental conditions such as inadequate nutrition, poor sanitation, recurrent infectious diseases, drug abuse, and inappropriate health habits in general. All of these factors have some bearing on the strength of the immune system, possibly setting the stage for infection by the AIDS virus.

One of the most intensively studied co-factors, commonly found in the medical history of AIDS patients, is repeated exposure to various germs. Previous infection by either cytomegalovirus or Epstein-Barr virus has been associated with the onset of Kaposi's sarcoma and AIDS-related lymphomas, respectively. Recent studies by American scientist Stephen S. Caiazza, M.D., and his colleagues from West Germany show that syphilis plays an important but hitherto unrecognized role in AIDS.[24] Using highly sophisticated tests, the researchers have found that most AIDS patients belonging to high-risk groups harbor the *spirochete* bacteria linked with syphilis. When these individuals were treated for syphilis with penicillin, the AIDS symptoms were often dramatically reduced.

These and other studies suggest that various organisms infect the bodies of persons at risk for AIDS and function as synergistic co-factors with the AIDS virus. It is important to recognize, however, that these organisms can be prevented from infecting and harming the body by making the immune system strong. Rather than try to wipe out these co-infections with drugs, we should first seek to eliminate them naturally by supporting the immune system through health-promoting diet and life-style. If doctors treat the hidden infections with tetracycline or other conventional drugs, they may end up weakening the immune system further. In some cases, along with balanced nutrition, it may be helpful to use small amounts of antibiotics or other less extreme drugs to treat the co-infections.

Genetic variation has also been proposed as a possible co-factor since genetic differences in susceptibility to infectious diseases are a well-known biological phenomenon. In a recent article in *The Lancet*, British scientists reported the first bit of evidence of individual genetic differences in susceptibility to HIV infection.[25] Examining blood samples from 375 homosexual men, some of them HIV carriers and some not, the researchers found that people with a particular genetic variant of the same protein were more susceptible to AIDS infection and disease. The protein, called *group-specific component* or *Gc*, comes in three forms: *Gc 1 fast* (*Gc 1f*), *Gc 1 slow* (*Gc 1s*) and *Gc 2*. Men who had repeatedly had intercourse with AIDS patients, and had become infected, were far more likely to have Gc 1f in *homozygous* form (no other variants present). Conversely, men who had not gone on to develop AIDS were far more likely to be homozygous for Gc 2. Interestingly, the Gc protein is a carrier for vitamin D and also a mediator of calcium metabolism. The potential role of vitamin D and calcium in the development of AIDS has not yet been determined.

The British findings, however, have since been contradicted by several studies which reported the absence of a significant association with the Gc protein.[26,27] The discrepancy may be explained by different methods used to study the Gc protein, to ethnic admixture in the British population, or to differences in ecological health factors—diet, smog, drugs, and so on. It is important to recognize that the expression of our genetic material is largely contingent upon environmental conditions. Every one of the body's trillions of cells is constantly influenced by biochemical factors such as nutrients, food additives, toxic drugs, heavy metals, carbon dioxide, and radiation.

Recent research shows that our primary genetic material—the DNA contained within the nucleus of the cell—is not impervious to common environmentally induced biochemical changes. Free radicals, generated by excessive oxidation of fatty acids and by ionizing radiation, can directly alter the DNA.[28] Vitamins B_{12} and D, and folic acid (another B vitamin), are essential in the proper synthesis of nucleic acids making up our genetic material.[29] Vitamin B_6 deficiency can cause impaired DNA and protein synthesis, which subsequently produces a depressed immune response.[30] Thus even diseases which implicate inheritable factors are fundamentally acquired; we cannot separate the biological functioning of the host from its environmental context.

As discussed before, a central part of the multifactorial development of immunodeficiency is antigen overload, whereby repeated exposure to foreign substances (antigens) overstimulates and eventually depletes key components of the immune system. Some substances in nature are more antigenic than others—that is, they stimulate the immune system to respond more actively, producing more antibodies and immune cells. Antigenic stimulation comes from myriad sources, including infectious organisms, drugs, food additives, dairy products and other foods. The standard American diet is replete with high-antigen substances, particularly cow's-milk protein and chemical additives. Over the long run, constant exposure to these foods may result in depletion and imbalance in the reserves of immune cells and antibodies, perhaps setting the stage for greater susceptibility to disease-causing viruses and bacteria.

Antigen overload and dietary imbalances work in a synergistic way: inappropriate or poor-quality nutrition may be unable to support an immune system confronted with antigen overload.[31] Such immune overload is aptly reflected in various high-risk subpopulations, including drug addicts and their offspring, prostitutes, hemophiliacs, and chemotherapy recipients in the West, as well as Africans and Haitians in their own countries. Populations adopting Western life-styles experience higher rates of cancers and other chronic diseases, and this suggests the possibility of diminished immune functioning among these groups.[32]

In the most definitive "risk" study to date, reported in the January 8, 1987 *New England Journal of Medicine*, scientists found several factors which may help identify people with the AIDS virus who are at greater risk of developing the syndrome. The study of 1,853 men compared 59 who developed AIDS with the infected men who remained symptom-free.[33] The researchers found the following factors to be closely associated with the subsequent development of AIDS:

(1)   A decreased level of T-helper cells and an increased level of T-suppressor cells. One possible explanation is that a healthy or normal T-helper/T-suppressor ratio may indicate a decreased risk of developing AIDS, or greater resistance toward the potential effects of HIV, the AIDS virus. If this ratio becomes inverted, even temporarily, it may allow the virus to wreak havoc in the body.

(2)   A low level of antibody to HIV. This suggests that antibodies may confer some degree of protection against the progression of immune deterioration and AIDS. People who show a vigorous antibody response are probably more resistant to AIDS than those who show only a small response.

(3)   A history of sex with someone in whom AIDS later developed places the individual at greater risk. In this case, people may become infected with a more virulent strain of the virus, or earlier infection may have taken place.

Unfortunately, the study failed to list among its "suggested determinants of risk" the possible contribution of diet, drugs, and medications. But the finding of more neutralizing antibodies in healthy carriers who remained healthy compared to those who contracted AIDS suggests that the body has its own means to protect itself from the pathological effects of HIV.

Commonsense observations of the life-style patterns of major high-risk groups supports the value of the multifactorial view. Gay men, for example, tend to have a greater history of sexually transmitted diseases (STDs) and repeated drug exposures. This group shows a high prevalence of hepatitis, cytomegalic virus, herpes, gonorrhea, syphilis, candidiasis, intestinal parasites, and other infectious diseases. By over-stimulating the immune system, recurrent infections may promote—as well as reflect—compromised immunity and enhanced susceptibility to infectious microbes. In addition, these men often receive immuno-suppressive drugs (steroids, antibiotics, and antifungals) to combat such infections, and also tend to indulge in recreational drugs. As discussed later in this chapter, many of these men also engage in anal intercourse, a sexual practice which exposes the intestinal tract to toxic substances which weaken the immune system.

Some of the environmental factors implicated in immune breakdown may operate gradually throughout the lifetime of high-risk individuals. Dietary and metabolic imbalances are the most overlooked yet perhaps the most essential influence on one's susceptibility to AIDS. The rich, highly refined American diet as well as alcohol, tobacco and other substance abuse common among gay men and IV drug users helps complete the multifactorial profile of greater susceptibility to AIDS and other infectious diseases.[34]

Other environmental factors may exert a profound influence during prenatal and early development. Breast-feeding, for example, appears to play an important role in establishing strong immunity in the developing infant. According to one survey of sixty gay men with either ARC or AIDS, all had been bottlefed as infants with the exception of one, who had been breast-fed for less than three months.[35] This may be more than mere historical coincidence. While bottle-feeding did become more popular in the fifties and sixties, nevertheless the overall message remains clear: these men had received formula milk during a critical period of immunological development. One could even say that such individuals would be less well adapted to the detrimental effects of formula milk. Thus cow's-milk formula may be an integral component of the multifactorial picture of AIDS.

With research pointing both toward and away from the virus as the primary causal agent, medical science has arrived at an important crossroads in its overall perspective on AIDS. This basic fact has split the scientific community in two. Many scientists contend that HIV is the necessary and sufficient cause of AIDS, and invest their energies accordingly—toward interfering with known viral mechanisms. Others argue that the virus may be necessary but is not the sole or sufficient cause, and that its effects may depend on an immune system previously compromised by other factors. Dr. Robert Gallo, of the National Center Institute, has himself acknowledged that long-term overstimulation of the immune system by foreign substances may be an important co-factor in the development of AIDS.[36] Let us now examine some the environmental and life-style conditions by which co-factors may come into play in the genesis of AIDS.

Apocalypse in Africa: The Untold Story ——————————

If the word "plague" has been used rather loosely to describe AIDS in America and Western Europe, no other word seems as appropriate for the nation states of Africa. AIDS has swept like prairie fire through the midsection of this continent, leaving well over 90,000 dead in its path, with several million predicted to die during the next decade. The countries hardest hit by AIDS all touch on the Great Rift Valley of East and Central Africa: Zaire, Zambia, Burundi, Uganda, Rwanda, and Tanzania. Every day, 15 new AIDS cases are diagnosed in the largest hospital of Central Africa, located in the Zairian capital of Kinshasa.[37] In Uganda, the number of persons afflicted with AIDS is doubling every four to six months. According to Dr. Samuel Okware, a public health official directing Uganda's AIDS prevention program, by the year 2000, one in every two sexually active adults will be infected.[38] Widespread prevalence of AIDS at that time could decimate much of the African population. In short, the entire AIDS belt of Central Africa stands in the foreboding shadow of apocalypse.

Researchers have found conflicting rural, urban, and socioeconomic differences in the epidemiology of AIDS in African countries. For example, HIV infection appears to be more of a rural or small town phenomenon in Uganda and Tanzania, while the cities appear most affected in Rwanda and Zaire.[39] Researchers have also reported variations in HIV infection and AIDS rates according to socioeconomic status. These observations reemphasize the limits of our understanding of the social and cultural dimensions of HIV transmission in Africa.

AIDS affects both men and women in a nearly one to one ratio, and in most areas the average incidence is slightly higher among young women. It is clear that the disease in transmitted primarily through two-way, heterosexual contact. The more sexually active someone is, as in the case of prostitution, the more likely one is to become infected. Perhaps in part because of their interaction with prostitutes, AIDS is recognized as a disease of the urban elite—the more productive and educated segments of the African population. As in United States and elsewhere, sexual promiscuity appears to increase the risk of transmitting the AIDS virus. Conversely, however, typical heterosexual activities (vaginal intercourse) do not necessarily increase one's immunologic susceptibility to the disease itself. This leads one to speculate on unidentified risk factors among African heterosexuals, factors which could include nutrition, medical care, and other aspects of life-style.

Blood transfusions are another common vehicle for heterosexual transmission in Africa, since much of the blood supply is contaminated. The potential contribution of blood transfusions is suggested by the 5 to 10 percent or greater seroprevalence detected among blood donors in Central Africa, a figure which also reflects the high background of seroprevalence among adults in these areas.[40] Approximately 10 percent of AIDS cases in Kinshasa reported receiving at least one transfusion during three years prior to onset of illness. In addition, overprescription of blood transfusion is an important problem in Zaire, Nairobi, and Zambia. Studies have shown that in some areas, 90 percent of transfusions given in a hospital may involve only a single unit of blood—an amount too small to warrant a transfusion by Western standards. As discussed earlier, however, blood transfusions themselves may cause depressed immunity, even in the absence of the AIDS virus.

Medical injections (and possibly scarifications for religious ceremonies) appear to be an additional route of exposure to HIV. In most villages, group inoculations for childhood diseases are usually done with a single syringe, and clinics routinely use the same needle for standard injections. By recent estimates, about 25 percent of AIDS cases in Central Africa may be spread by transfusions and injections.[41,42] Throughout the continent there is a general lack of a blood-collection and distribution infrastructure which would be capable of screening donors or donated blood for HIV. Finally, financial or other practical complaints may lead to reuse of disposable injection equipment and to insufficient sterilization or use of contaminated needles and other instruments. All this complicates problems to safeguard the blood supply in Africa.

The typical African view of the origin of AIDS contrasts sharply with that among Americans and Europeans. Inhabitants of central Africa believe that the disease originated in America or Europe and was transported to Africa.[43] Foreigners are thought to have brought AIDS to Kenya's capital city, Nairobi, and foreign sailors are blamed for the epidemic in Dar Es Salaam, the capital of Tanzania. In both cities, prostitutes appear to be the primary vehicles for spreading AIDS from foreigners to natives. In Kinshasa, where one out of seven babies in the major hospital is infected with the AIDS virus, the influence of Western culture may play a prominent role in promoting immune susceptibility to AIDS.[44]

One study of people in Africa offers information compatible with the multifactorial concept of weakened immunity as a precondition for infection by the AIDS virus.[45,46] HIV infection has been observed in approximately 25 percent of people living in certain parts of Africa, as indicated by Elisa antibody testing. Among those studied, however, there were no signs or symptoms suggestive of AIDS. In fact, the viral infection among these African blacks never progresses beyond a mild flu. Two explanations are often presented. One is that this particular version of the AIDS virus may represent a mutant strain from Africa, as discussed earlier. Another explanation proposed by Dr. Gallo and others is that the Black genetic makeup may somehow confer natural antiviral protection. Blacks in America and Europe, however, fail to demonstrate any such immunity to the AIDS virus.

A third explanation is that these African sub-populations, found primarily in the more remote rural areas, have *acquired* some kind of immunity to the AIDS virus. Such resistance could be conferred by the primarily vegetarian, low-fat, low-protein diet consumed by these groups, as well as their more active, health-promoting life-style in general. Of course, it is also possible that the virus harbored by these rural inhabitants simply has a very long latency period. But even this could involve the unique ecological milieu—including nutritional patterns—with which these segments of the African population interact in daily life. Because these rural dwellers are eating a more wholesome traditional diet, they probably have stronger immune systems than their urban counterparts eating the modern "supermarket" diet.

Among the vast majority of Africans manifesting clinical AIDS, we find the following profile of susceptibility:
- Rural undernutrition in many areas due to drought and poverty conditions.
- Urban overnutrition, including high intakes of white sugar, dairy products, and highly processed foods such as condensed and powdered milk.
- Chronic parasitic and bacterial infections, notably malaria and tuberculosis.
- Recurrent STDs, especially among prostitutes and their clients.
- Frequent and often indiscriminate use of blood transfusions.

All of these factors may contribute to compromised immunity, rendering the individual more vulnerable to the AIDS virus. We must keep in mind, however, that Africa is a continent of many different countries, languages, social and economic structures, cultural ethics and religions. Despite the sheer size and diversity of African nations, however, some general observations can be made. In many rural and town areas, the standards for general health and nutrition are low, and both probably influence vulnerability to the AIDS virus. The ascertainment of AIDS among starving rural dwellers is difficult because many AIDS symptoms are virtually identical to symptoms of undernutrition. Even the immunological measures—such as numbers of T-cells—are quite similar in both circumstances.

The profile of susceptibility toward AIDS in Africa is best classified by basic variations in socioeconomic status and life-style patterns within the entire population. Based on our extensive ecologically oriented research, we propose two distinct profiles of environmental risk factors. Each of these profiles are characterized, in part, by extreme nutritional imbalances: (1) chronic undernutrition in some rural areas where poverty, drought, and famine are rampant; and (2) poor or imbalanced nutrition due to adoption of Western dietary practices such as high consumption of sugar, dairy, and processed foods.

Of course, this two-fold characterization is somewhat oversimplified, as numerous incidental factors may also come into play, such as the stress of overcrowding and insufficient sanitary services. By our view, however, nutrition may be considered the key determinant of immunocompetence because it determines the relative supply of organic substances making up the immune system. Other ecological factors and psychosocial stress tend to overlap with nutritional status and therefore play an important synergistic role.

The first of these African sub-profiles is easiest to substantiate. One of the most well-documented effects of chronic undernutrition, or *protein-calorie malnutrition*, is a profound weakening of immune functions. Proteins are the basic structural and functional components of the trillions of cells making up the body, including the many kinds of immune cells and antibodies.

African doctors frequently refer to AIDS as the "slim disease" because it often shows up as an extreme wasting syndrome, not unlike the emaciating signs of starvation seen throughout the drought-ridden areas of Africa. Indeed, so common are these symptoms that many people with AIDS die without ever knowing they had the disease. "Slim" is characterized by profound fatigue, chronic diarrhea, and extreme weight loss—sometimes as much as 40 percent over a period of several months! These individuals often exhibit one or more opportunistic infections, including a high incidence of tuberculosis. They also tend to present with fever and swollen lymph glands (*lymphadenopathy*). Most of the men, women and children with the wasting syndrome die within a year of diagnosis.

The similarities between starvation (protein-calorie malnutrition) and the "slim" version of AIDS are not purely coincidental. It has been known for a long time that severe or repeated infections are a common cause of malnutrition. This happens because infections increase the rate of metabolism and the breakdown of tissues, which creates a need for extra nutrients. At the same time, malnutrition or undernourishment itself contributes to both the incidence and the severity of infectious disease.[46,47] With an insufficient supply of nutrients—protein, carbohydrate, unsaturated fats, vitamins, and trace elements—we cannot sustain immunocompetence, and our natural resistance to infectious organisms is markedly reduced. Morbidity and mortality are the logical outcomes of this process.

The second sub-profile, overnutrition or excessive eating patterns, calls for a more detailed explanation. One of the most intriguing observations in Africa is the significant correlation between AIDS and upper-class status.[48] This strongly suggests a possible contribution by environmental factors. Urban centers throughout Africa have been increasingly infiltrated by Western technology, including the typical American diet of refined sugars and flours, meats, eggs, dairy products, food additives, and other foods. In the highly westernized city of Kinshasa, this dietary pattern is far more typical of urban people in the upper income bracket.[49]

It seems plausible that the rapid modernization of Africa's urban population, particularly for the upper class, may have set the stage for compromised immunity and thereby predisposed them to the pathogenic effects of the AIDS virus. Depending on the degree to which their lifestyles and medical care had been Westernized, the effect of declining immunity would apply to both urban and rural Africans. Conversely, in areas where famine is widespread, one would expect an entirely different set of enrivonmental conditions promoting vulnerability to the AIDS virus: again, the high degree of malnutrition and infectious diseases would be logically more conducive to such susceptibility.

In a study comparing common symptoms of AIDS with other illnesses in Kinshasa, it was generally not possible to distinguish seropositive from seronegative individuals on clinical grounds only. Of 111 patients having the typical signs and symptoms of AIDS, only 52 (47 percent) were actually HIV-positive.[50] Concurrent infection with tuberculosis was frequently found but not predictive of AIDS. Similarly, African researchers generally do not include lymphadenopathy—swollen lymph glands—in the standard case definition of AIDS because this "pre-AIDS" condition is just as common among seronegative as among seropositive people. Thus it is not a sign that can be used to readily distinguish AIDS from other clinical conditions in Africa. The balanced distribution of tuberculosis and lymphadenopathy among those with and without the HIV virus may suggest that some degree of immuno-depression exists in the general population regardless of HIV prevalence.[51]

Living conditions in the bustling urban community of Kinshasa, where AIDS is rampant, may be generally characterized by diverging patterns of the poor and the affluent. The city's tap-water is unfit for drinking, and the majority of the population live in unclean, slum conditions. The typical upper-middle class dietary pattern, however, is much like the typical American diet, along with some of the *haute-cuisine* of French and Belgian influence: imported red meats, eggs, white sugar, baked white-flour products, dairy products, hydrogenated oils, and imported fruits and vegetables. Heavy reliance on imported products has introduced high levels of artificial preservatives and agricultural chemicals to the urban elite's food supply. Clearly this is not the kind of diet one would expect to support resistance to infectious diseases.

By contrast, the average diet of the Kinshasan lower class still maintains much of the traditional dietary fare: locally grown fruit, *cassava* meal (a starchy root vegetable), avocados, tomatoes, and red onions. This dietary pattern also includes whatever animal protein is readily available: fish, poultry, monkey meat, and even grubs and caterpillars. Home-brewed beer and palm wine are common beverages, and fruits such as bananas, plantains, pineapples, and jackfruit, comprise a large portion of the native diet. They occasionally use the cassava leaves for a kind of vegetable meal and make it into a paste to be eaten as tapioca.[52] Hot spicy dishes of fish and poultry are an infrequent delicacy among these people. In sum, the typical diet of low-income Kinshasans is basically low in protein, low in fat, and high in complex carbohydrates and fiber. By nutritional standards, this type of dietary pattern would clearly favor strong immunity.

Since one finds considerable sexual promiscuity among *both* poor and wealthy in Kinshasa, sexual activity alone does not seem to explain the disparity in AIDS cases between the upper and lower classes. (The birth rate is just as high if not higher among the lower classes.) Sexual promiscuity only explains why the prevalence of antibodies to the AIDS virus is high in the general population. In terms of the risk of susceptibility, the major difference between rich and poor people in African cities is the former's adherence to Western dietary practices.[53] Like their Western counterparts, urban Africans of upper-class status may actually be overnourished—too much fat, sugar, and protein—which may predispose them to problems associated with weakened immunity.

In Nairobi, Kenya, AIDS seems to have emerged sometime during the early 1980s.[54] The initial spread is attributed primarily to prostitutes from Tanzania and emigrants from Uganda. To date, researchers have been unable to find any disparity in the distribution of AIDS among the upper and lower classes in Nairobi. It may be that the socioeconomic distribution is simply less well-defined than in the urban centers of Zaire and Rwanda, for example. In this regard, adopting an ecological perspective, there is generally more Western influence in Nairobi than in other urban communities of Africa.[55]

As in Kinshasa, the typical dietary pattern among upper-class Nairobi residents closely resembles Western dietary standards. Red meat, eggs, dairy, white sugar, and fruit, are readily available, though not always affordable. With a recent infiltration by the fast-foods industry, however, typical Western dietary items have become increasingly available to poor people living in slum areas; only the cheapest foods are eaten in a diet that is a mixture of the common traditional foods and low-priced Western food products.[56] Refined cereals have replaced less processed foodstuffs, so that cereal fiber intake may drop to one-fifth among these and other urban Africans.[57] Among both upper- and lower-class residents, refined sugar and salt intakes are high, owing to tastiness and low price, as is the consumption of fats if wages permit, although these are still somewhat low compared to average Western intakes.[58]

Over the past three decades, population pressures, changes in agricultural production, and inadequate food supply, have forced thousands of peasants to move from rural areas of Kenya and neighboring countries into Nairobi. With ongoing immigration and extreme overcrowding, a serious social problem has arisen in the slum areas, compounded by violence and alcoholism. The water supply is unclean, but apparently not as polluted as Kinshasa's.[59] It is well established that overcrowding under unsanitary conditions promotes an increased incidence of STDs and other infectious diseases, as well as a high infant mortality rate.[60]

In addition to the heavily refined dietary patterns characteristic of upper middle-class residents of Central and East African cities, there is some evidence of indiscriminate reliance on Western medical technological advances, including overuse of pharmacologic drugs, antibiotics, injections, blood transfusions, and other procedures known to result in *iatrogenic illnesses* (illnesses caused by medical treatments themselves). Popular attitudes towards medicine-taking foster strong consumer demands for medication in these cities. Further, a strong preference is often shown by patients for parenteral rather than oral therapy, and there tends to be excessive use of parenteral treatment. In addition, injections may be administered by a range of medical, paramedical, and other practioners who might not be aware or trained in antiseptic techniques. All of these practices could contribute to stress on the immune system.

It is both plausible and probable that dietary factors play a major role in promoting susceptibility toward infectious diseases—including AIDS, tuberculosis and many parasitic diseases—in Africa. Regarding African cities, we may posit a possible relationship between gross socioeconomic and environmental changes on one hand, and rising trends in certain infectious and degenerative diseases on the other. We propose two basic areas of AIDS risk for the urban elite of African nations: (1) an immune-weakening affluent life-style, including psychosocial stress, inadequate exercise, and, above all, a diet rich in refined sugars, animal fats and protein, and low in fiber, complex carbohydrates, and trace elements (see next chapter); and (2) sexual promiscuity, especially by interacting with urban prostitutes, who are high-risk carriers of the virus.

The picture of AIDS in Africa may offer grounds for concern about a potential rise in heterosexual AIDS in other areas of the world. Part of the reason for widespread incidence of heterosexual AIDS in Africa is the generally higher prevalence of HIV and other infections agents throughout the African population in the context of unsanitary living conditions. A more profound reason may be maladaptation to Western influence in the cities, and starvation conditions in rural areas. In time, unless public health programs are able to halt transmission among heterosexuals, the same high level of prevalence could conceivably exist in postindustrial countries. Constant adherence to harmful dietary practices (either excessive or deficient in nutrients), together with a huge infiltration of artificial and toxic substances in today's food and water supply, could alter our biochemical milieu enough to weaken immunity and encourage activation of the deadly retrovirus.

The alternative to prompt and comprehensive preventive action may be widespread dissemination of the virus throughout Africa, with the consequent addition of yet another large health burden on the African population. Prevention of transmission of the AIDS virus in Africa, either through sex or transfusions, will require unprecedented and creative education and communication programs. The problems of medical injections and blood transfusions illustrate the difficulties which will arise in attempting to translate scientific information into effective prevention programs. From a multifactorial perspective, Africa may offer important lessons for the United States and Europe, especially in those African cities which have been heavily influenced by Western technologies.

The Haitian Connection ————————————————

Haiti is by most estimates the poorest country in the Western hemisphere. With a colonial history important to America's early development, Haiti has for nearly two centuries been identified as a country of little strategic or economic significance. Desperate for a better quality of life, hundreds of thousands of Haitians have sought escape from a home beset by destitution, disease, deforestation, illiteracy and violent political chaos. Many of us recall the mass exodus of poorly clad and forlorn Haitians in leaky boats bound for the shores of the United States in the mid-seventies. At that time, the plight of the Haitian "boat people" aroused much sympathy from the American people. But since the arrival of AIDS, which is thought to have been carried through Haiti from Africa, Haitians emigrating to the United States have been received instead with much scorn and derision, as if the people themselves represent the dreaded syndrome.

In July of 1982, about one year after AIDS was identified in the United States, the Centers for Disease Control published a report from the University of Miami describing opportunistic infections and Kaposi's sarcoma in 34 recently immigrated Haitians, including four women. The pattern of disease observed in this group was remarkably similar to AIDS-related conditions seen previously in U.S. homosexual men and intravenous drug users. Many speculated that AIDS might have been introduced into the U.S. homosexual community by men who had been infected while vacationing in Haiti. Upon questioning, however, none of the 30 Haitian men acknowledged previous homosexual involvement and only 1 out of 26 questioned gave a history of intravenous drug use. Some researchers have accused Haitian interviewees of lying about previous sexual orientation because of cultural taboos against homosexuality. But others say the taboo against homosexuality is not any stronger among Haitians than among Americans and Europeans.

It was later discovered that AIDS was also apparently new in Haiti. By mid-1983, approximately 5 percent of domestic cases of AIDS were occurring in persons born in Haiti who resided in the United States, and this percentage has persisted.[61] Taken together, these findings suggest two possibilities: (1) that Haitian nationality itself carries an enhanced risk of AIDS; and (2) the existence of some unidentified risk factors for AIDS among Haitian heterosexuals.

The inclusion of Haitians as an independent risk group has been a heated source of debate for both scientists and politicians. On the surface, the group does not seem to fit into any of the conventional risk models for AIDS. Many researchers now concur that it is probably not Haitian nationality itself that manifests the risk but that typical Haitian life-styles, cultural factors, and medical histories play a more important predisposing role. According to this view, possible predisposing co-factors include heterosexual promiscuity, unsterilized needles for medical purposes, histories of repeated parasitic infections, excessive use of antimicrobial agents, inadequate nutrition, and voodoo practices.[62]

Is it possible that living in Haiti confers a greater risk of contracting AIDS than living in other areas of the world? What about other regions in the Caribbean Basin? When we look at the total number of cases of AIDS occurring in individual Caribbean nations, the largest number of cases has been observed in Haiti. As of 1986, for example, Trinidad and Puerto Rico each had less than half the Haitian prevalence number, and other Caribbean nations showed much smaller numbers.[63] However, when the cases are standardized according to the population (number of cases reported per 100, 000 people), a very different picture of the distribution of AIDS in the Caribbean Basin Region emerges. Based on this standardized view, the situation appears considerably worse in Bermuda and the Bahamas than in Haiti.

Distribution of AIDS in the United States and Caribbean
Basin Regions as of 1986

Region	No. of Cases Reported	Population $(\times 10^{-3})$	Cases/100,000 Population
United States	24,169	234,249,000	10.3
Bermuda	42	55,000	76.3
The Bahamas	68	223,000	30.5
Trinidad/Tobago	108	1,149,000	9.4
Haiti	501	5,590,000	8.8
St. Lucia	10	119,000	8.4
Guadeloupe	11	315,000	3.5
Puerto Rico	81	3,197,000	2.5
St. Vincent	3	134,000	2.2
Martinique	6	308,000	1.9
Grenada	2	111,000	1.8
Barbados	4	251,000	1.6
Dom. Republic	62	6,248,000	1.0

Source: Lange, W. R., and J. H. Jaffe (1987) "AIDS in Haiti," *New England Journal of Medicine*, 316(22): 1409–10.

Although distribution of cases in Haiti has many features in common with that in Central Africa (such as malaria and tuberculosis), the overall incidence of disease is considerably lower in Haiti. By contrast, there appears to be an unusually high incidence of AIDS among people recently emigrated from Haiti to the United States. This again suggests a possible contribution of environmental factors. Psychosocial stress may play a role, as most of the Haitians, upon arriving in the United States, suddenly find themselves in an entirely new sociocultural context with little or no food, shelter, or financial security. On top of all this, these people have had to withstand the unfounded stigma as potential vectors for AIDS.

According to one study, a large proportion of the AIDS cases among Haitian immigrants originate in Carrefour, a suburb of Port-au-Prince, and known as a major hotbed for male and female prostitution.[64] This may indicate that prostitution serves as a major mode of transmission for heterosexual AIDS in Haiti. But again, too much emphasis upon transmission tends to overshadow the issue of susceptibility. In the crowded city of Port-au-Prince, for example, clean water is extremely difficult to come by, with slum conditions closely resembling those of Zaire. It may also be that the actual infection *does* take place in Haiti but that the disease itself is triggered by environmental conditions in the United States. If so, this could explain the disparity in AIDS incidence between immigrants and home-bound Haitians. In any case, more attention should be given to the potential impact of environmental factors to help explain why the syndrome afflicts recent Haitian immigrants to such an appreciable degree.

AIDS should prompt us to broaden our humanitarian focus beyond the plight of the Haitian boat people to the condition of Haiti as a whole. Haitians come from a country where poor nutrition is the norm, and chronic parasitic and tubercular infections are widespread.[65] According to the Cousteau Society, three out of every four children in Haiti are malnourished, and the incidence of infectious disease is three times higher than in neighboring islands. Haitians must also deal with the stressful living conditions of extreme overcrowding. (Haiti is one of the most crowded of the Latin-American republics, averaging more than 400 persons per square mile.) Furthermore, most of the food supply is imported, and, for the vast majority of the population, dangerously low and contaminated. Only one in five Haitians have access to safe drinking water; the others are compelled to draw water directly from urban sewage run-off during the all too frequent dry spells.[66]

The landscape of Haiti is dominated by rivers and mountains. Areas of level, arable land are limited in size and hemmed in by mountains or the sea. Most of the level land is now densely populated by impoverished rural dwellers who make their living from farming. Among the chief agricultural products today are sugar cane, bananas, cacao, coffee, and cotton. Some crops and livestock are also raised, but in recent years the country has relied increasingly on foreign food imports. The primary foods eaten by rural inhabitants include rice, corn, sweet potatoes, beans, cassava, cane sugar, and many varieties of tropical fruits. In Port-au-Prince, Haiti's largest and capital city, there is considerably more fish and imported food such as red meats, poultry, white sugar and heavily processed food products. This is typical of the country's other urban centers as well.

Until recently, Haiti's most important natural resource was its arable land. Today, however, much of the original vegetation has been removed because of overcrowding and poor ecological awareness. The more accessible forests have been heavily exploited for lumber and firewood, which, in turn, has brought about excessive soil erosion and desertification. Soil erosion causes the loss of essential minerals and overall reduction in soil fertility, thus diminishing the nutritive value of food.[67] With the wetter portions of the country rapidly drying out, much of the land is now unsuited for agriculture. Finally, because of economic pressures, many farmers have converted their land to growing sugar cane and coffee beans. This has forced a heavy reliance on food imports from the United States, Cuba, and other Latin-American republics. It has also sparked the massive movement of rural dwellers to towns and cities in recent years.

The hot climate and crowded living conditions would be conducive to a high incidence of bacterial and parasitic infection among native Haitians. On top of this, the people frequently receive immunosuppressive drugs to treat the frequent parasitic and bacterial infections, such as for tuberculosis. By further compromising the immune system, indiscriminate use of these drugs could intensify the vicious cycle of infectious disease experienced by many in Haiti. Another aspect of the Haitian profile of depressed immunity is the stress of crowded living conditions. Research on laboratory animals has revealed that the stress of overcrowding can bring about significant immunodepression and greater susceptibility to infectious diseases.[68] The problem is compounded further by the effect of nutritional patterns on brain chemistry, psychological functions, and immune responsiveness.[69,70] (These relations are discussed in chapter three.)

The widespread presence of AIDS in Haitian immigrants coming to

American merits closer attention. Haitian immigrants who came to America after 1978 were 40 times more likely to have AIDS than those who had immigrated prior to 1978.[71] In 1984, researchers concluded that the prevalence of AIDS in Haitian immigrants was probably due to exposure to its causative agent, the AIDS virus, and not some sort of genetic deficiency.

As said before, Haitian immigrants in the United States are generally living at the poverty level, consuming junk-food diets, and experiencing all variety of recurrent infections. Some researchers propose that AIDS has been transmitted among many Haitians as a result of covert homosexual activity, use of contaminated intravenous needles or sexual contact with infected prostitutes. The use of shared needles for voodoo practices has also been suggested. These aspects of transmission, however, are only part of the overall picture. The profile of susceptibility must also be considered.

In sum, it is plausible that Haitians as a group would tend to be more susceptible to insult by the AIDS virus because of their previous living conditions, their history of inadequate nutrition and recurrent infectious diseases. These characteristics strongly suggest a profile of weakened immunity, resulting from the complex interplay of multiple environmental factors: excessive use of antibiotics imbalanced nutrition, polluted drinking water, overcrowding and other psychosocial stresses. The Haitian profile also suggests a relationship between antigen overload (drugs and infectious entities) and susceptibility to AIDS. Finally, because AIDS in Haiti is primarily a heterosexual problem, the social and biological background of Haitian immigrants may comprise an important set of previously unidentified risk factors for heterosexual AIDS in general.

The Risk to Recreational Drug Users

As the problems of our modern world intensify, our society as a whole has responded not with constructive thought and action, but instead with malaise and apathy. Consistent with these general attitudinal trends is increased "psychoactive" drug use—uppers, downers, and whatever else alters one's mood artificially. We have turned into a nation of addicts hooked on substances such as alcohol, tobacco, headache tablets, and even junk foods. Addictive tendencies also carry over into other aspects of life such as work, sex, and money. *Addiction* itself, the obsessive attachment to some form of substance or activity, is a social and biological disease. At the core of this disease is the desire to escape from the pressures and challenges of daily living, and to seek happiness from outside ourselves. Until we honestly face this fact head on, recreational drug abuse will continue to escalate and contribute to the deterioration of our social and economic systems.

Intravenous (IV) substance abuse has been implicated as a way of spreading AIDS. Among heterosexuals in developed countries, IV drug users show the greatest risk of AIDS. Over half of all female AIDS cases have occurred among intravenous drug abusers.[72] Evidently, a needle contaminated with bodily fluids carrying the virus may enable transmission between people sharing the same needle. This is surely an important concern for preventing further spreading of AIDS, especially when one considers that there about 200,000 IV drug users in New York City, and another 36,000 patients in drug treatment. Of these, 60 to 70 percent, or about 150,000, are estimated to be infected with the AIDS virus.[73]

The other side of the coin, however, is that most recreational drugs do more than affect brain and nerve cells: they can also weaken the immune system. We can see this by comparing cases associated with blood transfusions to those associated with IV drug abuse. The number of cases associated with transfusions prior to the blood-screening programs was suprisingly lower than would be expected. This is noteworthy when we recall that individuals receiving a transfusion are probably receiving a far higher dose of HIV-contaminated blood, while IV drug users would be expected to receive only small amounts of contaminated blood. Thus, prior immunodepression due to repeated drug use may be necessary to place an individual at risk for developing AIDS. Morphine derivatives such as heroin parallel the immune-suppression of spermatic fluid and markedly alter the mechanisms of natural immunity.[74]

A growing body of research has documented varying degrees of compromised immunity resulting from repeated use of marijuana, cocaine, amphetamines, barbiturates, and even such common substances as tobacco and alcohol.[75,76,77] Thus habitual drug use may render individuals more susceptible to infection by infectious microbes or to the degenerative effects of cancer cells. Alternatively, these substances may encourage activation of a latent AIDS virus.

Habitual opiate users show a distinct array of abnormalities in their lymphocytes, or white blood cells. The opiates bind to and alter the functioning of lymphocytes, and, in particular, significantly reduce the number of T-cells.[78] Heroin addicts are now known to have an increased frequency of infections and a tendency to develop pronounced immunological dysfunction. Altered and numbers of various types of circulating immune cells and components pertinent to AIDS.[79] Not only narcotic drug users, but people who take opiates for prescribed relief of chronic, severe pain should be aware of the potential immunosuppressive effects of these drugs.

One of the leading proponents of the role of drugs in producing susceptibility to AIDS is Cesar Caceres, M.D., of Washington, D.C. Accoring to his calculations, derived from data of the Centers for Disease Control, 79 percent of those with AIDS in the United States should be categorized as habitual drug users.[80] Collating this data, Caceres has found that about half of those with AIDS use as many as five street drugs in a year. Of those with a history of drug abuse, 93 percent smoked marijuana, 97 percent used poppers, 68 percent took some form of amphetamine, and 70 percent took one or more IV drugs. This information seems suggestive at the very least. In addition, Dr. Caceres emphasizes that heavy cigarette smoking and alcohol consumption, particularly in those with previous lung (from long-term smoking) and liver damage (from hepatitis), may play a major role in encouraging susceptibility to AIDS.

The habitual use of *poppers*, a nitrite-inhalant drug which has been prominent in the gay male life-style since 1972, is associated with anemia, strokes, lung damage, and compromised immunity, and is suspected of predisposing one to Kaposi's sarcoma and possibly other cancers.[81] (In addition, the nitrites and nitrates used as preservatives in packaged meats and found in other animal products are known to cause cancer in laboratory animals.) However, because of conflicting reports, no one has yet determined whether the association with Kaposi's sarcoma is more than mere coincidence. Since poppers suppress the immune system, we can only *assume* that they would predispose one to *all* kinds of infectious microbes, HIV included. Common sense dictates that these drugs would be doing more harm than good to an individual exposed to the virus.

One study of 12,000 opiate addicts in Iran found much higher rates of bladder cancer among opiate users who smoke tobacco than among smokers who do not use opiates. In this case, the researchers suggest that the opiate either potentiates the carcinogenic effect of the tobacco or reduces the immune-system activity of the T-cells toward the cancer cells, or does both.[82] Another study found that lymphocytes of opiate addicts have a reduced capacity for repair of certain types of damage to DNA, our primary genetic material.[83] One intriguing possibility is that such an effect could have some bearing on susceptibility to the AIDS virus at the level of infiltrating our cells' genetic material and upsetting the DNA's normal functional integrity.

It is of interest that the typical profile of illicit drug abusers throughout the modern world shows a high incidence of both STDs (syphilis, chlamydia, and gonorrheal cystitis) and tuberculosis. In each of these conditions, the usual course of treatment involves strong antimicrobial drugs. Hepatitis and other forms of liver disease are also generally part of the profile of the intravenous drug user, which may suggest the contribution of weakened liver functioning as a predisposing factor in AIDS.[84]

In sum, the use of mood-altering drugs such as heroin, cocaine, marijuana and various other opiates, as well as poppers and amphetamines, tend to compromise the human immune system and predispose users to pathologies associated with the AIDS virus. Other aspects of the average drug user's life-style are likely to negate health as well, such as inadequate diet and exercise patterns. The drugs may interfere with metabolism and further worsen nutritional status. The overall implication of this multifactorial scenario seems clear: among drug abusers a compromised immune system probably plays a key role in their underlying vulnerability to AIDS and other diseases.

The Risk to Homosexual Men

The group most seriously afflicted by AIDS at this time in the United States and much of Western Europe is the gay male population. Among homosexual and bisexual men in some cities, as many as 70 percent may be infected. Thousands of these men, many of them accomplished artists and successful business professionals, have died since the disease was first recognized. Education on preventing transmission through "safe sex" seems to have slowed the epidemic, but many thousands may already be infected and continue to contract the disease. With an actual failure rate of over 10 percent, condoms are not entirely reliable in preventing HIV transmission via typical homosexual practices.

If HIV has been around for at least 40 years, why is it so prevalent in our gay community today, and why did it strike this segment harder than any other segment of the American population? Several explanations have been offered. One suggests a link between the introduction of the experimental hepatitis vaccine into the homosexual population and the occurrence of AIDS in that population. Widespread infection of homosexual men may have taken place through HIV-contaminated blood which was disseminated throughout the gay community by hepatitis vaccine testing of 1978. The vaccine was tested on homosexual populations principally in New York City and San Francisco, and AIDS was detected soon afterward.

According to Dr. J. Anthony Morris, a noted virologist from the National Institutes of Health, the hepatitis vaccine in question was derived from the blood of homosexual men who were infected with hepatitis.[85] Today the commercially marketed vaccine is prepared in the same manner, but HIV-contaminated blood is screened out with methods developed in 1985. Unfortunately, there is no way of telling how many people may have been infected by HIV prior to 1985 through the hepatitis vaccine. This situation is reminiscent of the polio-virus vaccine first developed by Dr. Jonas Salk. Dr. Salk screened his vaccine for all viruses which could be detected at that time. Some years later, however, scientists discovered an agent that could not be detected by Dr. Salk's techniques, and this agent was subsequently linked with several kinds of cancer.[86] The apparent safety of the Salk vaccine was based on techniques available to detect known infectious agents; however, these techniques could not detect unknowns. The same lesson may apply to the hepatitis vaccine and may explain, at least in part, why AIDS is so prevalent among male homosexuals in the Western world.

Because AIDS has spread more rapidly among members of the male homosexual community, they are regarded as the primary infecting agents of our society and have been heavily stigmatized. Such homophobia is devoid of any rational basis. Casual transmission of the AIDS virus does not occur, so an infected gay man cannot transmit HIV to another person by sneezing or coughing. More important, the fear of being exposed to infected homosexuals tends to obscure one of the more fundamental aspects of the problem: the relative contribution played by compromised immunity, which may be a significant part of the typical gay male's profile of susceptibility. Now that AIDS has begun spreading through heterosexual transmission, the crisis compels us to look beyond the modes of transmission to the biological consequences of certain life-style patterns which may weaken the immune system and lower our resistance to viruses and microbes, toxins and cancer cells.

As early as July 1983, Dr. Jay Levy and colleagues reported in the British medical journal, *The Lancet*, and again in December 1986 in the *New York Times*, that there are some members of the gay community, previously exposed to the AIDS virus who seem to remain symptomless for very long periods of time. This may suggest that certain individuals acquire some degree of resistance to the virus. In New York, at least

13 men who volunteered in 1978 for the hepatitis-B vaccine were already infected with HIV, yet have lived for nine years without developing AIDS.[87] An astonishing finding of this study is that the immune systems of all nine of these men are functioning normally, with no deficits in any of the white blood cells or other components linked with AIDS. A small San Francisco study found that of 155 homosexual men infected for seven years or longer, 29 have not developed AIDS.[88]

These and other studies suggest differences in individual susceptibility and resistance to the AIDS virus. A careful viewing of ecological health factors in the gay community reveals a background of stressful, immune-weakening life-styles and practices. Many of the health-negating areas of the male homosexual life-style also exist among male heterosexuals, but these aspects tend to be magnified among gay men. For instance, one finds rampant abuse of alcohol and recreational drugs in urban gay communities. Alcoholism among homosexual men and women is about three times the national average, with between 20 and 30 percent of homosexual men considered alcoholic or at risk of turning alcoholic.[89] Excessive use of recreational drugs such as marijuana, amphetamines, cocaine, LSD, and barbiturates is also common to the life-style pattern of homosexual men.

In a study of 87 gay men with AIDS by Dr. Harry Haverkos and co-workers of the Centers for Infectious Diseases, the following levels of drug usage were recorded: nitrite inhalants (poppers), 97 percent; marijuana, 93 percent; amphetamines, 68 percent; cocaine, 66 percent; qualudes, 59 percent; ethyl chloride, 48 percent; barbiturates, 32 percent; heroin, 12 percent; and any drug used intravenously, 17 percent. These men had been diagnosed with AIDS in 1981 and early 1982. Multiple drug usage was the rule, with 58 percent of all subjects using five or more different street drugs on a regular basis. Furthermore, the amount and frequency of each drug used in this group was very high—at least high enough to pose a toxic burden on the body and greatly increase the likelihood of depressed immunity.[90]

Why is substance abuse so widespread among homosexual men? Most psychologists agree that alcoholism and drug abuse have their roots in poor self-image and the distress it brings into our lives. In this way, low self-esteem may be a precursor to many self-destructive tendencies associated with the development of AIDS and other major diseases. Gay men must often deal with the added burden of self-doubt and insecurity, both personal and professional, which stems from an oppressive up-bringing and a long-standing sense of alienation. To protect themselves emotionally from the unresolved pain of those growing-up years, they are compelled to hide in the closet. With the emergence of AIDS, male homosexuals feel even more compelled to hide out, to shield themselves from the complex array of pains and pressures confronting them daily. This "closet" mode of existence seems to encourage health-negating habits in daily life. Tom O'Connor, author of the superb book *Living with AIDS*, writes that ". . . shielding ourselves from pain [of social discrimination] brings a new kind of pain altogether: the pain of denial. It hurts to deny our self-worth and dignity as gay men and women; thus, some of us turn to alcohol, drugs, and even sex in order not to feel that pain."[91]

Wealth and material gain are often the means by which gay men choose to prove themselves as equals or "normal" in the modern business world. However, continually barraged by prejudice and discrimination, they must learn to distrust a society intolerant toward homosexuality. The will to succeed is itself a complex source of tension and insecurity. In time, the insecurity and underyling sense of rejection turn into anger, and the constantly thwarted desire for social acceptance becomes frustration. As there is often no way to constructively focus or channel these intense negative emotions—other than say, competent psychological counseling and support groups—the anger and resentment tend to turn back on oneself and produce self-destructive behaviors such as alcoholism and habitual drug use. This complicated pattern of low self-esteem and self-abasing behavior is actually common among all minority groups, not just homosexual men.

The one recreational drug which sets the gay male community apart from the heterosexual drug-using community is poppers, the amyl and butyl nitrite inhalants commonly used to heighten sexual enjoyment. These drugs are a liquid mixture of various chemicals, packaged in small bottles under such names as "Rush," "Thunderbolt," and "Crypt Tonight." Many studies have indicated that habitual use of poppers may increase the risk of developing Kaposi's sarcoma and depressed immunity.[92] Animal studies have shown a direct link between amylnitrite inhalation and severe depletion of the T-helper cells, and consequently, an inverted T-cell helper/suppressor ratio.[93] A 1985 case-control study of life-style characteristics of 31 homosexual AIDS patients found that nitrite inhalants were a significant risk factor for the development of AIDS, both for Kaposi's sarcoma and for opportunistic infections.[94] Other significant risk factors in this study were cigarette smoking, marijuana use, frequenting bathhouses, prior infection with syphilis, and fist-rectal sexual practices.

The homosexual practice of anal intercourse is now known to be a major mode of transmission. In anal intercourse, the semen carrying the virus is ejaculated into the rectum. Due to the high permeability of the colon's lining, the virus may pass through and enter the bloodstream. Any sexual act which might rub or abrade the thin tissue that lines the colorectal wall may enhance the likelihood of infection if the virus is present. A woman's vagina is much less prone to abrasion and absorption because of the tougher physical consistency and comparatively low permeability. Although transmission of the AIDS virus can occur from male to female through vaginal intercourse, the risk of this happening is clearly much lower than through anal intercourse.

One of the physiological functions of the spermatic fluid is to locally immunosuppress the female genital tract, thus insuring that the sperm is not rejected as a foreign protein. Studies have shown that repeated injections of a mouse with mouse spermatic fluid produces a generally immunosuppressed mouse.[95] Sperm is a concentrated protein containing numerous purines, which are components of our genetic material. These purines carry the ammonia (NH_3) radical and can be highly toxic when allowed to circulate freely in the bloodstream.

It is not surprising, then, that human semen itself, when internalized either by swallowing or anal intercourse and absorbed through the gut, may weaken and impair the human immune system.[96] This fact is further supported by Centers for Disease Control studies of anal-sperm recipients among twenty-six homosexual males, and in heterosexual females who routinely practice anal intercourse.[97] In addition to purines, another component in human semen, *prostaglandin E2*, seems to have a greater immunosuppressive effect on male than on female recipients of anal intercourse.[98]

As a group, male homosexuals also experience an unusually high incidence of repeated venereal diseases such as gonorrhea, syphilis, herpes, amebiasis and various other parasitic infections. These disorders often call for excessive use of strong prescription drugs such as antibiotics and antifungal medications. Collectively, these and the factors cited above may serve to seriously compromise immunity among homosexual men. If anal intercourse is performed frequently, and the various aspects of life-style mentioned are maintained, it could very likely make an individual more vulnerable to AIDS and other infectious diseases.

Broad, unqualified generalizations regarding the gay male's life-style are mostly inadequate, since this is not a well-defined homogeneous group. Every individual has a unique way of interacting with his social and biological environment. Some men eat more meat and fatty foods, while others eat more sugar and refined foods; however, the majority

consume a combination of animal products and highly refined foods—
the typical American way of eating.[99] In addition, the major psychosocial
stresses mentioned earlier may play a distinct role in weakening the
immune system.[100,101] Furthermore, some men exercise while others
exercise hardly at all. Those living in urban areas probably do not get
enough regular exercise. These basic aspects of life-style could contribute to the overall picture of susceptibility in gay men as well as the
population at large. The environmental conditions known to diminish
health—including chemically adulterated and refined foods, recreational
and pharmacologic drugs, and polluted air and water—provides the
"background of toxicity" which may promote weakened immunity and
vulnerability to AIDS.

Anal intercourse, the swallowing of sperm, and high incidence of STDs
are the three most easily identified common denominators among gay
men. Note that these are risk factors in a dual sense: they may increase
the risk of both transmission *and* susceptibility. Again, we emphasize
susceptibility because it is the most often overlooked factor and may
provide insight into effective prevention and relief for AIDS. Perhaps
one reason gay men have been so dramatically affected in the United
States is that these three distinctive risk factors amplify the toxic burden
already placed on the immune system by the health-negating life-style
patterns typical of most Americans.

The Risk to Infants and Children

One of the most tragic aspects of AIDS is its rising incidence among
infants and young children. According to the Federal Centers for Disease
Control, over 800 cases of pediatric AIDS were documented between
1983 and 1988, and two-thirds of these cases have died. The U.S. Public
Health Service counts over 2,000 children in the nation with AIDS-
related symptoms. By 1991, the number of afflicted Americans under 13
could climb as high as 20,000, and 1 in 10 children admitted to U.S.
hospitals may have AIDS.[102] The tragedy lies in the fact that these infants
have no control over the conditions by which they are exposed to the
AIDS virus and other factors contributing to AIDS; of course, these
conditions are entirely determined and regulated by the child's parents
before and after pregnancy.

In Western society, the majority of infants with AIDS are born to
women who are IV drug abusers. Prior to birth these fetuses are constantly exposed to the mothers' bloodstream, and the effects of these
drugs are passed on or "inherited." The developing fetus's whole body

is constantly exposed *in utero* (in the womb) to drugs taken by the mother. Tragically, many of the infants are stillborn; others are born as drug addicts, and, if not quickly diagnosed and treated, they die from abrupt drug withdrawal.

Studies reported in the July 30, 1988 *New York Times* found widespread abuse of drugs by pregnant American mothers. For example, at Boston City Hospital, the records of 1,600 women showed that 17 percent had used cocaine and 27 percent had smoked marijuana in pregnancy; at the University of California's Davis Hospital, 25 percent of 800 women showed urinary evidence of cocaine, amphetamines, or heroin use. It is now well established that all of these drugs can have untoward effects on the fetus, including many kinds of structural malformations, brain damage, and behavioral abnormalities.

The human infant's immune, digestive, and nervous systems are incompletely developed during the first two years of life, so it is particularly prone to infection during this time. Moreover, if the infant receives formula or cow's milk—both of which are highly stressful to underdeveloped immune systems—its immunity may become further compromised. In this case the infant fails to receive all the essential benefits of human milk in promoting the full development of its immune and other systems, and in providing passive protection through the IgA antibody, as those systems develop. The use of formula milk in bottle-feeding is known to promote IgA deficiency, and to upset the balance of harmful and beneficial intestinal flora; it has also been linked with a higher incidence of food allergy in young infants, which reflects, in part, the underdeveloped condition of the intestines in early human life.

Besides infants of IV drug abusing mothers, two other targets of infantile AIDS are: (1) babies of prostitutes who apparently received the virus from bisexual men or IV drug abusers,[103] and (2) babies of mothers who received blood transfusions from someone carrying the virus.[104] As to the first group, these infants would have been exposed to the same risk factors reviewed in the previous section's discussion of prostitutes. As to the second, mothers who were receiving blood transfusions may have transmitted the virus in utero to their infants, as well as via the milk during lactation. In addition, we may note that these mothers were in the category of "high-risk pregnancy," which implies the tendency toward complications of pregnancy and compromise of the developing fetus. Blood transfusions are also associated with complications at birth which can impair the infant's biological integrity and may render it more susceptible to immunological problems.[105]

In Miami, Florida, there has been an ever-increasing number of pediatric AIDS cases identified since 1980. A long-term, ongoing study has sought to define the natural history of AIDS in 92 Miami children representing 81 families.[106] The major findings are as follows:

- *Transmission mode*: All but three of the 92 cases have been perinatally transmitted; the three were associated with blood transfusions given to very young infants.
- *Parental status*: Fourteen of the mothers have AIDS, and ten have died; five of the fathers have AIDS, and three have died. Thus the majority of the mothers either have extremely mild symptomology or are totally without symptoms.
- *Racial distribution*: 92 percent of the cases are Black, four percent are Caucasion, and four percent are Hispanic.
- *Sex distribution*: 52 percent are female, 48 percent are male.
- *Mortality rate*: About 45 percent have died between 1980 and 1986. However, dividing this between those who have AIDS and those who have ARC, the ones with opportunistic infections related to AIDS have a very high mortality rate of 78.2 percent. Those with ARC show a low mortality rate of 10.8 percent.
- *Age at mortality*: About two-thirds of the children died before age two, so there is a very high mortality rate for the young infant. After this time, the prognosis looks considerably better.

One of the more encouraging aspects of this ongoing study is that there is a cohort of children with ARC who are long-term survivors—between five to six years since diagnosis, with the oldest child at this point being eight years old. (An April 3, 1988 *New York Times* article reports that teenagers seem more resistant to AIDS than either infants or adults.) However, failure to thrive is very common in this group and occurs in 65 percent; diarrhea is frequently found and there is an exceptionally high incidence of common recurrent bacterial infections such as *streptococcus pneumonia* and *hemophilus influenza*. Those children who show a definite failure to thrive frequently do not completely recover their ability to grow; by contrast, those presenting with protein-calorie malnutrition were all able to do good catch-up growth and actually had a very good prognosis compared with those children who had failure to thrive.

For the entire Miami group, both AIDS and ARC children, various clinical syndromes have been identified. The majority present with recurring infection (bacterial, yeast, and viruses); 41 percent with lymphoid interstitial pneumonia; 15 percent with *cardiomyopathy* (congestive heart failure and cardiomegaly, and hypertrophy of left ventricle); 10 percent with hepatitis (acute enlargement of the liver along with liver enzyme elevations, sometimes resulting in liver failure and death); 10 percent with encephalopathy; 8 percent with protein-calorie malnutrition; 7 percent with lymphadenopathy (presents very early in the first year of life, along with liver and spleen dysfunction); and a rising incidence of kidney disease such as proteinuria, renal tubular acidosis, and the nephrotic syndrome. This tends to be a later outcome and not an early finding in these children. Not all children manifest just a single syndrome, and all of the above percentages overlap to some degree. As one would expect, those children presenting with more than one syndrome tend to have a poorer prognosis.[107]

Most of the Miami children have shown very high levels of antibody specific for the AIDS virus. Two of the 92 children have maintained normal antibody levels, particularly IgG antibody throughout the course of the illness; four children were antibody-deficient (*hypogammaglobulinemic*). It will be interesting to see whether those children who are able to sustain high antibody levels will prove to be the longest survivors, and whether those fortunate individuals are eating and living in ways which strengthen the immune system.[109]

In developing countries, malnutrition and its consequences are the leading cause of death of children. The two main killers associated with malnutrition are respiratory diseases and gastrointestinal diseases involving bacterial, fungal, and parasitic infections. These childhood menaces owe their severity to immune systems severely compromised by lack of adequate nutrition. Young patients with malnutrition characteristically have a variety of different infections, including gastroenteritis, pneumonia, chronic hepatitis dermatitis, intestinal parasitism, tuberculosis, leprosy, and AIDS. The organisms implicated are multiple: E. coli, streptococcus, hepatitis B, candida albicans, measles virus, HIV, pneumocystis carinii, and others.

In the Zairian capital city of Kinshasa, malnutrition, gastrointestinal illness, pneumonia, and anemia are commonly seen in seropositive children, but are not peculiar to these individuals. It is likely that the poor overall health picture of millions of African children renders them more susceptible to AIDS and is at least partly responsible for the widespread incidence of AIDS. As stated earlier, the diagnosis of AIDS among children is difficult since many signs of malnutrition closely resemble AIDS, and other potentially AIDS-related conditions—pneumonia, lymphadenopathy, and tuberculosis—are frequently seen as well.

In both Africa and the United States, maternal infection is the single most important risk factor for HIV infection of infants and young children. But while a high rate of *perinatal transmission* (mother to infant during pregnancy) certainly exists in many areas, the efficiency of perinatal transmission is unknown. Among hospitalized children in Kinshasa, 80 percent of children born to seropositive mothers were also positive, while 20 percent were seronegative.[110] Another African study found 69 percent of children born to seropositive mothers were seropositive.[111] Based on several epidemiological studies, researchers at the Albert Einstein College of Medicine estimate that up to 65 percent of HIV-infected women may transmit the disease in utero to their infants.[112]

What prevented the other infants (at least 35 percent of those born from seropositive mothers) from becoming infected by their carrier mothers? These interesting observations have been replicated by other researchers in Africa and the United States. Perhaps the efficiency of perinatal transmission is simply lower than other modes of transmission, or that some unidentified risk factors are associated with perinatal infection. It may also indicate that the immunologic profile of mothers is important: that some percentage of the mothers have developed immunity to HIV and therefore did not expose their infants in utero to the virus.

There are many ways by which an infant's immunity is either supported or compromised, and unnecessary impairment of the infant's immune system may be more common than is presently realized. As noted in chapter one, congenital malformations have increased by a multiple of four since the 1950s.[113] The rising incidence of both birth defects and spontaneous abortions has ushered in an entirely new specialty called *neonatology*. This trend in miscarriages implies a diminished ability of young women to carry their pregnancies to term. Such trends may be associated with increased use of cigarettes, marijuana, antibiotics, over-the-counter drugs, alcohol and so on, as well as the consumption of heavily refined and fatty food items. Many of these substances are known to have toxic effects on the developing fetus. Chemicals ingested by the mother, either via diet or medications, may enter the mother's milk and are passed on to the infant. Most pediatric cases in America involve mothers (or fathers, or both) who have been drug abusers.[114] Perhaps more children would be surviving this dreaded viral infection if mothers took better care of themselves.

The Risk to Hospitalized Patients ─────────────

There are some remedies worse than the disease.

Pubilius Syrus, First Century, B.C.

Increased susceptibility to AIDS could also be related to the effects of common medical treatments. *Iatrogenesis*, from the Greek *iatros* (doctor) literally means "doctor-induced," and refers to any illness or injury that is the direct result of medical intervention. Iatrogenic causes of AIDS involve medical procedures which inadvertently harm the immune system and may contribute to the subsequent development of disease. Both prescription and non-prescription drugs may be regarded as possible co-factors in various immune-related conditions such as AIDS, cancer, candidiasis, and hepatitis B. Powerful anticancer therapies such as surgery, chemotherapy, and radiotherapy may place people at greater risk for various cancers later in life.[115] Some scientists suggest that Rock Hudson's major heart surgery (coronary bypass) in 1981 helped trigger the replication of the AIDS virus, leading to the full-blown syndrome.[116] Common sense dictates that people requiring such medical procedures are usually in poor health to begin with. This is certainly true of organ-transplant recipients, whose most common cause of death is infectious disease.

Since the fifties we have evolved into a pill-popping society, with a dangerous overdependency upon prescription and non-prescription drugs. Based on a 1987 report issued by the National Center for Health Statistics, more than 23.6 million prescriptions were written by doctors in the United States between March 1985 and February 1986: and drugs were prescribed or provided at three of every five visits to the doctor's office. Topping the list of drugs most often prescribed by doctors was *hydrochlorothiazide*, the generic name for a drug that helps the body get rid of excess fluid and hence reduce blood pressure. Unfortunately this diuretic also carries a number of undesirable side effects, including lowered potassium, abnormal heart-beat rhythms, and even an increased risk of heart attack. Several studies of hunter-gatherer populations indicate a curious association between low blood pressure (*hypotension*) and chronic infectious diseases.[117] Is it possible that a blood-pressure-lowering drug somehow increases one's susceptibility to infectious disease? As an aside, it is of interest that deficiency of potassium—a mineral now considered important to blood-pressure control—is commonly seen in people with AIDS.[118]

The body has natural protective mechanisms to remove foreign and potentially toxic substances such as drugs before they can enter the general circulation. This aspect of our so-called natural immunity is largely fulfilled by the kidneys and liver. The kidneys are the most important excretory organs for eliminating drugs and their metabolic by-products (metabolites) from the body. If the kidneys should become compromised, the use of drugs and medications could pose a toxic load on the body which would weaken the immune system. Lack of kidney function could result over the long term from excessive protein intake (meat, eggs, and dairy) or excessive drug intake, or both.

As the body's metabolic mastermind, the liver's primary function is to process nutrients and remove all toxic substances (e.g., drugs, pesticides, and food additives) absorbed through the intestines. Even commonly used and presumably safe drugs such as aspirin must be administered in a dose large enough to get past the liver. In addition to poor nutrition, such as a fatty and refined diet, repeated ingestion of any synthetic chemical—illicit or otherwise—would tend to have an adverse effect on this vital organ.[119] This in turn could lead to a buildup of toxins in the blood and eventual weakening of the immune system.[120]

Many forms of medical therapy may inadvertently weaken the immune system, thereby rendering people more susceptible to infection by the AIDS virus. Anyone with some degree of compromised immunity, from whatever cause, would be more vulnerable to all variety of potential disease-triggering influences, including opportunistic microbes and cancer cells. Let us now consider some of the iatrogenic factors relevant to increased risk for contracting AIDS:

• **Antimicrobial Drug Treatments.** Antibiotics have long been among the most frequently prescribed drugs, with amoxicillin, erythromycin, and penicillin topping the list.[121] Most people with a background of recurrent sexually transmitted diseases are likely to have taken large amounts of antibiotics—in many instances, millions of units of penicillin may have been taken by a homosexual man over a ten-year period. While penicillin itself is not highly toxic, many of its side effects have a negative feedback effect on immune responsiveness. Penicillin destroys a large proportion of intestinal flora—the *gram-positive* bacteria—which normally live in a balanced antagonism with the *gram-negative* bacteria. The latter are then capable of spreading and overwhelming the immune system, despite all further administration of antibiotics. People who have taken heavy and repeated doses of antibiotics may constitute an easy source for the AIDS virus because their immune systems have been markedly compromised.

A considerable body of medical research documents the adverse effects that commonly used antibiotics have on different measures of the immune response.[122] For example, *tetracycline*, the drug often used in treating gonorrheal and chlamydial infections, may upset at least four major components of immune responsiveness. The overuse of antibiotics can also cause serious imbalances in "friendly" bacteria and other organisms inhabiting the body. When the beneficial bacteria are killed off by antibiotics, certain disease-causing fungi, viruses, and bacteria are allowed to multiply and promote illness.[123]

According to Robert Tauxe, M.D., of the Enteric Disease Branch of the Centers for Disease Control, the recent outbreaks of salmonella may be attributed to overuse of antibiotics for medical purposes (e.g., ampicillin given for ear and throat infections) as well as antibiotics ingested indirectly through the typical American diet. It is worth noting that penicillin and tetracycline are routinely placed in poultry and cattle feeds to promote greater milk production by dairy cows and faster growth of meat-producing animals.[124] When these animal products are consumed regularly, the continual infiltration of antibiotic substances into the human body lays the groundwork for antibiotic-resistant bacteria and imbalances of the microbial flora.

In a 1983 study reported in the *New England Journal of Medicine*, a group of ten Haitian AIDS patients claimed to be heterosexuals and to have not taken any drugs.[125] Upon entering the clinic, six of the ten patients presented with tuberculosis. In all six, opportunistic infections developed weeks to months after initiation of therapy with the anti-tuberculin drugs, *isoniazide* and *rampathin*. Here again we have a group of people with a profile of poor nutrition, stressful life-style (poverty), and a history of recurrent infectious diseases. When these people were given immunosuppressive drugs, they subsequently developed the typical opportunistic infections of AIDS.

The pattern observed in these patients suggests that their immunity was already substantially weakened prior to administration of the anti-tuberculin drugs. The immune system was then further compromised and suppressed by the drugs, rendering these people highly susceptible to all variety of opportunistic infections. Besides drug-induced toxicity, another mechanism by which these drugs would cause compromised immunity is by upsetting nutritional balances. Of the twelve known compounds used as antituberculosis drugs, six have been shown to cause nutritional deficiencies—notably vitamin D and several of the B-vitamins—which could in turn feed the immune-depressed condition.[126]

Antiviral drugs also take their toll on the body's overall immunity.

Most of these drugs are directed toward interfering with genetic mechanisms, such as the enzyme involved in transcribing the AIDS virus's genetic material onto the host cell's. Since the genetic components are highly sensitive to such interference, these drugs tend to destroy or limit the functioning of the cells themselves. Twenty-five percent of all participants in the first trials for *AZT*, or *Retrovir*, developed red-blood-cell deficiency (anemia) and required blood transfusions. And yet AZT is deemed to be the least toxic of all antiviral drugs; the rest have all produced serious side effects and depletion of certain immune components. Since a vaccine for AIDS is not likely in the near future, antiviral drug use will probably continue as a major mode of therapy for AIDS and ARC. Such treatment could intensify the condition of anyone suffering from an immunodeficiency-related disease.

● **Tonsillectomies.** Removal of the tonsils no longer enjoys the kind of widespread popularity it had in the past, and many doctors are beginning to question the practice. In the first place, there are no clear guidelines to determine when tonsillectomies are justified. Some doctors perform them on children who have occasional sore throats, while others virtually refuse to do them. Some contend that a child with an history of severe, recurring sore throat stands a better chance of being free of difficulty if he has his tonsils removed than if he does not. But there is also good reason to believe that many children will get better even if they do not have the common but controversial operation. Among the children who do not have their tonsils out, there will be a substantial percentage who get better on their own and do not continue to have episodes of infection.

Tonsillectomy has been hypothesized as one of the factors that may predispose people to developing AIDS after exposure to HIV. It is notable that the age group with the highest prevalence of AIDS in the United States is 30 to 39 and consists of individuals who grew up in a medical era when tonsillectomy was a common surgical procedure in childhood. In a small pilot study by Steven McCombie, M.D., eight out of ten AIDS patients reported having had a tonsillectomy in childhood; all were males, nine had an initial diagnosis of pneumocystis carinii pneumonia and one had Kaposi's sarcoma. Since the tonsils and adenoids are important parts of the immune system, surgical removal of these lymph glands in childhood may increase the risk of developing opportunistic infections in later life. Along these lines, one researcher has remarked:

The possibility of an observed relationship between AIDS and tonsillectomies is due to the fact that individuals who have undergone chronic infections that reflect an underlying immunological abnormality that puts them at increased risk for AIDS . . . . A better understanding of the intricate relationship of the immune system to the development of viral malignancies may result from the study of the effect of lymphoid tissue removal on susceptibility to leukemia, lymphoma, and AIDS. (McCombie, S., 1986, "Tonsillectomy as a co-factor in the development of AIDS," Medical Hypotheses 19: 291)

Generally speaking, unless the individual has chronic breathing difficulty because his throat is often obstructed by swollen tonsils, tonsillectomy is ill-advised. The tonsil's are one of our body's natural immune components and provide added protection against disease, including a supportive role for the body's secretory IgA system. There is also some evidence that tonsillectomy may even serve as a prognostic indicator for Hodgkin's disease, although the data are conflicting.

Why should we part with something vital to our health? Instead, we should learn to take care of our tonsils by eating well (avoiding highly antigenic foods such as dairy products and foods containing additives), exercising regularly, and generally living in a more healthy way to support the functioning of our lymphatic system. If a problem with the tonsils arises, it would be far better to ride out the storm than to simply cut them out. The latter way is both primitive and foolhardy.

● **Blood Transfusion Recipients.** For the general public, the most feared source of AIDS is the blood and blood products transfused for surgery, hemophilia, and other reasons. This fear is out of proportion to the actual incidence of transfusion-related HIV infection: the risk of developing AIDS is about one in a million transfusions, while the risk of dying from a transfusion reaction is one in six hundred thousand.[127] Moreover, as HIV- screening methods improve, these risks will diminish further. During the window period between 1978 and 1985 when no testing of blood-bank donors for HIV was done, approximately 10,000 people may have been exposed to the AIDS virus through blood transfusions. This number could be a very conservative estimate, however, as no one is certain how long HIV has been in the U.S. population.

One of the more positive aspects of AIDS will be increased attention to the relative efficacy of blood transfusions with an evaluation of their overuse and misuse.[128] People requiring blood transfusions are frequently in poor health to begin with, as their own medical records usually reveal. This suggests that blood-transfusion recipients as a group might be generally more susceptible to infectious disease. But there is another dimension to the problem: blood transfusions themselves carry a substantial risk of long-range ill effects. Much of the blood in our nation's blood supply comes from donors in the lower income brackets of society, many of whom may be suspected of carrying microbial infections. Only AIDS, syphilis, and hepatitis B are screened out of the current blood supply, so there are probably other infectious organisms unaccounted for. Further, the quality of blood supply may be affected by the nutritional status of the donors, and low-income Americans are usually subsisting on nutritionally deficient, additive-rich diets.

The immunosuppressive effects of blood transfusions themselves provides another piece to the multifactorial pie. These effects are recognized as beneficial against organ-transplant rejection and reduce the need for immunosuppressive drugs during transplant surgery. But the fact is that suppressed immunity, usually transient, is part of the price of receiving blood products. Until Raymond Keith Brown, M.D., spoke up in his landmark work, *AIDS, Cancer and the Medical Establishment*, very few people—doctors included—were aware of the immunologic side effects of blood transfusions. Medical students are not taught such facts during their training, when it is assumed that the only potential danger of transfusions is contamination with unknown microbial components.

Adverse changes in immune responsiveness have been observed even after a single blood transfusion; previously such changes were only seen in patients undergoing multiple transfusions for hemophilia or uremia.[129] In this study of two groups of patients undergoing surgery for heart disease, a significantly reduced ability to generate T-cell colonies and produce lymphokines and antibodies was noted 10 and then 60 days following the operation. Still unknown is the reason for the shortened lifespan of cancer patients who receive blood transfusions after surgery compared to those who do not receive transfusions.[130] Dr. Brown suggests that these conditions may relate to *pleomorphic* organisms (cell-wall deficient), present but undetected in the transfused blood.[131]

A 1985 study in the *British Medical Journal* found an elevated recurrence rate of colon cancer when blood transfusion has been given at operation.[132] Of 197 patients with surgically curable colon cancer, tumors recurred in 6 of 69 patients who had not been given transfusion, compared with 56 of 129 who had. The researchers also found a significant association between transfusions and the time to recurrence of cancer.[133]

In March 1986, Dr. Roger Foster reported in *Cancer* that the five-year survival rate was 33 percent worse for cancer patients receiving blood transfusion compared to those who did not receive blood. One hypothesis to explain the apparent post-transfusion condition of suppressed immunity is that certain blood products, particularly those more highly processed and susceptible to temperature changes, or those stored improperly, might liberate iron and hemoglobin upon transfusion. A high level of free iron in the blood is toxic to the liver and immune system, and fosters the growth of many microorganisms and cancer cells.[134]

Anyone requiring frequent blood transfusions—while undergoing heart-bypass surgery, for instance, or during the course of treating other serious conditions—is going to be immunosuppressed for a period of time, possibly several months or longer. Successive blood transfusions are accompanied by progressive deterioration of immune-system functions. Based on these and other studies, it has been proposed that the blood transfusions may alter the response of T-cells to the AIDS virus, thereby rendering one more susceptible to AIDS. Blood and blood products may not only transmit HIV, but may also suppress the transfusion-recipient's immune response to the virus.

● **Organ and Bone-marrow Transplant Recipients.** In recent years, with the development of artificial organs and more sophisticated surgical technologies, much attention has turned to the role of the immune system in determining the survival of the transplant recipient. The primary obstacle to using artificial body parts or performing a transplant of any kind is that the immune system rejects them as foreign. Indeed, the success of transplantation has always depended heavily on the use of powerful immunosuppressive drugs that prevent rejection by inducing a generalized suppression of the recipient's immune system. The consequence, of course, is increased susceptibility to infection by viruses, bacteria, and other microbes.

Since the T-helper cells and cytotoxic T-cells are the key cells involved in tissue-graft rejections, the drugs must be able to suppress these cell types above all others.[135] Recall that the T-helper cell regulates all aspects of specific immunity, and both cell types play major roles in protecting against viral infections. Not suprisingly then, transplant-related suppression enables the growth or reactivation of viral infections (especially cytomegalovirus) within the transplant patient.[136] It is likely that the aforementioned effects of blood and blood products used during surgery may also contribute to the compromised immune condition.

One study of bone-marrow recipients supports the multifactorial theory of AIDS.[137] Seventeen people were receiving bone marrow transplants from compatible donors (relatives) for various cancers involving the hematological, or blood-making, system. All of the 17 patients demonstrated the same clinical picture of reduced immune functions seen in AIDS. They had abnormal antibody production and an abnormal ratio of certain immune cells, the T lymphocytes. Overall T-cell functioning and immune responsiveness was depressed. The clinical picture involved across-the-board susceptibility to the same opportunistic infections seen in AIDS. Notably, only 1 of the 17 demonstrated the presence of HIV, as well as antibodies specific for the virus. This person had received a blood transfusion in which the AIDS virus was present. For the other 16 patients, however, the symptoms were clinically identical with AIDS—all had the same opportunistic diseases commonly seen in people with AIDS, but none showed any evidence of the HIV virus.

These observations may provide a unique perspective on the profile of a person with AIDS. Each individual in this group had been medically immunodepressed to prevent rejection of their bone transplants. Each manifested symptoms in every way as any AIDS patient would, and yet this "syndrome" could not be attributed to the virus, only to the process of immunodepression. In other groups of the high-risk category, the same array of symptoms would have been attributed to the AIDS virus, but here no such explanation is possible. All that is clear in this case is a condition of depressed immunity which enabled the development of opportunistic infections seen in AIDS. Other studies suggest that the bone-marrow transplant itself has a suppressive effect on immunity if recognized as foreign to the body. By contrast, so-called *autologous* bone marrow, derived from the recipient's own supply, appears to be less harmful, although the question of long-term disease-free survival is still unanswered.[138]

In sum, iatrogenesis may play an important but hitherto unrecognized role in the spread of AIDS. Americans may be taking too many harmful medications and undergoing too many unnecessary surgeries, or unwittingly placing themselves in situations in which harmful conventional therapies become necessary (e.g., bypass surgery for acute heart disease). There is a common tendency among modern people to look for instant answers to complex problems. Most of these individuals are unwilling to assume personal responsibility for their health, and most receive their education about health from television advertisements and pop magazines. More than a hundred psychotropic drugs—sedatives, antidepressants, tranquilizers—are freely prescribed and sanctioned by American physicians, suggesting that the "normal" way is to let external forces take care of our mental and emotional life. The reality of iatrogenic disease should prompt us to reevaluate our conventional quick-fix approach. Failing to anticipate some of the longer-term repercussions of certain allopathic therapies may cost us our lives.

The Risk to Heterosexuals

Toward the end of 1985, experts studying the distribution of AIDS cases were surprised by a shift in the general pattern of new cases reported. Whereas AIDS had spread most rapidly among the homosexual population between 1979 and 1984, by the end of 1985 the largest number of new cases was seen among heterosexuals. Today there are at least 250,000 infected heterosexuals in this country, 90 percent of whom may be unaware of their own infection.[139] The proportion of infected heterosexuals is increasing steadily and will probably continue to do so, according to the Surgeon General's 1987 report and an article of January 1986, appearing in the *Annals of Internal Medicine.*

At least part of the decrease seen among homosexuals was due to dramatic changes in sexual and life-style practices, as advised by the Gay Men's Health Crisis and other educational groups working with the gay community. Primarily, however, the slower spread of AIDS among heterosexuals has occurred for these reasons: (1) the initial infiltration of the gay community simply took time to reach the heterosexual community (probably through bisexual contacts and shared needles among homo- and heterosexuals); (2) the greater susceptibility of most urban homosexual men to infections of all kinds, suggesting some degree of compromised immunity prior to infection by the AIDS virus; and (3) the AIDS virus is spread less efficiently through heterosexual modes of transmission, including IV drug use and low-risk sexual activity such as vaginal intercourse. In the United States today over 250,000 heterosexuals are thought to be infected by the AIDS virus.

Authorities at the Centers for Disease Control (CDC) predict that the gay proportion of the AIDS population will decline as the disease continues to increase among heterosexuals.[140] According to the CDC, 17 percent of all AIDS cases are heterosexual IV drug abusers who transmit the virus primarily by sharing contaminated needles. About 2 percent of AIDS suffers are heterosexuals who received blood transfusions carrying HIV before clinics began screening the nation's blood supply in mid-1985. Women infected by bisexual men make up 1 percent and 1 percent are children exposed before birth by IV substance-using mothers. An additional 4 to 6 percent do not fit any identified risk group—gay men, drug users, hemophiliacs, blood-transfusion recipients and female sexual contacts of bisexual men.

These trends need to be placed in perspective, however. According to the U.S. Department of Health and Human Services, only 1 percent of all AIDS cases have occurred among heterosexuals. These individuals are primarily either prostitutes or IV drug abusers. Of the 2,665 reported heterosexual AIDS patients with known risk factors in the United States, only 647 (24 percent) are women.[141] Most of the transmission has been male-to-female, although a few female-to-male cases have also been reported.

Intravenous drug users are currently the heterosexual population at highest risk for AIDS in the United States, comprising about one-quarter of all reported cases. In Africa, however, the picture is somewhat different, as revealed in a study of clusters of Kaposi's-sarcoma cases in Zaire.[142] In 23 heterosexual Zairians treated for KS, 9 were female and all claimed to have never used IV drugs. All showed the typical AIDS symptoms: severely depressed immune systems, weight loss, chronic fever, diarrhea, and extreme vulnerability to opportunistic infections. Researchers suspect that many of these cases are prostitutes or their partners, or are people with a background of malnutrition and chronic parasitic infections.

Sexual promiscuity clearly increases the probability of transmitting the AIDS virus among heterosexuals. Multiple sexual partners raises the frequency of exposure to the virus and thereby increases the probability of successful infection. A study of heterosexual promiscuity among Africans with AIDS seems to support this idea.[143] The researchers collected information on the sexual habits of 58 African men with AIDS or the AIDS-related complex (ARC); 33 were diagnosed in Kigali, Rwanda, and 25 in Brussels, Belgium. Compared with healthy controls, the patients had a significantly higher number of different heterosexual partners per year and also had more frequent contact with prostitutes. Of 42 African women in whom AIDS or ARC had been diagnosed, 10 (24 percent) were prostitutes, but none of these women reported previous use of IV drugs. Studies of Haitian men with AIDS in Miami and New York City have also shown a significant association of AIDS with a history of prostitute contacts.[144]

The picture of AIDS in African towns and cities may provide a model for the potential spread of AIDS among heterosexuals in affluent countries. Since sexual intercourse is a major mode of transmission for the AIDS virus, AIDS may eventually spread like other sexually transmitted diseases (gonorrhea, chlamydia, syphilis, and genital herpes). It appears that STDs affect different segments of the population in a successive way, hitting certain groups before other groups. Genital herpes, transmitted only through intimate sexual contact, was largely peculiar to the gay community throughout the sixties and seventies. Now it is found widely among young sexually active heterosexuals, particularly college students. Millions of STD cases are reported annually, which means that every few seconds an American is involved in a high-risk sexual practice minus a condom.[145]

Prostitution and brothel operations today reflect a new social phenomenon: young professionals who do not want to take time away from their budding careers to cultivate serious relationships—marriage or family life—and who seek to release sexual tension during the week. Many of the same young men who patronize urban prostitutes are those who frequent singles bars on other nights.[146] Surprisingly, although this situation provides an obvious hotbed for spreading AIDS, the business of prostitution has gone unscathed in most cities across the nation.

While repeated sexual contacts carry with them a risk of contracting the disease among heterosexuals, it may not determine *susceptibility* to AIDS. On the other hand, sexually transmitted diseases and subsequent exposure to medications for these conditions may increase susceptibility. Like many native Africans, American homosexual men have a greater tendency to develop tuberculosis and parasitic infections than their heterosexual counterparts, and such infections depress immunity, which may increase susceptibility to infection by the AIDS virus. In fact, a history of STDs is now generally considered to place people at higher risk for contracting AIDS.

One of the curious by-products of conventional thinking about AIDS is the notion that "risk" pertains primarily to the efficiency or effectiveness of transmission. People involved in activities that are known to readily transmit the virus are considered to be in the *high-risk category*, while those not involved in these activities are deemed to be at no risk. (For some reason, *low-risk* is rarely mentioned.) This viewpoint is problematic because risk is considered only in the relatively superficial terms of transmission. The reality of AIDS, however, as with any infectious disease, is that people are at varying degrees of risk which correspond to varying degrees of immunologic susceptibility to the AIDS virus and other pathogens implicated in the syndrome.

Since the conventional definition of "risk" precludes the role of diminished resistance or compromised immunity, it was inevitable that a separate group of heterosexual people "at risk" would be identified as part of the epidemiological picture. All AIDS cases who do not belong to any identified risk group—gay or bisexual men, IV drug users, hemophiliacs, blood-transfusion recipients and female sexual contacts of bisexual men or IV drug users—are considered to be in the *no-identified-risk* (NIR) category. By this classification, the vast majority of AIDS cases in Africa, Haiti, and other Caribbean countries would be labeled as NIR. However, the ecological profile of susceptibility outlined in previous sections clearly undermines any broad-sweeping classification of NIR among infected people in these Third World countries. For example, recall that protein deprivation, which is widely prevalent in Africa and Haiti, renders the immune system especially prone to opportunistic infections such as those seen in AIDS. This example clearly indicates the link between protein deficiency and susceptibility to AIDS, yet very few researchers have turned their attention to nutritional causes. This type of risk is more subtle and goes beyond transmission.

According to the Federal Centers for Disease Control, at least 8 percent of all AIDS cases in the United States may be classified as NIR.[147] While the incidence of NIR seems relatively small, the rate may be increasing due to transmissibility factors in heterosexual contact and to variations in individual susceptibility. The manifestation of disease may be delayed because the typical forms of heterosexual contact would transmit a smaller quantity of virus, thereby possibly prolonging the incubation period. Alternatively, this group may have a higher threshold of immunologic resistance toward Human Immunodeficiency Virus, bacteria, fungi, and other microbes involved in the development of AIDS.

Compared to infected people in the known high-risk groups, individuals in the NIR category may be less susceptible to AIDS due to differences in life-style or ecologic factors. For example they do not engage in immunosuppressive activities such as anal intercourse or the habitual use of strong drugs and medications. Instead, a number of other factors, currently unrecognized by medical science, may increase the susceptibility toward AIDS. The factors which may predispose these individuals are poor dietary practices, lack of exercise, heavy emotional stress, and excessive reliance on drugs, medications, vitamin pills, or other substances which may cause metabolic or nutritional imbalances. Accordingly, the NIR category would include the majority of people living in the United States and other postindustrialized countries.

Some scientists prefer to call this group the *no-risk* group, which implies that there are no other risk factors besides those already recognized, including the AIDS virus itself. According to the multifactorial model, however, there is a strong likelihood of many unidentified risk factors existing, some of which promote susceptibility to AIDS and are unrelated to transmission per se. Thus it is more appropriate to retain the classification of no identified risk (NIR), as agreed upon by scientists at the 1986 International Conference on AIDS.[148] Reasons for the existence and classification of a subset of AIDS patients as no identified risk may be listed as follows:

(1) There may be some unrecognized risk factors, operating in a more subtle (collective, synergistic and gradual) way to predispose one to AIDS. This of course could include dietary factors, synthetic chemicals (medications, antibiotics, food additives, etc.), and psychosocial stresses.

(2) There is not enough information available on the patient due to mental degeneration, early mortality, or inadequate medical record-keeping.

(3) The recognized risk factor may be present but denied by the patient; this is a common assumption of researchers toward Haitians and "closet" homosexuals. However, such assumptions often turn out to be unfounded.

(4) The patient does not have AIDS, but a similar condition. Some examples include primary immunodeficiency disease (genetic), atomic radiation sickness, or the side effects of heavy chemotherapy or radiotherapy for cancer treatment.

(5) The individual received the AIDS virus through heterosexual intercourse. Of course, this only explains the mode of transmission, not why one person would be more or less susceptible than another.

(6) There may be some unrecognized modes of transmission. (Note: this seems highly unlikely; the AIDS virus can *only* be transmitted through bodily fluids and is extremely fragile to temperature changes.)

While the precentage of AIDS patients categorized as NIR is small compared to the percentage of known risk groups, it is nonetheless real and worth pondering. It indicates that there are some unrecognized risks promoting either susceptibility or transmissibility or both. Some of these hidden or unknown risks may actually be overlapping or supporting the more established risk factors. Could NIR involve something so basic as our daily diet? Time will tell.

AIDS and Scientific Revolution ───────────

The historical development of modern microbiology, from the late 1800s to the present, seems to be nearing a major turning point. Louis Pasteur, the founding father of microbial chemistry, introduced the idea that microbes cause disease. His germ theory led to the widespread use of antibiotics and other forms of antimicrobial medication to treat infectious disorders. Claude Bernard, a pioneering theorist of homeostasis and Pasteur's primary intellectual protagonist, argued vehemently that microbes could only exert their effects if the conditions of the body were sufficiently altered. He saw the body as the ground or "terrain" in which various seeds (germs) were periodically scattered. Depending on the soil conditions of this terrain, certain seeds would germinate and thrive, while others would remain dormant and eventually disappear.

Pasteur's view is the basis for the single-agent theory of AIDS, while Bernard's view is the basis for the multifactorial theory. The first perceives the AIDS virus as an absolute threat to human survival, while the latter regards the virus as a danger relative to the internal condition or immunologic integrity of the body. Incredibly, Louis Pasteur's last dying words showed a radical shift in his outlook: "Bernard was right: the germ is nothing, the terrain is all." Unfortunately, Pasteur's profound intuitive turnaround has since gone unheeded, and the conceptual schism between virology, immunology, and nutrition remains to this day. The threat of AIDS may help us create some fundamental bridges between these fields. At the same time, a new view of health and disease may emerge, one which integrates both Pasteur's and Bernard's insights.

Everyone knows that AIDS can be transmitted from infected individuals through blood and blood products, as well as by intimate contact with bodily secretions. Unfortunately, people have continually ignored the distinction between *transmissibility* (how HIV is spread) and *susceptibility* (why it continues to spread and afflicts certain people more than others). Indeed, since HIV is the presumed cause of AIDS, the basis for susceptibility has been entirely confined to modes of transmission. This lopsided perspective has promoted widespread paranoia and prejudice toward minority groups, and has led to the spending of billions of dollars on research and treatment with little if any progress in eradicating AIDS. The transmission-oriented view overlooks the strong possibility that weakened immunity may predispose people to successful infection by the AIDS virus.

The importance of emphasizing the multifactorial development of AIDS is clarified by recalling that this retrovirus is one of the most primitive parts of our genetic structure, coming from within the human body in an originally benign form. Indeed, in light of this possibility and the apparent ease with which viral mutations can take place, it would seem that our internal milieu could serve critically in nature's decision of whether or not to render the virus pathogenic. This "decision" would hinge on two general kinds of influence: (1) changes in the biochemical milieu which evoke a genetic mutation and hence render the virus pathogenic, and (2) changes in the biochemical milieu which weaken immunity and render the body susceptible to the now pathological capacities of the virus.

Currently, we may well be witnessing the long-term effects of some forty years of technological "progress' now concentrated in this group of individuals who may have reached an unknown yet critical dose level that gives HIV its deadly virulence. Needless to say, the multifactorial approach merits more comprehensive exploration.

Immune deficiency does not mean AIDS unless its becomes persistent and progressive. According to modern medicine, there are many causes of immune suppression, including chemotherapy for cancer, intentional immune suppression in organ-transplant patients, and recurrent microbial infections of any kind. Medical science has yet to acknowledge that dietary practice, psychosocial stress, and other factors related to the ecological milieu of daily life, may gradually and collectively wreak havoc on the immune system. These factors should be given highest priority in medical research, and yet they are continually neglected due to the alluring monetary rewards offered to AIDS researchers by the pharmaceutical industry. It is a sad state of affairs, especially since the average layperson waits for science to determine what is true and what steps should be taken.

As we have seen, the biological ramifications of declining immune competence may shed light on the various patterns of disease emerging in different segments of the population in recent years and raise concerns for the future. In particular, we are witnessing an evolving profile for the heterosexual population which bears many similarities to that of the gay population: the trends in disease typically experienced by gay men are now being seen in young heterosexuals. The protocols for treatment of these disorders (steroids, antibiotics, etc.) have likewise paired off. In short, there is ample reason to be concerned about compromising the immune system in the heterosexual population as it has been compromised in the gay population.

Several decades of observations in clinical medicine have brought about an awareness of rising trends in diseases among the young adult population concomitant to dramatic changes in medical technology and affluent life-styles. Children are now being exposed to antigen-loads of unprecedented proportions, particularly cow's-milk protein and food additives. In addition, we see rising incidences of tonsillitis, ear infection, bronchitis, acne and the flu, with accompanying excessive use of antibiotics and other kinds of medication. The current epidemic among our adolescent and young-adult population of herpes and other sexually transmitted diseases, and the attendant overuse of antibotics, some of which are extremely toxic (e.g., *Flagyl*), evokes concern over the similarities between the high-risk group profiles and the young-adult heterosexual populations.

In the sixties the administration of antibiotics to infants only weeks old was considered a very serious matter and was more or less a rare situation. Today it is not uncommon for newborns to be diagnosed with infectious conditions at birth, and it is considered standard medical practice to administer antibiotics for infections at birth, as well as to infants only a few weeks of age. An added concern is the lack of healthy mother's milk and widespread reliance on immunologically bankrupt formula milk. These profound parental responsibilities can no longer be taken for granted.

The cumulative effects of antibiotics, medications, formula milk, tonsillectomies, and food and chemical antigens, have undoubtedly taken their toll on our immunological resistance. Many of these chemicals are toxic in varying degrees, and chronic exposure over a period of time would tend to weaken the host organism's immunocompetence, rendering it increasingly vulnerable to subsequent infection and disease. Repeated cycles of challenge-and-response over time may ultimately result in a progressively diminished ability to cope with the non-self, or external environment, appropriately. It is time we all assess this overall picture and the consequences to ourselves and our species. Disease cannot be prevented unless the long-term toxic effects of the environment are understood.

The science of nutrition is still floundering amidst a vast ocean of skepticism and uncertainty. Allopathic physicians are more inclined to advocate pain-relief tablets than whole, natural foods, and it is unlikely that medical science will support nutritional therapies and nutritional research until AIDS exhausts all research efforts toward an effective drug-oriented approach. Nutritional and other unconventional therapies have received little if any financial support from government or other funding sources. As long as research is biased along the lines of the single-agent hypothesis—that HIV is the sole cause for concern—a genuine cure for this syndrome may remain nothing more than a grand fantasy.

Only recently have we heard several statements by major scientific organizations that, after so many years and millions of dollars of research, we are still losing the battle against cancer. And only recently have the American Cancer Society and the National Cancer Institute acknowledged evidence demonstrating the associations and correlations between dietary factors and various cancers. (For example, lung cancer is now associated with low intakes of zinc, fiber, B-vitamins and the vitamin A precursor called beta-carotene, all ideally supplied by a combination of whole cereal grains and various leafy green vegetables.[149,150,151] There is also a slow but growing acceptance of the role of psychological influences on immune competence and the genesis of disease. These recent developments have set a compelling precedent for a more comprehensive, ecological view of the problem of AIDS.

Most scientists, however, are hard put to relinquish their specialized interests and former ties to mechanistic theories (AIDS virus causes AIDS) in order to avail themselves of the multifactorial view. Hence, proponents of the single-agent theory of AIDS will most likely condemn this book for its "unscientific assertions," "overly empirical focus," "ill-substantiated conclusions," and the like. This is to be expected. The conceptual intolerance underlying such criticism has always been part of civilization's intellectual evolution, as Thomas Kuhn relates in his landmark book, *The Structure of Scientific Revolutions*. According to Kuhn, new theories are usually espoused only after temporary periods of rigid unacceptance which eventually result in adoption of a new paradigm.

Kuhn defines *paradigms* as "universally recognized scientific achievements that for a time provide model problems and solutions to a community of practitioners."[152] Better-known examples of new paradigms include Aristotle's analysis of motion, Ptolemy's computations of planetary position, Lavoisier's application of balance, and Maxwell's mathematical explanation of the electromagnetic field. Paradigms can also be thought of as conceptual frameworks within which one analyzes, interprets and further studies various fundamental phenomena. In a sense, paradigms are a kind of lens on reality; how we look at something determines, to a large extent, what we look for and what we tend to regard as "fact."

A "paradigm shift" occurred early in this century with the advent of quantum physics, which began with Planck's proposal that light is radiated in quanta of action, whole units which do not, like waves, dissipate as they travel through space. This idea ran contrary to established thought and from the outset was widely resisted. Kuhn's comprehensive analysis of paradigm shifts throughout the history of civilization led him to conclude that competition between segments of the scientific community is the only historical process that ever consistently results in the rejection of one previously accepted theory or in the adoption of another. He says:

> Paradigms gain their status because they are more successful than their competitors in solving a few problems that the group of practitioners has come to recognize as acute. To be more successful is not, however, to be either completely successful with a single problem or notably successful with any large number. The success of a paradigm . . . is at the start largely a promise of success discoverable in selected and still incomplete examples. Normal science consists in the actualization of that promise, an actualization achieved by extending the knowledge of those facts that the paradigm displays as particularly revealing, by increasing the extent of the match between those facts and the paradigm's predictions, and by further articulation of the paradigm itself.[153]

Resistance among scientists toward new paradigms is often rooted in personal or egoistic attachment, not in an objective mode of thinking about one's particular field or specialty. These days much time, money, and effort is being invested in consolidating one's intellectual and technical prowess in a particular field of study. To shift one's fundamental orientation after such rigorous training is no easy task. According to Brunner's *Theory of Incongruity*, people are typically unwilling to adopt new paradigms until a new set of data emerges which is totally incongruous with the old data. At this point, the rational mind is confronted with such a high degree of contradiction that all personal biases must fall away and the old paradigm is either modified or discarded. Unfortunately, some scientists will not allow themselves even this much. It is known that a few physicists of the pre-quantum era committed suicide when it was revealed that all matter is ultimately a permutation of energy.

The multifactorial hypothesis is still not mainstream among medical professionals and AIDS researchers. It is far simpler to analyze one single agent (HIV) having a definitive role in the final stages of the syndrome than to ascertain several interactive factors operating in a gradual, developmental manner. Further, one of the most fundamental tenets of modern medicine is that germs or microbes directly cause disease. This tenet was aptly reflected by the logo for the 1986 International Conference on AIDS, which consisted of three red concentric circles and four arrows pointing toward the AIDS virus in the center. There is also an economic incentive to uphold the single-agent perspective, as large pharmaceutical companies provide huge funds for testing and developing thousands of antiviral drugs—all of which are aimed at HIV, the presumed root of the problem.

The numerous drug companies represented at scientific conferences on AIDS are testimony to the fact that serendipitous and ecologically oriented AIDS research is hard to come by. A sad commentary of the 1986 International Conference on AIDS is that Dr. Elinor Levy and colleagues of the Department of Microbiology at the Boston University School of Medicine, presenting their work on the therapeutic benefits of the macrobiotic approach to AIDS, were the only presenters asserting such an holistic orientation. Notably, theirs was the *only* report indicating a progressive, linear improvement in immune function of men with full-blown AIDS over a two-and-one-half-year period. It is also unfortunate that very little research in this direction has followed the encouraging preliminary report from Dr. Levy and colleagues published in *The Lancet* of July 25, 1985.[154]

The resistance of medical professionals toward holistic paradigms such as the multifactorial theory is reminiscent of the plight of Dr. Ignaz Philipp Semmelweis in the 1840s. Dr. Semmelweis observed for the first time a much higher incidence of morbidity and mortality among postpartum women tended by physicians versus those attended by nursing staff.[155] The mortality from the illness, known than as *purerperal fever*, was extraordinarily high among the physician-treated women. Considered unorthodox by his colleagues, Semmelweis adopted an epidemiological approach that was novel for his time: he sought to differentiate *all* possible variables in the two wards. The results seemed at first meaningless. Postpartum patients examined by physicians who had come directly from doing autopsies on deceased women (including pelvic exams) showed a higher incidence of morbidity and mortality than those patients treated by the nursing staff.

In those days there were no aseptic techniques practiced, and sanitation practices were rudimentary at best. Dr. Semmelweis observed that the nurses washed their hands between patients. Speculating that contamination from the autopsied corpses to the living patients was a key factor in the high incidence of purerperal fever, he suggested that the physicians wash their hands before examining their patients. The idea met with staunch opposition, and Sammelweis was heavily castigated by some of the top orthodox obstetricians of the day. Obsessed by his conviction that young women were dying unnecessarily, he continued to defend his ideas. In time, however, the opposition became too intense.

Probably owing to his sensitive nature, Sammelweis eventually suffered a nervous breakdown and died a martyr in a mental institution.

Although Semmelweis died before seeing the fruits of his labors, subsequent generations have benefited greatly by his dedication and commitment to promoting what was then considered an unorthodox and unproven approach. Similarly, much of what is presented in this book could be considered unorthodox or unproven at the present time, and yet one day may become accepted, scientifically valid fact. There is much existing evidence which indicates that our basic premise in approaching AIDS is reasonable: The natural integrity of our immune system is the alpha and the omega of our biological well-being and long-term survival. When this integrity deteriorates, sickness and premature death are the logical outcome. Any means which serves to re-establish this integrity should be employed in the approach to AIDS.

Let us reiterate the primary contention of this book: *there is a practical basis for susceptibility to AIDS.* This practical basis involves not only the recognized modes of transmission, but also the body's natural means of protection or resistance. AIDS originates long before viral infection and the manifestation of opportunistic diseases, and is rooted in the quality of the external factors we select and consume in our day-to-day life. Knowing that we can support our body's ability to protect itself to the AIDS virus, we need not resign ourselves to regarding AIDS as an inevitable pronouncement of doom for all humanity. We need to begin looking within ourselves and at our total context of daily living, for we cannot always rely on modern technology to save us.

Our hope for the future lies in the intelligence of modern humanity. To once again quote Emerson: "Intellect annuls fate. So far as man thinks, he is free." The efficacy of our response to the AIDS crisis will hinge on a renewed appreciation of complex ecological relationships, both microscopic and macroscopic, and on an ability to take full responsibility for our well-being. The alternative approach presented here and espoused by a growing number of health-care practitioners is grounded in highly dynamic, multidimensional thinking, whereby the phenomenon of health involves interdependent physical, psychological, and social aspects. This kind of thinking requires a blend of rational and intuitive, logical and aesthetic, analytic and holistic modes of thought.

History is testimony to this great intellectual challenge. According to acclaimed Chinese historian Joseph Needham, the people of ancient China developed highly sophisticated technologies in metallurgy and astronomy—all without graph paper, computers, and other high-tech innovations.[156] They did, however, have a unifying principle, derived from intuition and commonsense empirical observation, which enabled them to see the world in terms of qualities, patterns and dynamic processes. The time has come to embrace both sides, to adopt a whole-brain worldview.[157] Adopting this larger perspective, we can better understand how we create health and disease. In time we may all come to see AIDS as an opportunity for learning and evolving further.

[1] Silberner, J., "What Triggers AIDS?" *Science News* (1987), 131(14): 220.

[2] Friedland, G. H. et al., "Lack of Transmission of HTLV-III/LAV Infection to Household Contacts of Patients with AIDS or AIDS-related Complex with Oral Candidiasis," *N Eng Med* (1986), 314(6): 344.

[3] Kuhls, T. L. et al., "A Prospective Cohort Study of the Occupational Risk of AIDS and AIDS-related Infections in Healthcare Personal," International Conference on AIDS, *Epidemiology* No. 162 (Paris, 1986).

[4] Klein, R. S. et al., "Prevalence of Antibodies to HIV among Dental Professionals," International Conference on Aids, *Epidemiology* No. 163 (Paris, 1986).

[5] Salahuddin, S. Z. et al., "HIV in Symptom-free Seronegative Persons," *Lancet* (1984), 2: 1418.

[6] "Two Saliva Studies—Reassuring," GMHC Healthletter (New York City, May/June, 1986).

[7] Ibid.

[8] Mandel, I., "Immunological Properties of Saliva and the Prevention of Oral Disease," in Symposium: Nutrition and the Immune System, Columbia University College of Physicians and Surgeons (New York City, 4 Dec. 1986).

[9] Siberner, J., "No AIDS via Mosquitoes," *Science News* (1986), 130(16): 252.

[10] Stewart, G. J. et al., "Transmission of HIV by Artificial Insemination by Donor," *Lancet* (1985), 2: 581.

[11] Gallo, R., "Human Retroviruses, Now and the Future," International Conference on AIDS, Plenary Session V (Paris, 25 June 1986).

[12] Up Front, "Stopping Sperm May Block AIDS," *Discover* (1987), 8(10): 11.

[13] Maysfield, M. and T. Topousis, "Two Organ Recipients Get AIDS Virus," *USA Today* (24, May 1987).

[14] Scott, G. B. et al., "Natural History of HIV Infections in Children," International Conference on Aids, *Epidemiology* No. 1 (Paris, 23 June 1986).

[15] Bell, J., "The Thin Latex against Disease," *New Scientist* (26 Feb. 1987), p. 58.

[16] Ibid.

[17] Selye, H., "Homeostasis, the Staying Power of the Body," in *The Stress of Life* (New York: McGraw-Hill Book Co., 1976), pp. 12–3. The great French physiologist Claude Bernard taught that one of the most basic features of all living beings is their ability to maintain constancy of the internal environment—the blood, lymph, and other body fluids—despite changes in the sur-

roundings. Ostensibly, disease is not just suffering, but an attempt to maintain the homeostatic balance of our tissues, despite damage caused by the pathology itself. Bernard recognized cells as functional "units of life," surrounded and maintained by the blood and body fluids.

[18] Atkinson, K. et al., "Evidence That Immune Deficiency after Marrow Transplantation Is Not Caused by AIDS-associated Retrovirus," *N Eng J Med* (1985), 13(3): 182–3.

[19] Johnson, E. and P. Ho, "The Elusive Etiology: Possible causes and pathogenesis of AIDS," in *Understanding AIDS*, ed. V. Gong (New Brunswick, N. J.: Rutgers University Press, 1985), p. 82.

[20] International Conference on AIDS, Epidemiological reports −35% serpos mothers give birth to seroneg infants (Paris, 24 June 1986).

[21] Biggar, R. J. et al., Seroepidemiology of HTLV-III Antibodies in a Remote Population of Eastern Zaire," *Br Med J* (1985), 290(6741): 808.

[22] Gershwin, M. E. et al., "Nutritional Factors and Immune Ontogeny," in *Nutrition and Immunity* (Orland, Fla.: Academic Press, Inc., 1985), pp. 107–53.

[23] Merino, F. et al., "Antibodies to AIDS-associated Retrovirus in Drug Addicts in Vizcaya, Northern Spain," *AIDS Research* (1986), 2(2): 133.

[24] Caiazza, S. S., Press conference at Penthouse building (New York City: The Betsy Nolan Group, Inc. Public Relations, 12 May 1987).

[25] Eales, L-J. et al., "Association of Different Allelic Forms of Group Specific Component with Susceptibility to and Clinical Manifestation of HIV Infection," *Lancet* (1987), 1: 999.

[26] Gilles, K. et al., "Genetic Susceptibility to AIDS: Absence of an association with group-specific component (Gc)," *N Eng J Med* (1987), 317(10): 630; also see letter from S. P. Daiger et al., p. 631.

[27] Thyman, M. et al., "AIDS and the Gc Protein," *Lancet* (1987), 1: 1378.

[28] Todd, G. P., "Free Radical Pathology," in *Nutrition, Health, and Disease* (Norfolk, Va.: The Donning Company, 1987), p. 20.

[29] Kutsky, R. J., *Handbook of Vitamins, Minerals, and Hormones*, 2nd ed (New York: Van Nostrand Reinhold, Inc., 1981), pp. 197–243.

[30] Beisel, W. R. et al., "Single-nutrient Effects on Immunologic Functions," *JAMA* (1981), 245(1): 53.

[31] Gershwin, et al. (1985), Op. cit. See Introduction and "The Potential Impact of Nutritional Factors on Immunological Responsiveness," pp. 1–4.

[32] Trowell, H. and D. Burkitt, eds., *Western Diseases: Their Emergence and Prevention* (Cambridge, Mass.: Harvard University Press, 1981).

[33] Polk, B. F. et al., "Predictors of AIDS Developing in a Cohort of Seropositive Men," *N Engl J Med* (1987), 316(2): 61.

[34] Cottrell, M. C., Survey of 60 gay men with AIDS and ARC in collaboration with Elinor Levy, Ph.D. of the Boston University School of Medicine.

[35] Ibid.

[36] Gallo (1986), Op. cit.

[37] Nordland, R. et al., "Africa in the Plague Years," *Newsweek* (24 Nov. 1986), p. 47.

[38] Serrill, M. S. et al., "In the Grip of the Scourge," *Time* (16 Feb. 1987), p. 58.

[39] Mann, J. M., "Epidemiology of HIV in Africa," International Conference on AIDS, *Epidemiology* 3, Keynote paper (Paris, 23 June 1986).

[40] Ibid.

[41] Nordland et al., (1986), Op. cit., p. 47.

[42] Epidemiologic reports, International Conference on AIDS (Paris, 1986). Overuse of blood transfusions has been reported in areas of Central Africa. In most instances these transfusions have involved the use of only one pint of blood—an amount too small to be considered indicative of the need for transfusion. This leads one to speculate upon use of this modality in Africa as an exaggerated response to the potential benefits of Western medical technology. The spin-off result could be excessive reliance on antibiotics, immunizations, and other procedures as well, all of which might weaken the native African's immune system.

[43] Mead, J. W., "Observations from Three Months in Zaire, Tanzania, and Kenya" (Unpublished manuscript) (Plymouth, N.H.: Holderness School, 1987).

[44] Norland et al. (1986), Op. cit., p. 46.

[45] Bigger et al. (1985), Op. cit.

[46] Law, D. K. et al., "Immunocompetence of Patients with Protein-calorie Malnutrition. The Effects of Nutritional Repletion," *Ann Intern Med* (1973), 79: 545.

[47] Chandra, R. K., "Nutritional Status, Body Composition and Immuno-competence," in *Body Composition Assessments in Youth and Adults* (1985); see also A.F. Roche, ed., "Report of the Sixth Ross Conference on Medical Research" (Columbus, Ohio: Ross Laboratories), pp. 254–60.

[48] Van de Perre, P. et al., "Acquired Immunodeficiency Syndrome in Rwanda," *Lancet* (1984), 2: 62.

[49] Mead (1986), Op. cit.

[50] Nzilambi, N. et al., "HIV Seroprevalence among Tuberculosis Patients in Zaire," International Conference on AIDS, *Epidemiology* No. 6 (24 June 1986).

[51] Ibid.

[52] Cassava, a starchy root plant extensively cultivated in west tropical Africa, exists in two forms, bitter and sweet, and serves as a daily staple. The starch of the bitter cassava is made into tapioca. But since the sap of bitter cassava contains the highly poisonous hydrocyanic acid, the root cannot be eaten in a fresh condition. Exposure to heat dissipates the poisonous principle, and the concentrated juice is used and added to food as a sauce, mainly as cassareep. Cassava roots are preserved for use by drying or pounded into manioc or cassava meal, used for cassava cakes. The sweet cassava is inoccuous and thus employed as a standard table vegetable.

260

53 Davidson, S. et al., *Human Nutrition and Dietetics* (London: Livingstone-Churchill Publications, 1979), p. 4.

54 Piot, P. et al., "Retrospective Seroepidemiology of AIDS Virus Infection in Nairobi Populations," International Conference on AIDS, *Epidemiology* No. 3 (Paris, 23 June 1986).

55 Mead (1986), Op. cit.

56 Ibid.

57 Lubbe, A. M., "A Comparative Study of Rural and Urban Venda Males, Dietary Assessment," *So Afr Med J* (1971), 45: 1289.

58 Trowell and Burkitt (1981), Op. cit., p. 21.

59 Mead (1986), Op. cit.

60 Trowell, H., "Urban Slums," in *Western Diseases*, eds. Burkitt, D.P. and H.C. Trowell (Cambridge, Mass.: Harvard University Press, 1981), p. 20.

61 Barry, M. et al., "Haiti and the AIDS Connection," *J Chronic Dis* (1984), 37: 593.

62 Marmor, M., "Risk Factors," in *AIDS: A Basic Guide for Clinicians* (London: W.B. Saunders Co., 1985), p. 48.

63 World Health Organization, "AIDS Cases Reported to WHO as of September 12, 1986" (Geneva, 1986).

64 Nichols (1986), Op. cit., p. 18.

65 Vieira, J. et al., "AIDS in Haitians: Opportunistic infections in previously healthy Haitian immigrants," *N Eng J Med* (1983), 308(3): 125.

66 Cousteau Society, "Haiti," Educational Film Documentary, NBC.

67 Hamaker, J. D. and D. A. Weaver, "The Decline of Soil Minerals and the Rise of Malnutrition," in *The Survival of Civilization* (Burlingame, Calif.: Hamaker-Weaver Publishers, 1982), p. 104.

68 Borysenko, M. and J. Borysenko, "Stress, Behavior and Immunity: Animal models and mediating mechanisms," *General Hospital Psychiatry* (1982), 40: 59.

69 Leprohon-Greenwood, C. E. and G. H. Anderson, "An Overview of the Mechanisms by Which Diet Affects Brain Function," *Food Technology* (Institute of Food Technologists, 1986), 40(1): 132.

70 Pert, C., "Brain and Biochemistry No. 10" (Rockville Pike, Washington D.C., 1986), cited in "Neuropeptides Link Brain and Immunity," *Brain/Mind Bulletin*, 11(4): 1.

71 Quinn, T. C. et al., "Serologic and Immunologic Studies on HTLV-3 and Other Infections in African and U.S. AIDS Patients (abst)," International Conference on AIDS (Atlanta, Ga., 14–17 Apr. 1985), p. 84.

72 Up Front, "AIDS Epidemiology: Women and drugs," *Discover* (June 1987), p. 12.

73 Stone (1987), Op. cit., p. 38.

74 Brown, R. K., "The Ninety Percent," in *AIDS, Cancer, & the Medical Establishment* (New York: Robert Speller Publishers, 1986), p. 23.

75 Dunnett, B., "Drugs That Suppress Immunity: Drug users have a new reason to kick the habit," *American Health* (1986), 5(9): 43.

[76] Glassman, A. et al., "Effects of Ethyl Alcohol on Human Peripheral Lymphocytes," *Arch Pathol Lab Med* (1985), 109: 540.

[77] Nutrition Update, vol. 1, No. 2.

[78] "Heroin Addiction and T Cell Depletion," *Science News* (1981), 119: 6.

[79] Merino et al. (1986), Op. cit.

[80] Fettner, A. G., "AIDS & Recreational Drugs," *Utne Reader*, No. 17 (New York: That New Magazine Inc., 1986), pp. 78–9.

[81] Lauritsen, J. and H. Wilson, "Death Rush: Poppers and AIDS" (New York: Pagan Press, 1986).

[82] *Science News* (1981), Op. cit.

[83] Ibid.

[84] Glasgow, B. J. et al., "Clinical and Pathological Findings of the Liver in AIDS," *Am J Pathol* (1985), 83: 582.

[85] Null, G., "Medical Genocide: The AIDS panic" (Distributed at a Press Conference in New York City, 12 May 1987), The Betsy Nolan Group Inc. 215 Park Ave., Ste. 1602, New York, N.Y. 1003.

[86] Ibid.

[87] Altman, L. K., "AIDS Mystery: Why do some infected men stay healthy," *New York Times* (30 June 1987).

[88] Ibid.

[89] Solis, D., "Gays Band Together in Workplace to Help Careers, Battle Prejudice," Wall Street Journal CCVII (1986), (49): 37, cited by T. O'Connor in *Living with AIDS* (San Francisco, Calif.: Corwin Publishers, 1987).

[90] Haverkos, H. W. et al., "Disease Manifestation among Homosexual Men with AIDS: A possible role of nitrites in Kaposi's sarcoma," CDC AIDS Research (Center for Infectious Diseases, 1985). Abridged version published in *Sexually Transmitted Diseases* (Dec. 1985), p. 103.

[91] O'Connor, T. and A. Gonzalez-Nunez, "Recreational Drugs and Alcohol," in *Living with AIDS* (San Francisco, Calif.: Corwin Publishers, 1986), p. 96.

[92] Lauritsen, J. and H. Wilson, *Death Rush: Poppers and AIDS* (with annotated bibliography) (New York: Pagan Press, 1986). Extensive documentation of studies showing the immunsuppressive effects of nitrite inhalants.

[93] Oriz, J. S. and V. L. Rivera, "The Effect of Amyl Nitrite on T-cell Function in Mice," presented to the American Public Health Association Convention (Nov. 1985).

[94] Newell, G. R. et al., "Risk Factor Analysis among Men Referred for Possible AIDS," *Prev Med* (Jan. 1985), p. 81.

[95] Brown, R. K., "The Problem of AIDS," in *AIDS, Cancer and the Medical Establishment* (New York: Robert Speller Publishers, 1986), p. 22.

[96] Mavligit, G. M. et al., "Chronic Stimulation by Sperm Alloantigens: Support for the hypothesis that spermatozoa induce immune dysregulation in homosexual males," *JAMA* (1984), 251(2): 237–41.

[97] Ibid.

[98] Kuno, S. et al., "Prostaglandin E_2 Administered via Anus Causes Immuno-

suppression in Male but Not Female Rats: A possible pathogenesis of AIDS in homosexual males," *Proc Natl Acad Sci* (1986), 83: 2682.

[99] Cottrell, M. C., Survey of 24 homosexual men with AIDS in New York City, in collaboration with E. Levy, Ph.D. of Boston University School of Medicine (1986).

[100] Mehrabian, A. and M. Ross, "Quality of Life Change and Individual Differences in Stimulus in Relation to Incidence of Illness," *Psychol Rep* (1977), 41: 367–78.

[101] McFarlane, A. H. et al., "A Longitudinal Study of the Influence of the Psychosomatic Environment on Health Status: A preliminary report," *J Health Soc Behav* (1980), 21: 124–33.

[102] Monmaney, T., "Kids with AIDS," *Newsweek* (7 Sept. 1987), p. 52.

[103] Van De Perre, P. et al., "Female Prostitutes: A risk group for infection with HTLV-III," *Lancet* (1985), 2(8454): 524.

[104] Ziegler, J. B. et al., "Postnatal Transmission of AIDS-associated Retovirus from Mother to Infant," *Lancet* (1985), 1(8434): 896.

[105] Salk, L. et al., "Perinatal Complications in the History of Asthmatic Children," *Am J Dis Child* (1974), 127: 30.

[106] Scott, G. B. et al., "Natural History of HIV Infections in Children," International Conference on AIDS, *Epidemiology* No. 1 (Paris, 23, June, 1986).

[107] Ibid.

[108] Ibid.

[109] Ibid.

[110] Mann, J. M., "Epidemiology of HIV in Africa," International Conference on AIDS, *Epidemiology* No. 3, Keynote paper (Paris, 23 June 1986).

[111] Davachi et al. (1986), Op. cit.

[112] Rubinstein, A., "The Clinical and Immunological Spectum of Pediatric AIDS," International Conference on AIDS, Communication 19: S 8K (Paris, 1986).

[113] According to the CDC in Atlanta, there has been a four-fold increase in congenital malformations since the 1950s.

[114] CDC Update, "Morbidity and Mortality Weekly Report" (1984), 33: 661–4.

[115] Tucker, M. A. et al., "Bone Sarcomas Linked to Radiotherapy and Chemotherapy in Children," *N Engl J Med* (1987), 317(10): 588.

[116] Slaff, J. I. and J. K. Brubaker, "The 100 Most Important Questions about AIDS," in *The AIDS Epidemic* (New York: Warner Books, 1985), p. 75.

[117] Fries, E. D., "Salt, Volume, and the Prevention of Hypertension," *Circulation* (1976), 53: 589.

[118] Kotler, D. et al., "Body Composition Studies in Patients with AIDS," *Am J Clin Nutr* (1985), 42: 1255.

[119] Ballentine, R., "Pollution: External and internal," in *Diet and Nutrition* (Honesdale, Pa.: The Himalayan International Institute, 1978), p. 329.

[120] Weiner, M. A., "What Makes Immunity Fail?" in *Maximum Immunity* (Boston, Mass.: Houghton Mifflin Co., 1985), p. 149.

[121] National Center for Health Statistics, "Highlights of Drug Utilization in Office Practice" (1987); cited in Naunton, E., "Diuretics Are in Vanguard of Pill Parade," *The Hatford Courant* (18 June 1987).

[122] Hauser, W. E. and J. S. Remington, "Effect of Antibiotics on the Immune Response," *Am J Med* (1982), 72: 711.

[123] Truss, C. O., "The Role of Candida Albicans in Human Illness," *J Orthomol Psych* (1981), 10: 228.

[124] "Antibiotics in Animal Feeds: Threat to human health?" *Science News* (1972), 101: 348.

[125] Vieira et al. (1983), Op. cit.

[126] Holdiness, M. R., "A Review of Introgenic Nutritional Deficiencies Induced by Antituberculosis Drugs," *Nutr Res* (1987), 7: 891.

[127] Brown, R. K., "The Problem of Blood," in *AIDS, Cancer and the Medical Establishment* (New York: Robert Spellers Publishers, 1986), p. 30.

[128] Ibid., p. 31.

[129] "Single Blood Transfusions Shown to Cause Immunologic Changes," *Oncology Times* (Apr. 1986).

[130] Stockwell, S., "Blood Transfusions Decrease Survival in Cancer Patients," *Oncology Times* (1985), 7(6): 1.

[131] Brown (1986), Op. cit., p. 91. Pleomorphic organisms are classical bacteria, fungi, and protozoa which adapt to physical and chemical agents (antibiotics, enzymes, acid-base balance, etc.) by defensively losing their cell walls.

[132] Blumberg, N. et al., "Relation between Recurrence of Cancer of the Colon and Blood Transfusions," *Brit Med J* (1985), 290(6474): 1037.

[133] Ibid.

[134] Weinberg, E. O., "Iron in Neoplastic Disease," *Nutrition and Cancer* (1983), 4: 223.

[135] Hall, B. M. et al., "T Helper-inducer Cells Mediate Rejection without T cytotoxic-suppressor Cells?" *Transplant Proc* (1985), 17: 233.

[136] Bach, F. H. and D. H. Sachs, "Current Concepts: Transplantation immunology," *N Engl J Med* (1987), 317(8): 489.

[137] Atkinson et al. (1985), Op. cit.

[138] Kersey, J. H. et al., "Comparison of Autologous and Allogeneic Bone Marrow Transplantation for Treatment of High-risk Refractory Acute Lymphoblastic Leukemia," *N Engl J Med* (1987), 317: 461.

[139] Slaff and Brubaker (1985), Op. cit., p. 5.

[140] Castleman, M., "AIDS Goes Hetero," *Medical Selfcare* (1985), 30: 18–20.

[141] CDC, Morbidity and Mortality Weekly Report, "Heterosexual Transmission of Human T-Lymphotropic Virus Type III/Lymnpadenopath-associated Virus" (1985), 34(37): 1–2.

[142] Greenwood (1984), Op. cit.

264

[143] Clumeck, N. et al., "Heterosexual Promiscuity among African Patients with AIDS" (correspondence), *N Engl J Med* (18 July 1985), p. 182.

[144] Castro, K. G. et al., "Risk Factors for AIDS among Haitians in the United States," International Conference on AIDS (Atlanta, Ga.: 16 Apr. 1985).

[145] Smiligis, M. et al., "The Big Chill: Fear of AIDS," *Time* (1987), 129(7): 53.

[146] Leishman, K., "Heterosexuals and AIDS," *The Atlantic Monthly* (Feb. 1987), p. 39.

[147] Baldwin R. and R. J. Chloupek, "AIDS Debate: Round two," *Discover* (1987), 7(11): 104.

[148] Lifson, A. R. et al., " 'No Identified Risk' Cases of AIDS," International Conference on AIDS, *Epidemiology* No. 1 (Paris, 23 June 1986).

[149] Biomedicine Report, "Smoking out B-vitamins' Role in Lungs," *Science News* (1986), 130(24): 377.

[150] Kvale, G. et al., "Dietary Habits and Lung Cancer Risk," *Int J Cancer* (1983), 31: 397.

[151] Hinds, M. H. et al., "Dietary Vitamin A, Carotene, Vitamin C, and Risk of Lung Cancer in Hawaii," *Am J Epidemiol* (1984), 119: 227.

[152] Kuhn, T. S., *The Structure of Scientific Revolutions*, vol. 2, No. 2, Preface of *International Encyclopedia of Unified Science* (Chicago: University of Chicago, 1970), p. viii.

[153] Ibid.

[154] Levy, E. M. et al., "Patients with Kaposi's Sarcoma Who Opt for No Treatment," *Lancet* (1985), 223.

[155] Garrison, F. H., *History of Medicine* (Philadelphia, Pa.: W.B. Saunders, 1968), pp. 435–7.

[156] Needham, J., *Science and Civilization in China*, vol. 2 (Cambridge, Mass.: University Press, 1956).

[157] Wonder, J. and P. Donovan, "The Split-brain Theory," in *Whole-Brain Thinking* (New York: Ballantine Books, 1984), pp. 3–10.

4. Lessons from the New York Study

Achieving the stage of acceptance indicates that the patient has formed a new, stable identity . . . Individuals in this state accept their approaching deaths but also take charge of the life they have left to live. They are likely to feel less victimized by life and to be less egocentric than before. They often find meaning in altruistic and community activities, and may find a sense of mission and important roles to fill. They take responsibility for their state of health, perhaps indulging in such holistic practices as positive imaging, macrobiotic diets and meditation, and are likely to exhibit a "fighting spirit" toward their illness and their caretakers. Many patients summarize these changes as becoming the type of person they had always wanted to be.

—Dr. Steven E. Nichols, Plenary Address,
1986 International Conference on AIDS,
Paris, France

A Pilot Study in New York City

The above statement by Stephen Nichols, M.D., psychiatrist of New York's Beth Israel Medical Center, reflects the medical profession's growing awareness of the value of holistic approaches, including macrobiotics. At the same conference, a group of Boston researchers were presenting their findings on the effects of the macrobiotic approach on the immune systems and overall health of 20 men with AIDS. One year before, in the esteemed British medical journal, *The Lancet*, these scientists had published a brief report assuring the medical community of a "no treatment" approach to AIDS. In their letter, the researchers stated that these men with Kaposi's sarcoma ". . . who have chosen not to enter conventional treatment protocols . . . seem to be surviving at least as well as patients who have been treated . . . their T4/T8 ratio, which reportedly correlates with survival, is higher than that reported for patients with KS . . . . Survival of these men who have received little or no medical treatment appears to compare very favorably with that of KS patients in general."[1]

The seeds of this study were cast in 1983, when the message of macrobiotics had only begun to make inroads into New York City's gay community. Lawrence H. Kushi, D. Sc., a graduate of Harvard University's School of Public Health, arranged with Boston University and with his father, Michio Kushi, to do a blood research program in New York. They approached a small group of men who had been attending macrobiotic educational activities at the Macrobiotic Center of New York and practicing macrobiotics as a way to manage their condition. These men then formed a support group, meeting periodically to share meals and discuss their experiences. Dr. Kushi, then a postdoctoral epidemiologist at the University of Minnesota School of Public Health, sought the assistance of Elinor N. Levy, Ph. D., and John C. Beldekas, Ph. D., of the Department of Immunology and Microbiology at Boston University's School of Medicine, and finally Martha C. Cottrell, M.D., who consented to serve as clinical coordinator for the study.

In May of 1984, the research team began monitoring the immune responses for 10 men who had adopted the macrobiotic approach. Blood samples and clinical observations were obtained biweekly from this group. A questionnaire provided medical histories, aspects of their psychological profile, and the extent of their previous and ongoing practice of macrobiotics. The opportunity was also given to discuss with the clinical coordinator any particular concerns they might have regarding their condition. The men were also encouraged to make arrangements for consultation with other physicians who had been involved in monitoring their conditions, or who were cognizant of the effects of dietary changes.

After observing significant clinical improvements in the group of ten and reporting their findings to *The Lancet*, the researchers opted to expand the study to 20 men, all with Kaposi's sarcoma, who agreed to adopt the macrobiotic approach. Between 1984 and 1986, this group has shown a significant increase in the total number of T-lymphocytes, which may indicate an improved prognosis for AIDS. Contrary to what might be expected, the number of T4 (T-helper) cells has increased over the first two years after diagnosis. For all surviving members, the T4 and T8 counts had either stabilized or increased. Some men even doubled their lymphocyte counts during the two-year period, and most have seen their total counts return to the normal range. Despite the remarkable improvement in T4 cells counts, however, changes in the T4/T8 ratios—which are typically abnormal in AIDS—have not been statistically significant.

After two years, Drs. Levy and Beldakas sent the following report to Michio Kushi:

> The results of our ongoing study of men with AIDS are encouraging. We have been studying the men sequentially since May 1984 to follow certain parameters. At present, the data suggests a stabilization of the percentage of T4 positive cells and of lymphocyte number in about 50 percent of the group. The general pattern with people with KS is a steady decline in the percentage of T4 and of total lymphocyte number. This is thought to be a significant indicator of morbidity. Therefore, the ability to stabilize these parameters in so large a proportion of our study group is a hopeful sign.

As one of the first records of the fact that AIDS can be successfully treated through changes in diet and life-style, this report seemed favorable enough to continue the study and to consider more carefully the potential value of macrobiotic dietary practices in the treatment of AIDS.

The positive changes in the immune systems of these men have been accompanied by favorable survival rates. As reported in the second and third sessions of the International Conference on AIDS, survival rates in this group are comparable to those of AIDS patients receiving medical treatment. Normal life expectancy for people with Kaposi's sarcoma is 22 months after diagnosis. As of June of 1986, the average survival in this group was approximately 25 months. As of June, 1987, eight of the twenty men had died; their median survival was 19 months. Among those alive today, four have survived at least four years since their diagnosis with AIDS; two have survived about six years. At the time of this writing (April 12, 1988) these long-term survivors appear to be in sound health.

In addition to the measurable biological effects of the macrobiotic diet, feedback from the men themselves has indicated a marked improvement in their personal attitudes, energy levels, and overall vitality. None of these men are bedridden, and all report great improvement in their quality of life. All have maintained physically and mentally active lives, with a large proportion participating in community and educational

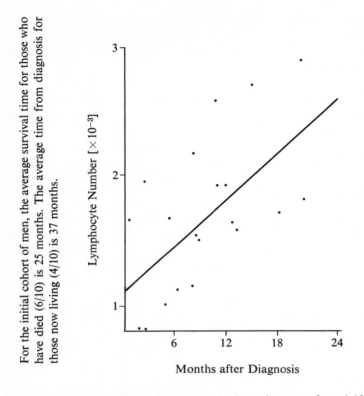

For the initial cohort of men, the average survival time for those who have died (6/10) is 25 months. The average time from diagnosis for those now living (4/10) is 37 months.

The average calculated lymphocyte number/mm increases from 1,122 at diagnosis to 2,584 two years later. The calculation is based on all the data points available.

activities. As a group, these men seem totally distinct from conventionally treated AIDS patients, who are chronically tired and ill, cannot work, and who are generally consumed by feelings of helplessness and despair. Says Dr. Levy, "The men in our study seem to enjoy a quality of life, rare if not unknown, among other men with AIDS."[2]

The stabilized lymphocyte counts, together with marked clinical improvements and fair survival rates, suggests the possibility that the nontoxic, noninvasive approach of macrobiotics may be a favorable alternative to conventional treatments. In their 1986 report in Paris, Dr. Levy's group stated, "The relative stability of lymphocyte number and distribution in this group as compared to reports of other groups suggests the possibility that certain treatments may contribute to the decrease in lymphocyte number associated with the progression of AIDS."[3] While drug treatments may further compromise the already fragile immune systems of people with AIDS, the macrobiotic approach seems to enhance the functioning of the immune system in AIDS. Moreover, certain unique compounds found in miso soup, sea vegetables, whole grains, and leafy green vegetables, may even help eliminate residual toxicity resulting from previous drug therapy or from extensive opportunistic infections.

Our observations suggest that those men who have shown the greatest improvement are those who have minimized or avoided medical treatments and adopted macrobiotics soon after diagnosis. These same men have generally adhered very closely to their dietary and life-style recommendations, at least during the first two years of practice. By contrast, those men who have fared poorly came to macrobiotics as a last-ditch alternative, some literally on their last legs, after trying drug treatments. Some men had a difficult time sticking to the dietary guidelines—having been habituated to a very rich diet with lots of sweets, pastries, and oily foods. Some oscillated between their macrobiotic regimen and drug therapies. Some avoided contact with the macrobiotic community to shield themselves from potential discrimination or from potential criticism by their peers and physicians.

Education has played a key role in how accurately men follow the macrobiotic recommendations. Those men who showed steady improvement over time were committed to studying the macrobiotic approach and communicated closely with macrobiotic teachers concerning dietary adjustments as their conditions changed. Other men, however, were not studying macrobiotic principles and acted impulsively during periods of toxic discharge. These men often resorted to allopathic procedures such as drugs for pain relief, and antibiotics for minor infections. These were personal choices usually sought without guidance by either physicians or macrobiotic teachers, and without considering the experiences of participants who had successfully worked through these periods of discharge with the aid of nontoxic holistic therapies.

This is not to say that conventional medical approaches were not applicable in some cases within the group. Conventional medical care was sought in certain life-threatening cases, such as for Kaposi's-sarcoma lesions of the gums, enlarged lymph nodes which compromised vital structures (e.g., impaired respiratory function), or pneumonias in which immediate relief was necessary. The men who have dealt best with these medical interventions are those who have sought guidance from experienced teachers and physicians cognizant of macrobiotic principles, who have provided invaluable information on timely dietary adjustments and ways of reducing the extent of radiotherapy and chemotherapy to minimize toxicity of these treatments.

The Psychological Component

> Denial's the name of the game. Blaming God or nature is profound denial of the human role in health and disease, life and death.
> —Rudy, June 1987, New York City

As reported by Dr. Elinor Levy at the Third International Conference on AIDS (in Washington, D.C., June 1987), the relative success of the macrobiotic approach to AIDS seems to have a major psychological component. Dr. Levy and her co-workers had previously noted that, in general, the men in the New York study seemed to have exceptional vitality, good sleep patterns, and were more optimistic about the outlook of their prognosis than other AIDS patients. Indeed, in overall appearance, many of these men appear healtheir than the average American!

Dr. Levy's 1987 report included a subset of approximately half of these men who had filled out psychological questionnaires, including the Beck Depression Inventory and McNair's Profile of Moods. The results suggested that these men "are generally less depressed . . . less anxious . . . and feel more energetic . . . than has been reported for other cohorts of men with AIDS. The psychological profile associated with this group is hypothesized to have a beneficial effect on the clinical course of their disease."[4] In addition, the same report noted "some striking correlations between certain psychological measures and immune variables, particularly T4 number."

These last observations—that positive psychological traits correlated with increases in T-cell numbers—make it clear that the therapeutic effects of macrobiotics extend beyond the possible immune-enhancement afforded by balanced nutrition. Moods and attitudes may be equally important. As Dr. Levy's group proposed in their letter to *The Lancet*, the "choice to forgo conventional medical therapy may indicate a strong, independent psychological makeup which could enhance survival." Part of this makeup, for example, could involve the belief that healing must be effected from within through changes in attitude, diet, and lifestyle.

Another important element may be the sense of group cohesion. All of the men in the New York study have shown strong support of each other in times of physical and emotional crises. Moreover, rather than isolating themselves as an AIDS study group, most have integrated themselves into the macrobiotic community. Several of the men are active in other community efforts to address the concerns of men with AIDS. Other members of the group have provided active support—including cooking and emotional support—for those who were in need of hospitalization early on in the study.

Some of these men have emphasized their spiritual awareness and growth as an integral part of their healing process. They have spoken repeatedly of a growing vision and awareness of their personal lives. This has resulted in their becoming increasingly involved with others on a more meaningful level as well as involved in service to the community. Says one member of the group, a designer and professional cook: "If anything, I have too much energy. I'm very busy in my work. I swim every day, I go out dancing twice a week. I live a typical New York life, plus I have really come to terms with the illness. I feel that I understand it and that ultimately I am in control. And I see a similar attitude in my macrobiotic friends. Their whole emotional tenure is very positive."[5]

The psychological findings from the New York study are nothing truly revolutionary. In fact, they are quite consistent with research in the new medical synthesis called *psychoneuroimmunology* (PNI). According to PNI proponents, the *neural* (nerve) and *endocrine* (hormonal) pathways by which the body responds to ordinary mental and physical challenges, as well as to situations perceived as threatening, are intimately intertwined with immune functions. Thus the immune system can be compromised by emotional stress, leading to a transient acquired immune-deficiency and greater susceptibility to disease.

A growing number of PNI studies indicate that thoughts and feelings may modulate the expression of immune-related diseases, from allergies to AIDS.[6] Thus medical scientists are discovering what folk medicine has taught for ages—that you can worry yourself sick and grieve yourself to death. For instance, recent research by Susan Kennedy and colleagues at Ohio State University's College of Medicine found that separated and divorced men had significantly lower immune-competence than married men matched for age and education.[7] This study is of particular interest because all the participants were infected by the herpes virus, a virus which spends most of its time in a latent or inactive phase. Separated and divorced men were more anxious and depressed than their married counterparts—and had higher levels of herpes-virus antibodies, indicating that the virus was probably more active or more prevalent in their bodies. This was one of the first controlled studies to confirm the link between herpes reactivation and psychological stress. In similar research but with the opposite sex, separated and divorced women experienced both lower immunocompetence and increased mortality from disease.

The cells of the immune system respond to a wide variety of social upsets. Pressure and instability in the social world—from final examinations to bickering in-laws to missed job deadlines—show strong links with depressed immunity. Medical students at certain high-pressure times of the school year may exhibit varying degrees of depressed immunity. In five different studies, employing 20 different immunological tests, there was a significant, albeit transient, decrease in various parameters of the immune system during medical school final examinations.[8]

Another dimension to the anxiety-immunodepression link was illuminated by the work of John B. Jemmot and colleagues, who divided a population of dental school students into two groups: those motivated to form and maintain close relationships and those who were driven primarily by ambition or power. Dr. Jemmot found that when the "power motivated" group was placed under stress of exams and the rigors of curriculum, they experienced decreased levels of *immunoglobulin-A* (IgA, the antibody that protects against viruses and toxins along the digestive and respiratory tracts). By contrast, the group who were more relationship-oriented experienced higher levels of IgA during stress, and following the stressful periods tended to recover lost IgA more quickly than did power-oriented people. This observation has since been corroborated by other studies as well.[9]

In their report before the 2nd International Conference on AIDS, Dr. Levy's team noted strong correlations between the number of T4 cells and certain psychological measures, including vigor, depression, anxiety, and curiosity (inquisitiveness, imagination). The researchers also noted an "interesting association" between T4 counts and the *ability to express anger*—a psychological variable referred to as *anger-out*. Of eight men studied, those who measured more strongly for *anger-in* had less improvement in their T4 counts. On the other hand, anger-out seemed to exert a positive influence on the T4 cells.

Previously, the relationship between repressed anger and disease has been limited to heart attack. In the context of the present study, the possible connection between repressed anger and depressed immunity may involve the prevailing psychosocial milieu of the gay community. Our society has developed certain taboos against feeling and expressing anger. Angry women, for example, are frequently dismissed as irrational or worse, and male homosexuals may be scorned similarly for expressing anger. Anger is kept repressed at the cost of feeling guilty, depressed, and self-doubting—all disempowering emotions which, as Dr. Harriet Lerner explains in *The Dance of Anger*, keep us from taking action except against our own selves, making us "unlikely to be agents of personal and social change."[10]

Anger presents itself as both a boon and a bane to our personal well-being. Dr. Lerner describes the functional importance of anger as follows:

> Anger is a signal, and one worth listening to. Our anger may be a message that we are being hurt, that our rights are being violated, that our needs or wants are not being adequately met, or simply that something is not right. Our anger may tell us that we are not addressing an important emotional issue in our lives, or that too much of our self—our beliefs, values, desires, or ambitions—is being compromised in a relationship. Our anger may be a signal that we are doing more and giving more than we can comfortably do or give. Or our anger may warn us that others are doing too much for us, at the expense of our own competence and growth. Just as physical pain tells us to take our hand off the hot stove, the pain of our anger preserves the very integrity of our self. Our anger can motivate us to say 'no' to the ways in which we are defined by others and 'yes' to the dictates of our inner self.[11]

Dr. Lerner points out that we learn to fear and repress our own anger ". . . not only because it brings about the disapproval of others, but also because it signals the necessity for change. We may begin to ask ourselves questions that serve to block or invalidate our own experience of anger: 'Is my anger legititmate?' 'Do I have a right to be angry?' 'What's the use of my getting angry' 'What good will it do?' These questions can be excellent ways of silencing ourselves and shutting off [repressing] our anger."[12]

Like hunger, anger is a real feeling that cannot be denied too long, and that should not be swept under the rug of abstraction. It exists for a reason and always deserves our utmost respect and attention. We all have a right to *everything* we experience—and our anger is no exception. Constructively expressed, however, anger can be a source of personal transformation and can challenge the transformation of others. In Dr. Lerner's opinion the goal is not necessarily to get rid of our anger nor to doubt its validity. The goal is to gain greater clarity about its sources and then learn to take a new and different action on our own behalf.

Venting our anger is not necessarily a good strategy either, however. If we continually vent anger toward other people, groups, or institutions, we may only further maintain or rigidify old themes and behaviors and, in so doing, "fail to exercise our power to clarify and change our own selves."[13] Inappropriately expressed, anger-out can perpetuate feelings of depression, low self-esteem, self-betrayal, and even self-hatred unless we also choose to change our circumstances and live in a way that is consistent with a positive worldview and positive image of ourselves. This is where the macrobiotic philosophy comes in, as discussed later in this chapter. Also, according to traditional Oriental medicine, anger dition of chronic irritability produced by excessive consumption of animal products and oily foods, and by overeating in general.

By the macrobiotic view, we are far less inclined to accumulate pent-up emotions if our physical body is functioning harmoniously and if we maintain awareness of our constantly changing biological needs. In addition, healing must be strongly emphasized on the attitudinal level, since beliefs and attitudes may be promoting negative emotions which may impede physiological improvement. However, we should be wary of any exclusively mental approach when dealing with anger or other forms of emotional distress. Positive thinking surely has its place, but is generally too symptomatic and superficial to be applied to the deeper processes that determine chronic emotional patterns.

Many people today carry a tremendous amounts of emotional trauma and memories in various parts of their bodies. Repressed anger may reveal itself periodically through firey outbursts toward those we interact with in day-to-day life, or, less noticeably, as a chronic tightening in the shoulders, chest, and arms. By contrast, unresolved grief—perhaps related to loss of a family member during early childhood—may express itself through respiratory disorders and tightness in the upper back. Such psychosomatic manifestations may be effectively resolved through a combination of dietary changes and holistic, mind-body approaches (see appendixes).

Self-esteem and Attitudinal Healing

Most forms of human behavior reflect one's personal identity. How we perceive and feel about ourselves often influences the way we habitually live and respond to our environment. If we are happy and content in our existence, we will generally tend to live in ways which preserve and reinforce that positive state of being. If we are unhappy and discontent, we tend to live in more self-destructive, health-negating ways. The desire to preserve one's sense of total well-being is the driving force behind all enduring behavioral changes which promote health and happiness. Thus, how we take care of ourselves directly reflects our self-image, or how much we truly value ourselves.

The problem of diminished self-esteem, so pervasive among today's younger generations and minority groups, has much to do with the pressures of modern life. Children and minorities are especially vulnerable to the impact of current social values and growing economic pressures. Many young people, regardless of nationality, have early in life developed a powerful association between self-esteem and external factors. In school, this may involve being "in" with the right people, getting good grades, or being competent in athletics. Outside of school, the externalized self-esteem may take the form of material success and job status. In either context, with feelings about self so intimately linked to factors outside themselves, these people are vulnerable because they feel that they cannot control what they need to maintain positive self-esteem.

Low self-esteem and poorly defined sense of self are also common aspects of the male homosexual's psychological orientation.[14] If one's sense of self is contracted or small, one tends to experience the world as an oppressive, threatening, or foreboding place. Minority discrimination may trigger feelings of powerlessness, self-doubt, and insecurity—feelings which usually go unrecognized or are somehow repressed. Under more personal circumstances, such as the breakup of a relationship, a person may feel let down, dejected, and deprived. The perceived lack of power, together with a sense of personal ineptitude (negative self-esteem and helplessness), seems harmful to the immune system.[15] Negative self-esteem may also perpetuate self-destructive behaviors such as drug abuse, alcoholism, or workaholic tendencies. These behaviors could weaken the immune system and hence reinforce the effects of the negative emotions themselves.

Feelings of helplessness or powerlessness often accompany the unpredictability of the physical course of AIDS. In many cases, prolonged periods of relative stability may be interrupted by sudden episodes of disease. The rapid weight loss and physical wasting associated with severe opportunistic infections leads to dramatic changes in body image. The capricious nature of these periodic infections and setbacks tends to bring up all the issues we have about feeling in control and all the helplessness that is born out of the feeling that the disease is "invariably fatal."[16] Such feelings might compel one to seek out extreme measures of external support, such as experimental drug treatments or radical chemotherapy, both of which may further compromise the immune system. Alternatively, such feelings may quell all initiative for therapeutic action. In its most rigid, deep-seated form, such apathy may only seal one's death sentence.

Not everyone with AIDS succumbs to feelings of hopelessness and helplessness. Some take the attitude of a spiritual warrior and use this period for self-reflection and the establishment of more life-sustaining priorities. Gary, one of the New York study participants, said in an interview, "It's almost like the diagnosis suddenly gave me a reason to live. It gave me something to hook on to, something to get me going in a positive mode. I'm a much more positive and happy person now, and despite my situation, I enjoy my life to the fullest. I do a lot more things than I never did before. I really enjoy my life a lot more now." Thus for some, AIDS may serve as a spark to live life more fully and to break out of long-standing patterns of health-negating behaviors.

Those persons with AIDS who improve often experience the process as becoming a more integrated human being and feeling more in control despite external circumstances. The term "control" has a dual significance here. This beneficial kind of control is at once a sense of personal discipline and, paradoxically, a relinquishing of control. Oscar, a long-term survivor from the New York study, told us, "It's been very hard for me *not to be in control*. There are certain things you have to give up, like fixed ways of thinking. It's hard to trust the universe and just go with the flow. The first four weeks of dropping drugs and stimulants were absolutely torture." Several members of the New York group believe macrobiotics has helped them feel more flexible, more open to new possibilities (like recovering from AIDS), and generally more willing to let go of fixed ideas and behaviors.

Control, in this sense, is the ability to flow with change, to withstand great challenges, or to respond appropriately in the face of unforeseen difficulties. As long as we realize that our actions and responses make a difference in every situation, we can maintain a sense of personal autonomy, inner peace, and spiritual freedom. These attitudes are the basis for a more disciplined and orderly way of life. Fear and anxiety arise when we try to control an unpredictable situation. Feelings of depression and helplessness result when we experience a situation as out of control. The healthy sense of control connotes a faith in one's ability to heal and live more fully, as well as a willingness to make mistakes. It is referred to as an "inner locus of control." It is now recognized as one of the key factors for promoting sound immunity.

The basic link between self-esteem and immune status suggests that more attention should be directed toward enhancing one's sense of self.

Attitude, Behavior, and Immunity

ENHANCES IMMUNE FUNCTION	DEPRESSES IMMUNE FUNCTION
Daily Behavioral Pattern	
Appropriate, balanced nutrition	Inappropriate, poor-quality nutrition
Regular, moderate exercise	Inactivity or erratic exercise patterns
Relaxation, meditation	Emotional stress, frequent anxiety
Simple pleasures and entertainment	Habitual substance abuse (e.g., drugs)
Regular, paced breathing practice	Smoking and shallow breathing
Regular, adequate sleep	Insomnia, somnolence
Approach to Life and Health	
Active, self-responsible approach	Resigned, helpless approach
Optimistic, positive outlook	Pessimistic, cynical outlook
Humorous, light orientation	Overly serious, heavy orientation
Curiosity, inquisitiveness	Boredom, closemindedness
Sense of purpose, commitment	Apathy, aimlessness, myopic outlook
Change seen as opportunity to grow	Change experienced as personal threat
Internal equanimity, stability	Agitation, restlessness, volatility
Strong social support system	Isolation, lack of close friendships
Involvement, social integration	Alienation, lack of integration
Warm rapport with family	Poor rapport with family
Psychological Parameters	
Internal locus of control	External locus of control
Positive self-esteem	Negative self-esteem
Happy, positive attitude	Depressed, negative attitude
Moderate self-confidence	Too much or too little self-confidence
Personal autonomy	Strong needs for dependency
Ability to express anger	Inability to express anger

The macrobiotic approach seems to have a marked effect on this aspect of the psyche. Positive changes in body image, usually followed by improvements in self-esteem, often arise after an initial detoxification period when one adopts a balanced diet and health-promoting life-style. Moreover, taking better care of oneself serves as a powerful metaphor for affirming or furthering one's self-worth. The possibly key role of positive self-esteem in the context of AIDS seems aptly reflected in the profiles of long-term survivors in the New York study.

The individual's ability to develop and sustain meaningful personal relationships—with family, friends, lovers, and co-workers—is a critical ingredient in the recovery of health. Conversely, a sense of isolation or alienation from others, as well as from the natural environment, is antithetical to the healing process. What is called for instead is an active sense of relationship and involvement in all situations, personal and impersonal. In our interview with Adam, who was diagnosed with AIDS nearly six years ago, he discussed how his range of sociability had expanded since beginning macrobiotics. He said that he had developed a more relaxed and fulfilling rapport with women, and that his attraction to men had taken on a more spiritual significance. Overall, macrobiotics had helped Adam "feel more whole as a person" and "more connected to people and experiences."

This introduces another component in the psychological profile: the individual's spiritual orientation, as revealed by those aspects of daily life which are most meaningful, or which experiences are most valuable, nurturing, and sustaining. Some experiences are primarily self-oriented, others are more altruistic or socially oriented. In any case, the spiritual outlook or "philosophy of life" serves as a dynamic perceptual tool in daily living and provides reference points for decision-making.

A Philosophy for Life and Healing

What do you think has become of the young and old
   men?
And what do you think has become of the women
and children?

They are alive and well somewhere,
The smallest sprout shows there is really no death,
And if ever there was it led forward life, and does not
wait at the end to arrest it,
And ceas'd the moment life appear'd.

All goes onward and outward, nothing collapses,
And to die is different from what any one supposed,
   and luckier.
                              —Walt Whitman, "Song of Myself"

Perfect love casteth out fear.
                              —I John 4: 18

One insight gained from discussions with participants of the New York study was that an individual's worldview, or personal philosophy of life, may play a profound role in one's ability to maintain good health. While every individual had a slightly different outlook, they all held similar attitudes which seemed to reduce the anxiety normally evoked by AIDS. Positive, life-enhancing attitudes arose spontaneously in the course of recovery. It was as if any sign of improvement—from the clearing of facial complexion to a pronounced increase in stamina—gave one a new lease on life. The process of living in the context of life-threatening illness became an opportunity to widen one's focus from a narrow set of goals or desires to a greater emphasis on relationships, the beauty of nature, and a greater appreciation for the simple fact of life itself.

Some positive changes in attitude and philosophical outlook arise naturally through the study of macrobiotics. By this inherently optimistic worldview, the universe is seen as a harmonious, orderly organism operating for the benefit of all creatures within it. Illness is considered an imbalance within the organism. Understanding the totality of this imbalance enables one to direct one's way of life toward the recovery of balance. Illness is not seen as a matter of chance, morality or divine punishment, but merely as a reflection of one's ignorance of natural order, and thus as an opportunity for learning, growth, and enlightenment. In particular, the experience of disease (*dis-ease*) affords the possibility for expanding awareness of the relationship between self and environment, which in turn underlies the responsibility for one's entire well-being.

Such personal responsibility encompasses one's sense of empowerment and ability to transform one's condition from sickness to health, imbalance to balance. This concept contrasts sharply with the common view of the individual as a victim of cruel fate—*struck* by the mysterious AIDS virus or by so-called terminal cancer—a view which actually disempowers and leaves one fearful, confused, and impotent.

Through the process of renewing health by simple life-style adjustments, this perspective eventually shifts from a mere concept to become an integral way of understanding and *experiencing* the world. It becomes the lens of the mind's eye, giving accent and depth to all experiences, positive and negative. Sickness and health, life and death, are recognized as dynamic, complementary aspects of a divine order which is inseparable from the events and activities of daily life.

By the macrobiotic view, everything in the universe is composed of energy or vibration. All matter is a permutation of the same energy which courses throughout the entire universe, producing all phenomena and governing all processes of change. Since energy is constantly moving, all is in constant flux. Every atom, molecule, and cell in our bodies is changing from moment to moment. As each cell in the body is created, another is being broken down. The balance between creation and destruction is maintained by the orderly patterning of the universal "life-energy" which surrounds us and interacts with the energy fields we generate by virtue of our organic quality—the composition of our blood and tissues. The smooth flow of energy through the living body determines our relative condition of health. Every aspect of our biochemical make-up merely mirrors this subtle, magnificent dance of energy on which our life depends and by which all life processes are essentially animated.

Given that all is flux and movement, we could also say everything is alive. Hence what we call "dead" is actually but an abstraction, a construct of the human mind. Chief Seattle, a great visionary of the native Americans, once said, "There is no death, only a change of worlds." In the language of modern physics, the law of conservation dictates that energy is neither created nor destroyed. Thus all energy exists eternally. Since we too are energy, we never really die in the ultimate, vibrational sense. Only when we allow our three-dimensional reality to be the *only* reality does death appear as an absolute end. But quantum physics has revealed that the three-dimensional reality is organized by an imperceptible, multidimensional reality, the so-called implicate order, which exists beyond the realm of the five senses. From this extremely subtle realm unfolds the tangible, explicate realm of physical matter. In the implicate realm, there is only eternal movement and change; there is only order and wholeness, an implicit perfection underlying and interconnecting the perceptible realm of separate objects and events.[17]

True healing means to make whole, to reestablish a profound sense of affinity with the universe, hence our desire to preserve and enhance our life. But most people think of healing as the elimination of physical signs and symptoms. This is considered the only measure of therapeutic success over the ravages of illness. Conversely, death is perceived as personal failure. This concept permeates society, from the level of individuals to that of institutions, from patients to the medical establishment. The language used in the care of ill people is one of winning or losing battles in the vicious fight against disease. Agents assigned the role of causing disease are viewed as invaders to be killed or conquered. The invading microbe and malignant tumor are the enemy to be vanquished, while the physician treating disease is the ally without which victory is deemed virtually impossible.

This basic attitude has profoundly influenced the quality and intensity of modern medicine's approach and the patient's role in dealing with disease. Allopathic treatments—drugs, medication, radiation, and surgery—are in large part designed according to their degree of aggressiveness against a particular disease entity, often to the extent that they involve drastic levels of toxicity which diminish the individual's sense of well-being and ability to recover. Excessive reliance on powerful pharmacologic drugs is largely the product of this conquest-oriented mentality. The physician is driven to avoid failure with his patients and must, at all costs, avoid losing the battle, often-times at the cost of losing his patient. The patient, on the other hand, surrenders his power by abdicating responsibility for the resolution of the condition, having been indoctrinated by the cultural notion that we are victims of circumstances beyond our control, outside ourselves. Because illness is viewed primarily in this way, the entire process is not appreciated beyond its gross physical manifestations.

With microbes and malignancies posing as the enemy on one side, and the medical establishment posing as the defending army on the other, the patient himself becomes the battleground. He becomes removed from, in a sense, the power of participation. The patient is seen as—and perceives himself as—standing between that which is attacking him and that which will save him. Stripped of his own sense of personal autonomy and self-regenerative ability, he is overwhelmed by a sense of total vulnerability, entirely at the mercy of either the invading organism or his own "defending army," or both. This engenders the so-called *victim mentality*, a way of thinking rooted in a sense of fear and separateness from the natural world. The victim mentality feeds into feelings of anxiety, resentment, and apathy, all of which tend to undermine the possibility of healing.

Under these circumstances, there can be no real victory for the patient. The entire outcome of the battle is placed, literally, in the physician's hands. Armed with the best of medical technology, the physician strives to avert death. At the same time, however, the physician can borrow the power rendered by the patient's fear of death. Thus, for the physician, death represents both ally and adversary. His encounters with the patient become enshrouded in an ominous power struggle which affects the ulimate course of therapy. As discussed by Jay Katz in *The Silent World of Doctor and Patient*, the physicians' dual orientation toward death "casts a dark shadow over another covert struggle between physicians and patients: how life is to be lived. Life, including the life of illness, can be lived in myriads of ways, and not only according to the views of physicians." Katz also points out that "doctors view death as a personal defeat rather than an eventual inevitability to which they, like their patients, must submit."[18]

If the symptoms of disease are successfully eradicated by drugs or medical procedures, the patient's role in health and illness goes undervalued and unappreciated. In most cases, rather than embrace an orientation that promotes life and health, the individual upholds the former attitudes and behaviors from which the previous disease conditions originated.

The problem here seems rooted in our fundamental view of health and disease, and in our tendency to deny ourselves the *experience* of these phenomena. We have forgotten that disease, like health, is a natural process. Like birth and death, pleasure and pain, health and illness are opposite poles of life to be understood through experience and self-reflection. As Larry Dossey, M.D., states in *Beyond Illness*, to deny illness is to undermine our understanding of the nature of life itself.

> We do not know how to savor health because we have lost the vital connections between health and illness. One cannot replace an organic relatedness with the world with antibiotics, surgical procedures, and promissory immortality without destroying something that is vital, something that is health itself. It is not that modern interventions are "bad," but that they are no substitute for the wisdom of "the way things are" . . . Technology is not wisdom of itself; it is no guarantor of the experience of health.[19]

Dossey points out that excessive reliance on medical technology has cost us much of our sense of connection to the natural process of living, which includes both health and disease. It has blinded us from the fact that birth and death, health and sickness, are inseparably related in the flow of life. Ironically, it is largely through our fear of death and disease that we end up becoming sick more often and more severely and dying prematurely. As long as we view disease as something which controls us, which constitutes an exclusively external threat to our survival, we cannot succeed in the process of healing. We remain the victim of our own beliefs and perceptions of life.

Even when a medical crisis is "resolved" on the gross physical level, the fear remains that it can happen again. In this case the individual feels out of control and usually adopts a cynical and hypercritical view of self-healing methods. As noted before, this creates fertile ground for an intensified disease process or for the recurrence of disease. Unfortunately, most medical procedures bring only the illusion of success. While the immediate episode has been eliminated, the overall process of disease continues. If successive treatments fail, the physician's battle is considered lost, and nature's evil forces again become the victors. At this point, if all medical attempts have failed, many literally resign themselves to dying. *Joie de vivre* no longer seems to be an option as one becomes overwhelmed by the doomsday scenario portended by grim statistics and gloomy newscasts.

Sometimes, however, while facing a so-called terminal illness the individual may choose to step back and reevaluate the situation. He may choose to see illness as an opportunity for learning and enlightenment through which healing ultimately takes place beyond and not limited to the physical dimension. He develops an appreciation for that which may be accomplished through reasonable, self-directed means (health-oriented life-style adjustments), as well as a guarded awareness of inappropriate means (toxic, experimental drugs). This creates an environment in which the condition and welfare of the whole person is gauged not only in physical terms, but also in emotional and spiritual terms.

Confronted with the possibility of imminent death, some people acquire a profound sense of appreciation and gratitude for the simpler and often taken-for-granted things in life. In her superb book, *Minding the Body, Mending the Mind*, Dr. Joan Borysenko reports a Japanese study, headed by Dr. Yujiro Ikemi, which focused on a small group of survivors from cancers usually considered incurable.[20] Dr. Yujiro Ikemi noted that each survivor's initial response to the diagnosis had been one of sincere gratitude for life. They were grateful for what had passed before, for being alive in the present, and for whatever life they might have remaining. Also, in all five patients, the cancer had appeared at a time of great existential crisis. Rather than yield to fear, cynicism and apathy, each patient had decided to regard the crisis as an opportunity for resolving the issues that had created them. Each person chose to view the crisis as a positive spiritual challenge and was willing to accept responsibility for the situation. Lastly, each patient had completely and sincerely availed themselves to the will of God or infinite order.[21]

Gratitude for difficulty can serve as the spiritual antidote to fear, which is the ultimate block to all healing. When we allow ourselves to focus on our glass as being half full rather than half empty, the process of healing is greatly enhanced. This kind of gratitude enables us to appreciate more fully the myriad vicissitudes of life, the ebb and flow of daily experience. In climbing a mountain, the more we experience hardship, the greater our joy when we reach the top. In fighting a war, the more misery we experience, the greater our appreciation of peace. In suffering from illness, the more serious the illness, the greater our spirit of appreciation when we restore health. Difficulties are paradoxically the cause of happiness, and avoiding them is the root cause of our unhappiness. In order to be happy all the time, we should continue to avail ourselves to difficulties as they arise, while at the same time carefully attending to our physical health.

Sickness may therefore present the opportunity to appreciate greater health. During the healing process, one experiences a release of tensions, stressful conditions, and behavioral patterns which have brought about physical and spiritual degeneration. In the resolution of these fundamental issues, the toxicity or pathogenic aspects of the disease and their effects on the immune system are lifted and the natural process of healing is suddenly free to take place.

Macrobiotics helps the individual realize his or her place as part of a larger life process. By placing the vast multiplicity of all phenomena in the context of universal balance and unity, the macrobiotic perspective removes the stigma of fear and helplessness, the mystical threat of invading organisms, and the ever-present reality of cellular disintegration or physiologic dysfunction. In addition, awareness of universal order enables one to see one's personal life from a broader perspective and allows one to make choices that have harmonious rather than chaotic consequences. This, in turn, instills a sense of control over one's destiny and thereby promotes a more confident and positive movement toward personal wholeness. The entire process is supported at a most fundamental level by the organic healing power of a natural, vegetable-quality diet and harmonious life-style. These integral components work collectively in the restoration of order on all levels, from cellular to psychic, from self to society.

Each of us is part of a larger whole, which functions for the benefit of all its parts. The idea that we are an integral yet infinitesimal part of the universe, and the concept of the ephemerality of all things within this eternal order, enables us to see both the relative insignificance of this fleeting lifetime and the critical importance of each passing moment. Through awareness of the value of being fully present, one comes to focus on the experience of each moment, and thus chooses those things which will continually enhance the quality of life. This, in turn, creates the opportunity for living, growing, and evolving toward the highest human achievement—the awareness of the connectedness of all things and the infinite order of life.

The process of healing is never entirely uniform; each individual experience has its own peculiar rhythm. In time, the individual with AIDS comes to see that what matters is not the outcome of the healing crisis, but the *process* and our experience of each moment within that process. The activity itself thus affords the individual an opportunity for spiritual growth and greater awareness. Our awareness of each moment in the present is the key element here, for such awareness inevitably leads to a greater willingness to risk, to *choose* to change, and thus leads to the capacity for self-regeneration, personal well-being, and increased lifespan.

As expressed by Larry Dossey, M.D., in *Beyond Illness*, the principle of complementary opposites has a fundamental bearing on our mental and emotional well-being. Beyond the physical plane, opposites exist as abstract, relativistic concepts belonging to the realm of thought. By the very acts of focusing our attention on any one concept, we create its opposite. Thus light could not exist without dark, male without female, health without sickness, birth without death. Awareness of the unity of opposites then leads to the experience of life as a dynamic, orderly interplay of polarized tendencies. It leads to the profound realization that order prevails even amidst chaos, that all apparent antagonisms are complementary as well.

In this state of awareness, one appreciates the whole of nature as observed through the cyclic movements of summer and winter, light and dark, birth and death, happiness and strife, acceptance and denial, wholeness and fragmentation. In acknowledging the truth of this endless, orderly flow of change and extending this sense of truth to our own lives, we are better able to appreciate our personal events and experiences as necessary for evolution toward greater wholeness. Acceptance of the rightness and fairness of natural order frees one from regret over past mistakes or fear of future tribulations and can heighten one's ability to create joy and harmony in daily life.

Paul, another of the study's participants, said that his appreciation for life had come out of the recognition that he had basically two choices: live or die. He decided ". . . to have the joy for living and to appreciate things more. For the first time when I was confronted with this life-or-death thing, I actually chose to be positive and put all the wonderful energy that I had put into negative living into positive living."

On the psychosocial level, awareness of universal order fosters an appreciation of all people and interpersonal events as essential nourishment for personal growth and spiritual evolution. As one gives to others, so also does one nurture oneself by expanding one's sense of self, for by showing compassion for the world one frees oneself from the bondage and loneliness of the ego. Some 2500 years ago this basic truth was proclaimed in the negative by Buddha: "Do not do unto others as you would not have them do unto you." Following him, the same truth was expressed in the positive by Christ: "Do unto others as you would have them do unto you." A more recent interpretation may include Pogo's remark: "We have met the enemy and it is us." The flip-side of this statement is that, once we recognize our ability to create our experience or reality, we become our own allies and take control of the situation at hand.

Considered in this light, illness is no longer a devastating end in and of itself, but instead serves as a vital bridge to recovery of greater personal and interpersonal freedom and awareness. Moreover, as we recognize our true wants and needs, and as we learn to focus on what is of real importance in each moment of life, the experience of illness opens up opportunities for establishing meaningful relationships with others.

Serious disease may sometimes compel us to confront the imminence of death. In doing so, we may suddenly glimpse the true meaning of life on a cosmic scale, as well as the ephemerality and relative insignificance of our own personal life. By expanding our sense of self in this way, we can better let go of the fear of dying and are better able to prevent premature death. In other instances illness may reveal to us the appropriateness of death and enable us to direct our remaining life toward resolving old conflicts which lay hidden or seemingly beyond reach. The process of one's individual life—the period between birth and death—is part of an immense continuum of continual evolution toward higher spiritual awareness and ultimate perfection. To live life fully requires accepting the reality of death.

Cultivating an appreciation for natural order is a crucial step toward fully recovering our natural birthright of inner peace and harmony. Furthermore, by letting go of fear, guilt, judgments, resentment, low self-esteem, and all other negative or disruptive emotions, we make available the energy necessary for healing mind and body, and greatly enhance the potential for recovery from disease or other hardship. The process can be further supported by realizing our ability to choose our responses to these aspects of our emotional life, as well as to the environment as a whole.

Rather than imprison ourselves with self-destructive emotional habits and attitudes toward life—which are themselves merely reflecting our ignorance of natural order—we can learn to regulate and transform them into their opposite tendencies. Techniques such as meditation, yoga, tai chi, music, visualization, and dance, are all viable options, and each may be explored to determine which is (are) most appropriate for individual needs. By instilling a sense of inner peace and order in daily life, these practices will reinforce the calming effects produced by following a simple grain-and-vegetable-based diet.

The recognition that one is solely responsible for oneself and one's world does not mean that one has literally created the world, nor that the world is merely a figment of one's imagination. It means, rather, that the meaning of the world, its events, objects, and people, are all determined by one's mode of perception—one's own worldview or paradigm. Moreover, it means that one knows oneself to be the cause and context of this mode of perception. Werner Erhard, founder of EST, calls this "being at cause." If one feels discontent or unhappy, it is ultimately due to a distorted perception and dualistic interpretation of the situation at hand: one has assigned false or fragmentary meaning to the presumed "cause" of one's unhappiness. For example, a woman suffering from frequent fungal infections slips into deep depression and associates the condition with her sexual relations. As long as she blames her problem on external influences—in this instance, her boyfriend—the infection persists. Instead, attention should be turned to the practical aspect of daily patterns of living, including dietary practice.

Changing one's negative emotional state may therefore entail two steps: (1) working through the emotional energy in a positive, constructive way (meditation, movement, playful activities, psychotherapy, etc.); and (2) making a fundamental change in one's total perspective, as illustrated by several of the men interviewed from the New York study. It is this latter step to which macrobiotics makes its greatest contribution in the area of psychosocial problems. Macrobiotics offers us a profound perceptual tool for seeing our world as a benign and orderly home, to be respected and honored. As Jesus said in *The Gospel According to Thomas*: "The Kingdom of Heaven is spread upon the earth, yet men do not see it."

Relaxation, Pleasure, and Self-discipline —————————

> There is no need to run outside
> For better seeing
> Nor to peer from a window. Rather abide
> At the center of your being;
> For the more you leave it, the less you learn.
> —Lao Tze, *Tao Te Ching*

One of the simplest and most powerful ways to induce the *relaxation response*, the body's natural stress-reducing response, is the practice of meditation. Beyond its practical function of counteracting anxiety states, meditation may be seen as a natural process of self-reflection, or a harmonious attunement with all of our thoughts and feelings, whether based in the past (e.g., guilt, grief), in the present (e.g., anger, depression), or in the future (e.g., fear, anxiety). The basic aim is not to suppress these mental and emotional processes, not to analyze or judge them, but to simply observe and gently let go of them as they arise.

Although there are many styles of meditation, the basic form involves sitting quietly with eyes closed, shoulders relaxed, and posture straight. One commonly recommended practice is centering awareness on the rhythmic flow of breathing. We simply allow ourselves to notice how the breath goes in and out, without trying to control it in any way. The breathing tends to get slower and shallower as the meditation progresses. This is one of the natural physiological effects of the relaxation response: as metabolism slows down, the body requires less oxygen. When we do this consistently on a regular basis, we usually begin to experience deep relaxation and peacefulness, the magnitude of which increases with practice. As the breathing slows, so does the mind, and yet we become more aware, more able to concentrate despite distractions, and more inclined to relax spontaneously in high-pressure situations.

Through the daily practice of meditation (twenty minutes, twice a day is highly recommended), we train the mind in the art of dynamic awareness. This awareness will carry over into our day-to-day experiences, affording us more clarity and flexibility in our choices and responses, and restoring our ability to enjoy the simplest of life's pleasures. Meditation can also be applied directly to various activities, such as a simple walk around the block, knitting a quilt, or cooking a delicious meal. Ultimately, the meditative mood becomes second nature to us. As Joan Borysenko, M.D., writes in *Minding the Body, Mending the Mind*, "The final goal of meditation is to be constantly conscious of experience so that relaxation and peace of mind become the norm rather than the exception."[22]

Dr. Borysenko, who is co-founder and director at the Mind/Body Clinic at New England Deaconess Hospital, pinpoints "mindfulness" as the active ingredient in meditation. By training ourselves to be fully mindful of the present, we can become more perceptive of deeper levels of meaning and of a more expansive reality. Mindful action means intent atertness to whatever enters our awareness in the present. This mode of being has been understood since ancient times and is still practiced in various parts of the world. It has been formalized in Eastern traditions, such as the ancient tea ceremony of Japan and the practice of tai ch'i chuan in China. Mindful action entails allowing yourself to open your attention completely, to gently focus on everything—thoughts, sensations, sounds, and feelings—as they enter your awareness. Mindfulness is meditation in action.

Meditation can exert a powerful influence on our sense of time. According to Larry Dossey, M.D., in *Space, Time, and Medicine* (Shambhala Publications, 1982), our mode of temporal awareness influences our capacity to cope with potentially stressful circumstances and thereby affects our state of health. Time is our measure of change, and yet change itself is an eternal process. The clock measures time in relation to human perceptibility, and the minutes and seconds ticking away on our clocks are convenient indicators of the passage of time. The classical perception of a fleeting time convinces us that linear time is escaping; time is "lost" or "running out," and the temporal flow of experience seems to be moving along an ever-tightening spiral.

If our sense of time is overly contracted, we tend to feel tight, anxious, and dissatisfied with life. We tend to feel helplessly closed off from the larger whole of existence, and our actions are more often based on egocentric attitudes. This contracted temporal awareness infuses our entire way of life with a restless energy that demands the utmost speed and efficiency. It usually reflects the way we see reality and is fundamentally based on fear. Often it manifests as the need for power which derives from *the fear of losing control.* The basis for this fear, as discussed by Michio Kushi in *Stress and Hypertension* (Japan Publications, Inc., 1989), derives fundamentally from two sources: our worldview and biochemistry, both of which are influenced by our daily way of life, including dietary practices.

For most of us in today's fast-paced world, learning mindfulness takes much patience and commitment. It is advisable to choose at least one activity each day to carry out mindfully, with full attention. For example, taking a mindful walk every day is an excellent practice. Learn to walk slowly while simply observing the sensations in your feet and legs as you move them each in turn. Observe the sensations in your body as a whole and in your breathing, which should become deep and relaxed. Maintain a relaxed gaze at some point in front of you. Learning to walk in this way is one of the most powerful tools for relieving tension and establishing inner clarity and stability.

Mindfulness may of course be applied to any activity, whether it be chewing food, scrubbing floors, or driving a car. For instance, if you are cutting vegetables, simply cut vegetables while absorbing yourself in the colors, scents, textures, and movement. If you are cleaning house in the morning, just clean house with full attention to the activity itself.

While the practice of mindfulness itself is easy, its effectiveness is relative to our spirit and intent. In the beginning, we may need to remind ourselves constantly so that it becomes a habit, for example, by putting small notes around the house or making regular affirmations of "I am mindful, I am present in this moment." Another excellent practice is learning to listen with full attention whenever engaged in conversation.

The practice of meditation enables us to establish total harmony within ourselves. It brings home the realization that, as Jesus said, "the Kingdom of God is within you." As a process of spiritual attenument, meditation helps us realize the infinite healing powers or qualities that lie within us: love, faith, humility, and gratitude. These four elements are the fundamental ingredients of all forms of enduring healing. They are the spiritual means by which we unveil our deepest, self-regenerative capacities.

A balance of moderate yet regular exercise and relaxation will promote the strength of the cardiovascular and lymphatic systems. There are a wide variety of relaxation methods to choose from. To realize the full value of meditation or visualization exercises, they should be carried out completely and consistently on a day-to-day basis.

Closely aligned with the need for relaxation is the need for pleasure. The pleasure we experience in our daily activities has an important place in healing and in our resistance to disease. Consider job satisfaction. Research suggests that those of us who derive a sense of personal fullfillment from our work tend to experience better health and longevity. As long as we maintain an attitude of balance and moderation—taking time to relax and attend to interpersonal needs—the desire to work hard at something we feel is meaningful or worthwhile will not be harmful.

A great deal of psychological healing can take place simply through a positive, pleasurable approach to life. The pleasure derived from caring for and about people draws us out of a narrow concern with ourselves into a larger involvement with life. The pleasure of studying and applying certain philosophies, mores, and customs, helps us to establish a sense of order and coherence in our lives. Joking, laughing, acting like a kid, or going to a funny movie are all valid ways of improving health. Just as gardening and cleaning house are beneficial forms of exercise, an orderly and pleasurable way of life is an invaluable form of self-psychotherapy.

The practice of macrobiotics helps instill the necessary clarity and flexibility to balance the stresses and conflicts in our lives with harmonious relationships and the taken-for-granted simple pleasures, such as breathing and walking. With the consistent practice of macrobiotics, and as one's condition becomes more stable and one's mental outlook more clear, pleasure itself seems to take on new meaning. As tastes and blood chemistry shift to a more even keel, former sensorial attractions (to exotic foods, loud music, etc.) become less extreme. Several of the participants in the study remarked that the food had become more delicious to them than they could have previously imagined. As their taste buds adjusted and their cooking skills developed, the macrobiotic way of eating became increasingly palatable—and pleasurable.

Getting to this stage of simple pleasure, however, is often quite challenging, requiring much self-discipline, self-confidence and personal autonomy. Rudy, another long-term survivor in the study, told us how trying the transition to macrobiotics can really be:

> Becoming macrobiotic was the hardest thing I ever did. I had to change everything—how I thought, how I ate, how I lived. First I had to take responsibility for my illness. I couldn't think of myself as just an innocent victim any longer. Then I had to give up all the foods I really enjoyed—cheese, ice cream, pastries, coffee, not to mention alcohol and other drugs. I already had given up sex because of the illness, so altogether most of my playthings in life were taken away. I had to go from being completely self-indulgent to being a semi-ascetic: from Hugh Hefner to St. Francis. Besides, I wasn't free any longer to medicate away my emotional problems and tensions. I had to deal with my self-loathing, my anger towards my parents and toward society, all without relying on drugs. I have had some pretty rough moments over the past two years.[23]

Rudy's experience indicates that the very act of tempering one's former desires usually causes one to look at those areas of life that have been denied or are in need of attention. Emotional issues come to the surface as one's orientation changes and attention turns toward caring for oneself. For others, the fine balance of pleasure and discipline takes on an altruistic significance that, in time, tends to annul any sense of deprivation, punishment, or denial. Of his experiences with adhering to macrobiotic principles in the New York study, Oscar said the following:

> I have learned not to look upon my restrictions as punishment. For a very long time, I thought that I was being punished, and macrobiotics was part of my payment....Now I know that's not the way it works, that's not the way I want it to be ... I look upon it more as simply trying to make the right decision from moment to

moment. I ask: what would be better for everybody involved? I feel part of something else. I don't divorce myself from the rest of the world. I go beyond thinking of ice cream or coffee as pertaining to the individual me. I see my life in a more universal way. If I look at it as complete, I feel part of a group and I am responsible to our being here. What can I do to make us better? If I mess up, it's we who are going to suffer . . . Although I'm an individual, I have to think as a collective whole.

Thus, rather than restricting his freedom, Oscar's efforts to maintain the discipline of a healing diet had become a form of self-renunciation which granted him profound inner fulfillment. He saw his healing as a larger process of social healing.

Empowerment and self-discipline are important themes to bring out in the course of counseling. Consider this statement by Max, a participant who began practicing macrobiotics three months after being diagnosed with AIDS in September of 1983:

I've gained tremendous respect for my vessel, this body of mine. Macrobiotics puts control where it belongs—back in your mouth, in your body. It gives us the capacity to say 'yes' and 'no' again, to choose the quality of our life, not just with food, but in all activities, with all stimuli. I really feel that it can pull gay people, individually and in general, out of isolation, give us a real universal viewpoint on our humanity . . . So many people are dying. We can't expect that this will be taken care of *for* us, it has to come *from* us.[24]

The paradox of a disciplined, orderly way of life that respects our physiological limitations is that, rather than inhibiting us, it enhances our sense of freedom. We become less attached to material means of gratification, less bound by our sensorial whims, and therefore more free in spirit. Peace and contentment are not in things; they are in us. The Buddha is said to have died laughing after eating a piece of meat. The typical Zen monk is portrayed with a broadly smiling face, revealing the gentle, playful nature of one who can appreciate the simplest pleasures in life—the humor and irony, the beauty and magnificence of each experience. With the right attitude, the discipline of balanced diet and lifestyle can even liberate us from the illusion of happiness through sensorial gratification. By living simply, attending to the basic necessities of health and well-being, we will naturally unveil the happiness that is our real nature.

Directives for Counseling and Therapy ━━━━━━━━━

The primary purpose of counseling is three-fold: (1) to help the individual accept the reality of the disease and its ramifications, including personal concerns such as self-image and attitudes, health concerns such as management of symptoms, and social concerns such as potential loss of job, family and peer support, and community resources; (2) to assist the individual in realizing that health and sickness, living and dying, are choices, conditions that are largely controllable; and (3) to guide the patient toward a health-promoting way of life, as well as appropriate modes of therapy for physical and mental health.

(1) Identification of Key Concerns. At the 1986 International Conference on AIDS, noted psychiatrist Stephen Nichols, M.D. (whose quote appears at the beginning of this chapter) described the psychological aspects of coping with AIDS. Based on his experience in treating several hundred persons with AIDS and ARC since 1981, Dr. Nichols outlined three stages of adjustment most commonly experienced: a crisis, transition, and resolution.

In the *crisis stage*, the individual reacts with strong denial of the condition and of one's fears related to the diagnosis. This denial is a normal reaction which serves to protect the individual from intense emotional pain. If maintained indefinitly, however, such denial may also engender complacency, apathy, helplessness, and profound anxiety. Family, friends, or peers tend to mirror this process by avoiding or distancing themselves from the disease, or from those who may have the disease. Because of homophobia and the popular idea of AIDS as a "gay disease," many people, even heterosexuals, may become isolated.[25]

According to Dr. Nichols, people in the crisis stage often have difficulty comprehending information and may distort what they are told regarding their condition. Prolonged denial instills an "emotional numbness" which alters their ability to discriminate between appropriate and inappropriate courses of action, such as opting for experimental, usually toxic, drug treatments.[26] For this reason, contact with supportive services such as macrobiotic counseling, support-group meetings, group therapy, legal and financial assistance, housing and self-healthcare education should be sought as early as possible. Many of these services are available through agencies in the gay community, such as the Gay Men's Health Crisis in New York City or the Shanti Project in San Francisco.

The *transitional stage* is the most turbulent expression of adjustment. This begins when the individual's denial is superseded by alternating waves of anxiety, anger, guilt, and self-pity. According to Dr. Nichols, this is "... a time of great distress, confusion, and disruptiveness. It often occurs as patients leave the hospital and encounter social rejection which further aggravates their distress ... everything seems to be changing. They don't know whom they can trust or depend on. Despite this chaos, however, patients are desperate for guidance and are especially accessible to professional intervention."[27]

This is also the stage at which tremendous anger and resentment may be evoked. Guilt regarding one's condition may give way to anger toward one's own person. Anger may be sparked further by confronting public hostility and prejudice. In most cases, however, this anger is repressed, perhaps because it is considered inappropriate or unfounded, or because the atmosphere surrounding one's daily life does not readily lend itself to such emotional release. According to Dr. Nichols, many individuals repress this anger through "bargaining," in which they "hope to be saved by being good." Instead of venting this anger, most express sadness, depression, or negative self-esteem. Suicidal tendencies are common during this stage.

To reach the next stage, the experience of *resolution*, the individual with AIDS must first come to *accept* his own person and illness. He must stop blaming himself and others. At the same time, this personal acceptance can be bolstered by the acceptance and consideration of his peers and family. Counselors can help patients and their families reach this stage by gently confronting the fear and emotional concerns connected with the symptoms and possibility of death. In addition to attending support-group meetings, integrative forms of psychotherapy such as Rubenfeld Synergy or other gestalt approaches are highly recommended to help one work through blocks to positive self-esteem.

(2)   Psychological and Spiritual Reorientation.   Many people with AIDS or ARC come to the initial phase of acceptance and then stop. Even though they have reconciled their personal crisis in their own minds, they still lack a sense of empowerment or control over their lives. The possibility of surival becomes a mere pipe dream, a fantasy beyond realization. Falling into resignation, guilt, and self-pity, they say things like, "Look what I've done to myself," or "Look what has happened to me." The individual develops his own belief system to fit his experience of the world and to explain his symptoms. Hearsay and statistics reinforce his pessimism or victim mentality. He believes that his condition will only get worse. Death presents itself as an escape from the pain and suffering, so he quietly chooses to die.

In the context of AIDS, acceptance is a spiritual imperative, demanding wisdom and insight—the clarity and intuition developed through mindfulness and an orderly way of life. For this we must boldly face all our fears. We must look at the world directly, honestly and comprehensively. We can look at ourselves and acknowledge that the discord is not just external, but also exists within ourselves. Rather than deny the painful or difficult aspects of life, we learn to embrace them by allowing our hearts to open to the full range of human experience: life and death, health and sickness, pleasure and pain, darkness and light. Even in the midst of tremendous suffering, we can experience harmony through acceptance of all that exists. Inner peace and contentment are established when we allow ourselves to face our fears, sadness, anxiety, and sense of inadequacy, when we exchange our attachment to seeing how things should be with the wonder and appreciation of things as they are.

Accepting the full scope of our illness serves to crystallize all hopes for recovery. Life and health are, to a large extent, personal choices, byproducts of the way we chose to live. When we are sick or suffering, we may come to realize that at some point we gave up on those choices; we gave our health over to our sensorial whims, or to the hands of fate, or to the expertise of the medical profession. Acceptance of our personal responsibility to life and health becomes the spark which ignites the "fighting spirit," the will that drives all affirmative action. One decides that living and healing are personal choices. People with AIDS may be encouraged to say, "Look what I can do for myself." Out of this simple attitude blossoms a way of living that supports rather than negates life and health. Life-style itself is a direct outcome of beliefs, attitudes, emotions, and motivation.

For every individual, there must be a higher purpose in living, something meaningful beyond the material plane of the five senses. This realm of meaningful experience may be called *spirituality*. The counselor can help people recognize what is meaningful and why it is worth living for. At the same time, the counselor can help one let go of personal judgments, negative self-statements, or a sense of personal inadequacy from not having attained certain goals. Ultimately, the counselor assists people in acquiring a more positive and more functional worldview or philosophy of life.

The philosophy of life provides various frames of reference; it is a kind of spectacles through which we view the world and create the meaning of things. The same set of facts or circumstances can look very different when viewed through another person's eyes. In one frame of reference, a person may see illness as a divine punishment for one's sins, while health represents a reward undeserved, at best an obscure possibility. In another person's frame of reference, however, health represents a resource for experiencing life more fully. It has everything to do with one's present attitude, diet, and activity levels.

The counselor or therapist can help illuminate the various frames of reference which give birth to negative or limited behavioral patterns. For example, if someone believes that dietary changes are the only requirement for recovering health, this can lead to neglect of other areas such as regular exercise and relaxation, both of which interact synergistically with balanced diet. Shifts in our mental attitudes and spiritual outlook can help us realize even deeper levels of healing, ensuring that a synergy of positive, health-promoting factors are brought into play.

By simply listening and being supportive in times of depression, confusion or anxiety, counselors serve primarily as people to talk with, as companions in times of personal need. Compassion, respect, acceptance, firmness, and acknowledgement of another person's gift—all of these are essential attributes of an effective counselor. In addition, the counselors should embrace a dynamic, monistic view of life and death, helping people see beyond the fear of dying to the joy of living in this moment. In this way, counselors can inspire people to take charge of their lives on all levels: physical, mental, emotional, and spiritual.

Counseling can help us expand our view and make life more bearable, even in the midst of personal crisis. The Chinese word for *crisis* is written by combining the symbols for the words "danger" and "opportunity." This reflects the enlightened view that difficult experiences can be either positive or negative, either beneficial or deleterious to one's personal well-being. Being responsible to all our experiences is the basis for realizing the profound growth potential provided by life-threatening disease. Once we have accepted our integral part in the matter, we can get on with the process of living and moreover of enjoying life—even up to the time of death.

Physical health and psychological health are inseparable. With a strong biological condition, we *feel* more alive and resilient, more willing to take on even the most difficult or threatening of situations. By renewing our native vitality, we feel more capable of managing the pressures of daily life, of coping with all forms of stress and tension. Internal dis-ease gives way to positive attitudes and spiritual well-being, and subsequent exposures to stress only serve to strengthen us further. Stress becomes a bright, positive force which makes us stronger and our life more fulfilling. Attention to the practical needs of daily life is just as important as attention to attitudes and overall mental outlook.

(3) Reorientation of Diet, Life-style, and Therapy. The macrobiotic approach addresses the totality of human needs—physical, mental, emotional, social, and spiritual. Dietary needs are determined according to each individual's constitution and condition, and to psychosocial and environmental conditions. By adjusting one's diet in accord with macrobiotic principles—eliminating fats, refined sugars, and toxins and emphasizing whole grains, legumes, and land and sea vegetables—positive physiological changes are effected which, in turn, promote positive psychological changes. After attending to the most controllable aspect of daily self-healthcare (diet), more direct attention can be applied to emotional healing.

Most illnesses associated with negative emotional states involve the repression or denial of feelings. Effective healing at this level demands a three-pronged approach: (1) addressing and being sensitive to the way pain or tension is being held or repressed, (2) identifying the kind of external stimulus or approach needed for its release, and (3) using appropriate techniques to elicit the release and promote a healthy response to emotions when they arise. The body's primitive reactive nature is normally geared to discharge energy before it becomes too concentrated. Through emotional release, such as having a good cry or appropriately releasing anger, one often establishes a more relaxed body that may be reflected in a more relaxed posture or more regular rhythm of breathing.

Research with biofeedback, guided imagery, and hypnosis, suggests that the mind can be trained to either suppress or enhance immunity. As feelings of hopelessness and helplessness decrease, emotional stress diminishes and immune functions show marked improvement.[28] Observations from the New York study suggest that through a combination of counseling, mind-body therapy, support-group activities, and dietary change, a considerable amount of anxiety and emotional trauma may be prevented or alleviated.

Most books on stress-related problems have primarily emphasized the effects or symptoms of stress—high blood pressure, erratic emotional states, headaches, muscle cramping and tension. The approaches suggested to combat stress include meditation, relaxation, yoga, massage, biofeedback, tranquilizers, psychiatric assistance, and simply "learning to cope with stress." Workshops on stress management have asserted that if people become aware that the stress they are under is limiting their performance or life experience, they can overcome the identified stresses through sheer effort. A similar theme is echoed in Dr. Herbert Benson's *The Relaxation Response* and other popular books which advocate specific techniques for reducing blood pressure and alleviating the symptoms of stress.

Simply learning the techniques for relaxation is usually not enough. Since this orientation addresses symptoms rather than underlying causes, in most cases it offers only a temporary or partial solution. The problem is neither the symptoms nor the external source of stress, but inappropriate perceptions and bodily imbalances that fuel the stress response. The real value of these skills will only be realized if they also help transform a person's perception of himself and what is important in life. Self-esteem and a meaningful philosophy of life tend to promote feelings of confidence and coherence, and, in our view, better health. As the main thrust of psychological counseling, this provides the grounding through which practical health concerns are more effectively realized.

While eating well *does* promote the elimination of internal toxins and the establishment of healthy physiological functioning, people will sometimes find themselves in situations in which it is difficult to eat well. Conflicting social or familial forces may induce feelings of self-doubt and fear of alienation, as in the case of someone being ridiculed by his peers for his dietary preferences. Lack of social support is probably the main reason most people opt to deviate from their macrobiotic practice. Infrequent bingeing or general inconsistency in one's dietary practice will slow down the detoxification and rejuvenation process. Here the need for discipline is paramount. In the New York study, those men who have adhered most closely to the dietary guidelines have also been the most clinically stable and required the least medical assistance. Of utmost importance was the avoidance of potential immune stressors in the diet, such as refined sugars, food additives, conventionally produced eggs and poultry, cow's-milk products, and red meats.

All of the men in the New York study chose a variety of holistic therapies to complement their macrobiotic dietary practice. These other "alternative" therapies include stress reduction, meditation, visualization, guided imagery, music and color therapy, exercise, and the constant affirmation of the powers of the mind, spirit, and will to live. In addition, instead of waiting for the body to clean itself gradually, some men have sought to speed up this process by applying various preparations and techniques commonly used for macrobiotic home-care (see *Macrobiotic Home Remedies* by Michio Kushi and Marc Van Cauwenberghe, M.D., Japan Publications, Inc., 1985). Other holistic practices requiring skilled professionals—acupuncturists, herbalists, homeopathic physicians, chiropractors, psychologists, Rubenfeld Synergy practitioners, shiatsu practitioners, and others—were also used. Most holistic professionals believe that, in general, their specialized methods are far more effective when the individual adheres to a natural, balanced diet such as macrobiotics.

In sum, since effective healing involves important changes in attitudes and relationships, as well as in the person's daily health habits, effective counseling for persons with AIDS must extend far beyond issues of transmission and the imminent possibility of dying. It helps to illuminate important biological, psychological, social, philosophical, and spiritual concerns. It teaches one how to live well for the remaining portion of one's life. On the theoretical level, competent counseling recognizes the integral relationships between: (a) mind and immunity, (b) nutrition and immunity, and (c) nutrition and mind (see Appendix E).[29] The abstract and the concrete complement one another. All factors related to health are considered integral to an individual's healing process. No one factor alone is more important than any other, though dietary practice affects us in a more enduring and general way—affecting both mind and immunity—and is more within the realm of control than others.

The Role of Group and Community Support ⎯⎯⎯⎯⎯

> People who love you will always love you. If people cannot support you, then they never really loved you to begin with. My real friends are with me no matter what. They accept all parts of me, including macrobiotics.
>
> —Adam

Since the original construction of AIDS as a "gay disease," and its later description as African and Haitian in origin, minority reactions to AIDS have ranged from silence to hysteria, from denial to rage. The government has proposed testing policies which seek to identify and further isolate marginal groups. Despite the fact that AIDS has begun to creep through the heterosexual population—including a growing number of no-identified-risk individuals—it remains a disease associated in the popular mind with intravenous drug abuse and deviant sexual conduct. Ongoing stigmatization of gay men, female prostitutes, and drug addicts, as well as Blacks, Hispanics, and Haitian immigrants, has magnified the importance of providing strong social support to people with AIDS. In addition, the social specter of this seemingly incurable disease has sparked a reevaluation of social identity and consciousness among male homosexuals and others labeled as high risk for AIDS.

It is important to realize that the psychosocial profile of the typical

American homosexual existed prior to the initial hysteria over AIDS, and may even have contributed to the profile of susceptibility. Among many urban gay men, we often see extreme competitiveness and insecurity, both personally and professionally, which leads to isolation and lack of trust. This may in turn perpetuate feelings of social rejection, alienation, and finally, anger and resentment. Since, in many cases, there is no way to focus, channel, or release this anger, it often turns back on the individual and manifests as self-destructive behavior. The unusually high level of recreational drug abuse in the gay community may be a by-product of this process. In any case, there is a paramount need to deal with repressed anger and other negative emotions so that self-destructive behaviors do not gain the upper hand.

Everyone desires social cohesion, and minority groups are the primary targets of social rejection. Inability to connect with the whole of society can lead to deep-seated frustration and resentment. The macrobiotic approach tends to draw the focus away from the social arena and instead directs attention to the realm of the inner self, to getting in touch with ourselves, renewing our energies, and finding peace within. Through healing ourselves, we begin to experience a greater affinity with the world around us—including people. Paradoxically, even though aspects of macrobiotic living seem far removed from the norm, we actually begin to feel *more* connected with society.

In the New York study, the regular support-group meetings have served an invaluable function. Rather than discuss drug protocols, medical research, or hospital treatment, the conversation usually centers around human relationships, spiritual concerns, the dynamic interaction of mind and body, the healing energies of food and meditation, and personal insights and experiences. Usually one or more doctors and macrobiotic teachers are present, and visitors are also welcome. The atmosphere of these gatherings is invariably light and upbeat. As one observer notes, "Everybody who is from the outside who comes to our meetings are always so knocked out by the positive energy in the room. Even the people who look like they are really close to death have a very positive attitude about their life and what they have chosen to do. So it is important that they try to get themselves involved as much as possible with other people who are thinking the same way."[30]

These meetings have provided a context in which people can express and recognize their fears and anxieties. In this friendly, informal setting, stress and tension are often more readily released than in the conventional psychotherapy setting. In the group context, an individual is exposed to others' emotional difficulties and holding patterns. By listening to others' experiences and sharing his own, he may come to recognize many similarities to his own experience. He realizes that he is not alone and that there are those who genuinely care. The successful, transformative experiences of others can inspire him to transform his own vulnerability into empowerment, his apathy into a more constructive, life-enhancing orientation. And the success of a single individual can rekindle the hopes and enthusiasm of the whole group.

A growing support network has helped many people take charge of their lives through macrobiotics. Most participants in the study have frequently interacted with other members of the macrobiotic community, including teachers and sympathetic physicians. Throughout these interactions, individuals with AIDS have felt accepted and respected without qualification. Says one participant, "If macrobiotics were required to change its name, I think it should be called 'friendship'. I've found friends in the macrobiotic community I never knew existed on this planet, and I'm grateful that AIDS came along because it has helped me acknowledge and understand my self-destructive tendencies. With macrobiotics I feel more [socially] integrated, and more into preserving and enhancing my life." Despite rumors that the Kushi Institute is homophobic, most members of the New York study have expressed similar gratitude for the support they have received from people both inside and outside the movement.

Conclusion

As word of the promise of macrobiotics continues to spread, more scientists are beginning to examine its potential efficacy in the treatment of AIDS. Insights gained from interviews and clinical observations in the New York study should prove useful to other people dealing with AIDS. The medical community has already accepted that positive attitudes and the will to live play an important role in healing. The Simontons' pioneering work with cancer patients has added a whole new component to healing. If a compassionate, caring attitude can positively influence recovery from cancer, might this also be the case with AIDS? Given the integral links between the immune and nervous systems, the placebo effect and other psychic phenomena can no longer be considered extraneous to the process of healing. It is possible that the softer, less objective changes in a person's condition—hope, confidence, curiosity, and humor—tend to precede the more quantifiable ones that show up in the blood. Healing reveals itself not only in quantities of cells and microbes, but also in the quality of a person's feelings, thoughts, and behaviors.

As of January 1988, 8 of the 20 men in this study have died. They will not be forgotten, nor will their courageous commitment and personal contributions to the understanding of AIDS and immunity be forgotten. These last four years have been a time of profound growth and learning for all involved in the New York study. Throughout this time, we have seen that a positive approach to health can be a blessing even to people on their last leg, even as they approach their final hour. Through our dying friends' trials and tribulations, hopes and disappointments, we have often been reminded of the delicate balance by which our lives are maintained.

Preliminary observations from the New York pilot study, despite the absence of a control group, are impressive enough to warrant serious consideration and further investigation. This study has been presented at the second and third sessions of the International Conference on AIDS, yet there has been little response by the medical establishment or popular media. Reports appearing in such widely read publications as *Newsweek* ("Preying on AIDS Patients," June 1, 1987) and *Medical World News* ("AIDS Patients Turn to Unproven Therapies," April 28, 1986) have reflected a mixture of negativity, indifference, and personal bias. Most commentaries imply staunch disbelief that such a simple course of treatment—minimizing the use of drugs and changing the menu—could stabilize and possibly improve the immune systems of AIDS patients. Many people remain rigidly bound by the belief that the ultimate solution to AIDS will come only from expensive therapies sanctioned by the federal government or medical establishment. That dietary changes offer a viable treatment for AIDS is, for most, sheer blasphemy.

The importance of a high-fiber, low-fat diet in preventing cancer has only recently been recognized by the National Cancer Institute and National Academy of Sciences. As with the long and costly war on cancer, diet will probably be the last place medical science looks to treat AIDS. But as Dr. John Beldakas, AIDS researcher of Boston University's School of Medicine has said, "If diet is responsible for affecting the courses of other illnesses, why not AIDS?"[31] Ultimately, the decision to adopt a healthy diet and life-style lies with the individual, not the experts. Here a change in social consciousness is needed, as relatively few Americans really attend to their nutrition, exercise, and relaxation needs on a daily basis. Further, while many public health programs urge avoidance of cigarettes, illicit drugs, and high-fat foods, such recommendations are limited and oversimplistic. A major shift in educational emphasis is imperative.

The optimum dietary plan addresses not only fat and fiber, but all nutritional aspects, from animal proteins to vegetable oils, from antioxidants to rare trace elements. Similarly, the concept of prevention must embrace as much as possible all factors that may overburden the immune system. The most sensible way to deal with AIDS may come not from medical technology, but rather from simply taking better care of ourselves.

Macrobiotics offers not the ultimate remedy, but rather a multifaceted approach to health that addresses the entire *process* of disease and hence aspires toward both prevention *and* correction. The goal is not merely to relieve sickness but also to restore health, to heal, to make whole. The solution to AIDS is the logical unfoldment of a comprehensive view of the integral relations between humanity and the environment, including viruses, drugs, stress, food, and people. It is not a fixed and prepackaged method for eliminating the terrible symptoms of AIDS, but a dynamic way of seeing and approaching the problem as a whole. In addition, by its prevention-oriented nature, macrobiotics strives for a healing of *all* individuals, with or without AIDS. Its message is global healing for global peace.

No advocate of the macrobiotic approach is claiming a "cure" for AIDS. Indeed, it would be ludicrous for *anyone* to make such a claim because the term is implicitly obsolete in the context of AIDS as it is officially defined. (The official definition includes presence of HIV antibodies in addition to various outward symptoms. These antibodies only indicate *previous* exposure, not that the virus is still present.) But if a person's overall state of health, including measurable components of the immune system, is an indication of recovery, then the macrobiotic approach offers grounds for hope. And if, in addition, positive outward changes such as increased vigor, optimism, humor, and curiosity can be regarded as "significant" indicators of a better prognosis, then the promise of macrobiotic healing goes beyond physical rejuvenation.

In its study of the effects of food and emotions on health, modern science is finally catching up with the ancient wisdom of traditional cultures. Through a deeper respect and understanding of our primordial bond with the natural world, we can all recover our natural birthright of sound health. By avoiding chemicals and considering the effects of individual differences, the changing seasons, and the various modes of food preparation, macrobiotics offers the dietary approach most finely attuned with nature. This approach, when consistently practiced, helps us establish the smooth and efficient mode of functioning for which our bodies were designed. Finally, the study of macrobiotics goes far beyond our daily bread. In its broader meaning, macrobiotics is simply a way of understanding our relationship to nature—including our human nature.

[1] Levy, E. M. et al., "Patients with Kaposi's Sarcoma Who Opt for No Treatment," *Lancet* (17 June 1985).

[2] Kotzsch, R. E., "Putting an Alternative to the Test," *East West* (1986), 16(9): 66.

[3] Levy et al. (1986), Op. cit., Dept. of Microbiology, Boston University School of Medicine, Boston, Mass., presented at the 2nd International Conference on AIDS, Paris.

[4] Levy, E. M., Cottrell, M. C., L. H. Kushi, and P. H. Black, "Patients with Kaposi's Sarcoma Who Opt for Alternative Therapy: Immune and psychological measures" (1987), Dept. of Microbiology, Boston University School of Medicine, Boston, Mass., Fashion Institute of Technology, N.Y., and the Division of Epidemiology, University of Minnesota, Minneapolis, Minn., presented at the 3rd International Conference on AIDS, Paris.

[5] Kotzsch (1986), Op. cit.

[6] See, for example, Locke and Hornig's large collection of medical abstracts in *Mind and Immunity*, Institute for the Advancement of Health (New York, 1983). *The Brain/Mind Bulletin* is another good source for PNI research.

[7] Biomedicine Report, "Worried Sick: Hassles and herpes," *Science News* (1987), 132(23): 360.

[8] Kiecolt-Glaser, J. and R. Blaser, reported by J.A. Miller in "Immunity and Crises, Large and Small," *Science News* (1986), 129(22): 340.

[9] McCelland, D. C., G. Ross and V. Patel, "The Effect of an Academic Examination on Salivary Norepinephrine and Immunoglobulin Levels," *J. Human Stress* (Summer, 1985), pp. 52–9.

[10] Lerner, H. G., *The Dance of Anger* (New York: Harper & Row Publishers, 1985), p. 3.

[11] Ibid., p. 1.

[12] Ibid.

[13] Ibid., p. 5.

[14] Levy, E. M. and M. C. Cottrell et al., Unpublished preliminary observations of 48 gay men with AIDS or ARC in New York City (1986).

[15] Laudenslager, M. L., "Coping and Immunosuppression," *Science* (1983), 221: 568.

[16] Borysenko, J., "Sam's Story," in *Minding the Body, Mending the Mind* (Mass.: Addison-Wesley Publishing Co., 1987), p. 193.

[17] Weber, R., "The Enfolding-unfolding Universe: A conversation with David Bohm," in *The Holographic Paradigm and Other Paradoxes: Exploring the Leading Edge of Science* (Boulder, Colo.: Shambhala Publications, Inc., 1982), pp. 44–104.

[18] Katz, J., *The Silent World of Doctor and Patient* (Free Press, 1984), p. 208.

[19] Dossey, L., "The Light of Health, the Shadow of Illness: A living unity," in *Beyond Illness*, New Science Library (Boston and London: Shambhala, 1984), p. 27.

[20] Borysenko (1986), Op. cit., p. 11.

[21] Ibid.

[22] Borysenko, J., "Getting Back in Control," in *Minding the Body, Mending the Mind* (Mass.: Addison-Wesley Publishing Co., 1986), p. 47.

[23] Kotzsch (1986), Op. cit.

[24] Cunningham, T., "Macrobiotics and AIDS: One study indicates that changing the diet may be the means of prolonging life for some people with AIDS," *The New York Native* (July, 1986). Quote of Max, a participant in *New York Study.*

[25] Nichols, S. E., "An Overview of the Psychological and Social Reactions to AIDS" (New York: Beth Israel Medical Center, 1986). A plenary address before the International Conference on AIDS (June, 1986). Gluckman and Vilmer, Elsevier, Paris, 1987.

[26] Ibid.

[27] Ibid.

[28] Johnson, J. H. and I. G. Sarason, "Life Stress, Depression, and Anxiety: Internal-external locus of control as a moderator variable," *Journal of Psychosomatic Research* (1978), 22: 205.

[29] Kushi, M., *Health and Education Series: Stress and Hypertension* (Tokyo and New York: Japan Publications, Inc., 1990).

[30] Snyder, M., "Macrobiotically Speaking: A candid conversation about AIDS," in *Changes*, vol. 2, Issue 1 (Baltimore, Md.: Macrobiotic Magazine, 1987).

[31] Cunningham (1986), Op. cit.

Epilogue: AIDS as Biological Degeneration

It is now 1989, and medical authorities around the world have proclaimed AIDS as the health catastrophe of the century. With the death toll increasing year after year, some believe this may be the greatest plague ever to hit the world. A recent World Health Organization (WHO) report entitled "AIDS and the Third World" speculates that, in time, AIDS may infect 50 to 100 million people. The Federal Centers for Disease Control estimate that by the end of 1991, over 200,000 Americans will have died from AIDS; by the end of 1992, more Americans may have died from AIDS than died in World War I, the Korean War, and the Vietnam War combined. If trends unfold according to projections, says *The Futurist*, AIDS may kill more people by the end of this century than have been killed by *all* of the wars of recorded history.

What guidance does recent research offer us to respond effectively to the AIDS threat? Unfortunately, a great deal of confusion still exists, as revealed by the October 1988 issue of *Scientific American*, which was devoted entirely to AIDS. Dr. Robert Gallo, of the National Cancer Institute, is still using reckless phrases like "no other risk factors present" in order to prove his claim that HIV is the sole and sufficient cause of AIDS—even though his list of risk factors precludes any contribution by dietary excess or emotional stress. And though researchers have found that a relatively nontoxic substance called CD4 may inhibit viral infection, there is still no definitive medical treatment for AIDS.

Fortunately more research has begun to focus on the immune system itself. In 1987, scientists reported that out of 1,000 homosexual men studied, 4 who initially showed antibodies to the virus slowly lost those antibodies; notably, the 4 men had no symptoms of disease, suggesting either that they had overcome HIV or that the virus had entered a latent phase and was undetectable (perhaps hiding in the nerve or bone-marrow cells). A 1988 study of 18 men carrying HIV found that some were infected more than a year before their bodies produced antibodies in response to the invading virus. Both studies may suggest that the immune system's responsiveness to HIV and other AIDS-related factors may vary widely. Whether the immune system prevails in the end may depend entirely on how well it is taken care of throughout life.

One of the shocking revelations of 1988 was that teenagers represent a population increasingly at risk for AIDS. As of September, more than 15,000 persons between the ages of 20 and 29 had been diagnosed. But since there can be as much as ten years between the time of infection and the onset of illness, many of the twenty-year-olds probably were infected as teenagers. And in this modern age of noncommittal sexual relations —of widespread skepticism about monogamy and ambivalence toward condom use—the possibility for HIV silently spreading among younger people is most worrisome. According to a large 1989 study of students visiting the infirmaries of U.S. college campuses, at least 1 out of every 500 college students may already be infected.

Every issue has two sides, however, and with AIDS the situation is no different. The fact that the onset of AIDS is slower among teenagers (*New York Times*, April 3, 1988), indicates that immunocompetence plays a key role in thwarting the disease process. The key, once again, is knowing how to keep the immune system vital, strong and competent —hence our focus throughout this book. It is time for departments of education to implement programs which teach students to look beyond HIV transmission to the behaviors which protect them from the disease process itself. It is time to learn the meaning of comprehensive prevention, to learn about strengthening our natural disease resistance. And in more than one sense, teenagers are ripe for such education!

As we age, the immune system's ability to protect the body from viral infections and other pathogenic influence begins to decline. According to Dr. Ranjit K. Chandra, reknowned authority on the relationship between nutrition and immune function, this lowering of immune-system strength is reflected by a progressive decline in cell-mediated immunity (T-cell function), along with an increased rate of cancer and infectious disease as people age. Curiously enough, another characteristic of people over 65 years old is the tendency to become malnourished, due to conditions which decrease food consumption, including emotional and motivational inhibitions, digestive and dental problems, and diminished taste sensitivity. The elderly often show decreases in lean body mass and diminishing blood levels of many nutrients. Dr. Chandra believes there may be a causal relationship between undernutrition and impaired immunity in elderly persons.

But what does aging have to do with AIDS? The connection is profound yet simple. AIDS may be regarded as a form of *accelerated aging* because both AIDS and aging involve excessive free-radical damage and progressive deterioration of the immune system. The analogy may also suggest something about the particular timing of AIDS at this time in history. We as a society appear to be aging much faster than our predecessors. This process may be reflected by the fact that cancer and heart disease, once considered "diseases of old age," are now seen with increasing frequency among our younger people. Premature aging among the younger generations, many of whom look five years older than their real age, is another sign of this process. Some premature aging may be induced by the growth hormones that are heavily concentrated in commonly consumed animal foods, such as beef, chicken, eggs, and dairy products. In addition, changes in skin tone and texture are directly linked with free-radical damage of body tissues, much of which, again, is caused by food items found in the typical American diet.

Free radicals, those highly unstable molecular fragments which damage cell membranes and cause disintegration of bodily tissues, are produced within the body throughout one's lifetime, but increase as people get older. Hence free-radical generation is thought to be a normal part of the aging process. The immune system's functioning is impaired by free radicals because white blood cells are especially rich in unsaturated fats (which are highly vulnerable to free-radical damage). Excessive free-radical production can also affect the immune system via DNA damage, which is an ongoing fact of life. All cells suffer genetic damage, but the more repair processes the body has to undergo the greater the likelihood for a mutation to occur. The free-radical generating character of the typical American diet may explain why people seem to be developing immune-related problems such as cancer and viral infections at an increasingly younger age.

Like the balance between microbes and immune cells in the body, a certain balance must be maintained between free radicals and natural "antioxidant nutrients." Just as one should strive to minimize microbial exposure through proper sanitation practices, one should strive to minimize free-radical damage by eating properly, exercising regularly, and keeping physically fit in general. At the same time, just as one should maintain a healthy immune system, one should maintain strong reserves of antioxidants, which may be considered part of our so-called natural immunity.

Antioxidants are found mostly in plant foods in the form of vitamins C, E, and beta carotene (precursor of vitamin A), and the trace minerals as zinc, manganese, and selenium. These micronutrients bind with free radicals in the body, thereby preventing cellular destruction and tissue disintegration. In fact, this is one of the key mechanisms thought to be involved in the immune-enhancing effects of these micronutrients. By preventing free-radical production, the immune system is allowed to function with all its components relatively intact—provided that other aspects of nutrition are also taken care of. The important role of anti-oxidant nutrients has recently been recognized by the National Cancer Institute and the American Cancer Society. This may explain, in part, why people following a macrobiotic diet often look far younger than their years—often ten or even fifteen years younger, depending on whether or not they smoke cigarettes (tobacco smoke causes additional free-radical damage).

Mother's diet during pregnancy and lactation may be extremely important in this regard, since fatty acids and chemical toxins in her blood could pass through the placenta, causing excessive free-radical exposure and thereby weakening the developing fetus. Refined-carbohydrate foods, such as white sugar and flour products, may contribute to genetic mutations via *glycosylation* (the cross-linking of glucose molecules to proteins and DNA), as discussed by Cerami and co-workers in their May 1987 *Scientific American* article, "Glucose and Ageing." This effect of sugar, together with those of fatty acids and chemical additives, may account for most of our "diseases of modern civilization," including AIDS.

Such effects may help us understand why diseases once ascribed to "old age" are now afflicting young people at an increasingly alarming rate. Our immune integrity has declined along with the crumbling of our genetic foundation. Consider the immune-system cell type called the natural killer (NK) cell, which declines in number as we age (Bowry, T. R., 1984, *Immunology Simplified*, Oxford University Press). NK cells, as discussed earlier, can directly disintegrate virus-infected cells, and can also eliminate *neoplasia* (cancer) because they are cytotoxic to many types of tumors at their first exposure. NK cells are detectable in the circulation and in the spleen, and they are not considered part of the specific immune system. Could the increasing incidence of cancers among younger people indicate a premature decline in the numbers of NK cells and other important immunologic parameters? If so, how might we account for this decline? Given what we now know about nutrition and other environmental factors, the answer may be as simple as the kinds of food we choose to eat.

This brings us to some of the areas of everyone's life-style that need reevaluating. Some of the serious degeneration evidenced in the American population at this time may be due to the incomplete development of our immune systems. In many cases this negative process starts in the early years with the refined, adulterated, and fatty diet typical of Americans. From day one, our immune systems are not only over-stressed, but improperly nourished as well, setting the stage for sickness in early life. It is not uncommon to see high-school and college students going to their daily classes with chocolate bars, cokes, and doughnuts in hand. This is obviously not supporting their biological needs, and it may well underlie the large prevalence of colds, sore throats, anemia, fatigue and premenstrual tension.

In addition, most of these young people have not been breast-fed, and thus have been denied the multiple benefits of this practice for immunologic development. They also tend to have high intakes of cow's milk in the form of cheese, butter, ice cream, and other dairy products. An examination of their medical histories reveals a high incidence of recurrent ear infections, throat infections, bronchial and sinus infections, and acne, resulting in repeated use of antibiotics, antihistamines, and over-the-counter drugs. When they reach adolescence and become socially and sexually active, there is usually use of recreational drugs plus recurrent sexually transmitted diseases and further use of antibiotics, each episode requiring stronger dosages and longer duration of treatment. Altogether these factors carry an increasing potential for adverse side effects. For example, such reliance on antibiotics undoubtedly disturbs the condition of the intestinal microflora, which is reflected in the recent widespread rise in the incidence of candidiasis. In recent years there has also been a rise in the incidence of herpes.

The overall picture of our young-adult heterosexual population suggests striking similarities with the adult homosexual population. Since these similarities may indicate a tendency toward reduced immunocompetence among the younger generations, they certainly deserve the attention of everyone concerned with the education and health-care of this population. It behooves us to take a broader look at the message of AIDS, for the message is both positive and negative. It is negative for obvious reasons and positive because it may motivate us to reevaluate our health-care system and personal responsibilities for our own well-being. Health does not come in pills or shots, in aerobics classes, or in avoiding hamburgers from time to time. It begins with an awareness toward the relative effects of our daily patterns of living over the long term.

Twenty-five years ago it was quite unusual to see venereal warts in the gynecological clinics. It was also rare to see herpes zoster in the younger age brackets or college-age people. The disease was known to afflict primarily the elderly, manifesting as a clinically depressed condition due to malnutrition, chronic disease, or various kinds of strong medications. Whenever herpes was present, physicians were suspicious of an underlying subclinical cancer.

Today the picture is quite different. In the young-adult population, herpes and venereal warts are very common. Fungal infections, mixed vaginitis, and various idiopathic infections—chalamydia being the most recent one—are rampant among the female population. Interestingly, the most commonly used drug for chlamydia is flagyl. This drug has been used for many years for parasitic infections in the gay population. We are now aware of its many toxic and immunosuppressive side effects. There also appears to be an increasing incidence of nonspecific urethritis in males and nonspecific vaginitis in females (both of which are now being defined as chlamydial infections). And since the early 1970s the number of trichamonis cases has escalated; again, the recommended treatment has been flagyl.

Thus we see a large percentage of our sexually active young adults presenting with sexually transmitted diseases, ailments which were once quite rare and obscure. Why have they begun to afflict us at this time in such a concentrated way? This is still an unsolved problem. Most medical authorities have attributed these rising trends to increased levels of sexual activity, based on both society's growing acceptance of promiscuity and the comparative ease of contraception, especially the pill. The implication of this view is that there is an inherent risk of infection involved in any casual sexual encounter. This view is only concerned with transmission of an infectious agent, and it completely ignores the issue of susceptibility or resistance. At best, resistance is viewed in terms of condoms or diaphragms, but never in terms of balanced blood chemistry and sound immunity.

How do these observations relate to the high-risk groups for AIDS? It is not uncommon for gay men to have a history of chronic herpes, venereal warts, gonorrhea, syphilis, and recurrent parasitic and fungal infections (in particular, candidiasis), and repeated stresses to the immune system in the form of strong medications and numerous antibiotic treatments. This is the profile presented throughout the medical literature for designation of the high-risk categories. It is also the profile which seems to fit best with heterosexuals who are getting AIDS. The combination of viral infections with the various taken-for-granted stresses of modern life—formula milk, imbalanced nutrition, lack of exercise, tonsillectomies, antibiotics and other medications—may ultimately bring about a substantial breakdown of the immune system. We deem this to be true for all people regardless of sexual preference.

Our immune system's intricate design is a beautiful example of natural order. The fine integration and complexity of this system has given some scientists a renewed sense of respect for the natural processes by which true health is ultimately maintained. At the same time, innovative research technologies, in revealing for the first time the innermost depths of the microscopic realm, have compelled us to reevaluate the classical paradigms that have guided scientific inquiry for centuries. Indeed, it may be time for a major paradigm shift in medicine. This, in a nutshell is the great intellectual challenge posed by the AIDS epidemic for modern society. AIDS presents an opportunity for learning, evolving and removing those things which no longer serve us in our evolution on Earth. It is always darkest before the dawn.

3

Dietary Guidelines
and Home Cares

Michio Kushi

1. Macrobiotic Food and Recipe Suggestions

Macrobiotic cooking is unique. The ingredients are simple and cooking is the key to creating meals that are nutritious, flavorful, and attractive. A cook has the ability to change the quality of food. Longer cooking and the use of pressure, salt, heat, and time makes the energy of the food more concentrated. Quicker cooking and less salt preserves the lighter quality of the food. A good cook manages the health and well-being of those for whom he or she prepares meals by adjusting these factors properly.

- *Methods of cooking and food preparation:*

Regular Use:
Pressure-cooking
Boiling
Steaming
Waterless cooking
Soup
Pickling
Oilless sautéing
Water sautéing
Pressing
Other traditional cooking
  methods

Occasional Use:
Sautéing
Stir-frying
Raw
Deep-frying
Tempura
Baking
Other traditional cooking
  methods

- *For variety, the following aspects of daily cooking can be changed:*
  1. The selection of foods within the following catagories: grains, soups, vegetables, beans, sea vegetables, condiments, pickles, and beverages.
  2. The methods of cooking: boiling, steaming sautéing, frying, and pressure-cooking.
  3. The way of cutting vegetables.
  4. The amount of water used in cooking.

5. The amount of seasoning and condiments used.
6. The type of seasoning and condiments selected for use.
7. The length of time that various dishes are cooked (do not over-cook or pressure-cook vegetables), or processed (such as the length of time for pickling).
8. The use of a higher or lower flame when cooking various dishes.
9. The combination of foods and dishes.
10. The selection of dishes to harmonize seasonal change.

Standard Macrobiotic Diet

The guidelines that follow are broad and flexible. The standard macrobiotic way of eating offers a wide range of foods and cooking methods to choose from. You can apply them when selecting the highest-quality natural foods for yourself and your family.

These suggestions are especially for people living in a temperate climate. Modifications are required if you live in a tropical or subtropical climate, or a polar or semi-polar region. It is also necessary to adjust diet when traveling to one of these regions, and to consider each person's individual needs and condition. For this reason, it is advisable to meet with a qualified macrobiotic teacher or participate in programs such as the Macrobiotic Way of Life Seminar presented by the Kushi Foundation in Boston, in order to receive individual guidance.

Whole Cereal Grains

Whole cereal grains are the staff of life and are an essential part of a healthful way of eating. For people in temperate climates, they may comprise up to 50 to 60 percent of daily intake. Below is a list of the whole grains and grain products that may be included:

Regular Use:
Short-grain brown rice
Medium-grain brown rice (in warmer areas or seasons)
Barley
Pearl barley (*hato mugi*)
Millet
Corn
Whole oats
Whole wheat berries
Buckwheat

Rye
Other traditionally used whole grains

Occasional Use:
Long-grain brown rice
Sweet brown rice
Mochi (pounded sweet rice)
Cracked wheat (bulgur)
Steel-cut oats
Rolled oats
Corn grits
Corn meal
Rye flakes
Couscous
Other traditionally used whole grain products

Occasional Use Flour Products:
Whole wheat noodles
Udon (wheat) noodles
Somen (thin wheat) noodles
Soba (buckwheat) noodles
Unyeasted whole wheat bread
Unyeasted whole rye bread
Fu
Seitan
Other traditionally used whole grain flour products

• *Selecting the highest-quality grains:* Cooked whole grains are preferable to flour products or to cracked or rolled grains because of their greater ease in digestion. In general, it is better to keep intake of flour products—or cracked or rolled grains—to less than 15 percent of your daily whole grain intake.

Although the whole grains available in most natural food stores are adequate for regular use, the highest-quality grains are organically grown, without pesticides or fertilizers, and are hulled just before use. A grain such as brown rice is surrounded by a hard shell or husk. The husk is normally removed after harvest. The outer layer, or skin of the grain, contains proteins, enzymes, vitamins, and minerals. The inside portion is made up of carbohydrate. When rice is polished, the outside skin is removed and white rice is left. In brown rice, the outer skin is left on.

The outermost layer of brown rice—the cellophane like, transparent skin—is very resistant to chemicals, but is fragile when it comes to physical attack. Brown rice grains are easily chipped, and once this has happened, oxidation occurs and the color and quality of the rice begin to change. The vitality and nutritional value of the grains are diminished.

The highest-quality natural rice available on the market today is called "paddy rice" and is purchased unhulled. The husk is removed at home just before the rice is cooked. Home rice-hulling machines are now available. Freshly hulled rice has an ideal balance of energy and nutrients. Rice-hulling machines do not crush or grind the grains in order to remove the husk. The grains are gently milled to preserve the outside skin. (Information on obtaining rice hulling machines is available from the Kushi Foundation, 17 Station Street, Brookline, MA. 02146, or call (617) 738-0045.)

Freshly hulled rice and other grains are especially recommended for restoring natural immunity.

Grain Recipes

There are two main methods for cooking grains: pressure-cooking and boiling. Either may be used as explained in the following recipes, although the way of cooking grains need not be limited to these methods.

Brown Rice: Pressure-cooking is the preferred method of cooking brown rice the majority of the time. Pressure-cooking allows the rice to cook thoroughly. Pressure-cooked rice is more easily digested, retains more nutrients, is a little less soggy, and has a stronger healing energy than rice cooked by other methods. There are several ways to pressure-cook brown rice. Two of the most often used are:

1. *Non-soaking*: Place the brown rice in a pressure cooker and add the appropriate measure of water. Do not cover. Place on a low flame for approximately 10 minutes. This is a pre-soaking period, which allows the grain to slowly expand, making it more digestible and sweet.

Add the appropriate amount of sea salt, cover and turn the flame to high. Bring to pressure. When the pressure is up, reduce the flame to medium-low and place a flame deflector under the cooker. Pressure-cook for 50 minutes, remove from the cooker, and serve.

2. *Soaking*: Place the brown rice and water in a pressure cooker and soak overnight or for 6 to 8 hours. Add the appropriate amount of sea salt after the grain has soaked. Cover, place on a high flame and

bring up to pressure. When the pressure is up, reduce the flame to medium-low and cook for 50 minutes.

Basic Pressure-cooked Brown Rice

2 cups brown rice, washed
2½–3 cups water
pinch of sea salt per cup of grain

Pressure-cook using either of the above methods. Remove the pressure cooker from the flame and allow the pressure to come down naturally. Remove the cover and allow the rice to sit for 4 to 5 minutes. Remove the rice and place in a wooden serving bowl.

Variations:
- 1½ cups rice and ½ cup barley (soaked overnight)
- 1½ cups rice and ½ cup millet
- 1½ cups rice and ½ cup sweet rice
- 1½ cups rice and ½ cup wheat berries (soaked overnight)
- 1½ cups rice and ½ cup rye (soaked overnight)
- 1½ cups rice and ½ cup hato mugi (pearl barley)
- 1½ cups rice and ½ cup chick-peas (soaked overnight)
- 1½ cups rice and ½ cup *azuki* beans (soaked overnight)
- 1½ cups rice and ½ cup black soybeans (dry-roasted)
- 1½ cups rice and ½ cup lotus seeds (soaked 3 to 4 hours.)
- 1½ cups rice and ½ cup fresh sweet corn
- 2 cups rice and ¼ cup sesame seeds
- 2 cups rice and 1 *umeboshi* plum (instead of sea salt)
- 2 cups rice and 1 strip *kombu* (1 inch per cup instead of salt)
- 2 cups rice and ½ cup squash chunks
- 1 ½ cups rice and ½ cup pre-cooked whole dried corn

There are hundreds of other combinations of grains, seeds, beans, bean products, vegetables and other items that can be cooked with brown rice. Please refer to the macrobiotic cookbooks listed in the bibliography for recipes.

Gomoku (Rice with Five Ingredients)

Gomoku is a brown rice dish made from roasted brown rice, vegetables, and various other ingredients. There are usually five items in this dish but it can also include more ingredients. Gomoku can also be made from unroasted rice. In this case, first soak the rice for several hours and then combine with vegetables, beans, bean products, or other ingredients. Roasting the rice gives Gomoku a drier texture. It has strong energy and can be enjoyed once a week or so.

> 2 cups brown rice, washed and dry-roasted until golden
> 2–3 pieces dried tofu, soaked and cubed
> 4–5 shiitake mushrooms, soaked, stems removed, and diced
> 2 Tbsp dried daikon, soaked and sliced
> 1 strip kombu, 2 inches long, soaked and diced
> ½ cup carrots, quartered lengthwise and cubed
> 2 Tbsp lotus root, diced
> ¼ cup sweet corn
> 2 Tbsp burdock, diced
> 3 cups water
> pinch of sea salt per cup of grain

Place all ingredients in a pressure cooker and cover. Bring up to pressure and cook for 45 to 50 minutes. Remove from flame and allow pressure to come down. Remove the cover and place in a wooden serving bowl.

Boiled Brown Rice

> 2 cups brown rice, washed
> 4 cups water
> pinch of sea salt per cup of grain

Place the rice, water and sea salt in a heavy cooking pot, cover and bring to a boil. Reduce the flame to medium-low and simmer for about 1 hour or until all the water has been absorbed. Remove and place in a wooden serving bowl.

Boiled rice can also be cooked using any of the variations listed for pressure-cooked rice.

Rice Balls (Musubi)

> 1 cup cooked short-grain brown rice
> ½ sheet toasted nori, cut in half
> ½–1 umeboshi plum
> pinch of sea salt

Dampen your hands in a small bowl of water with the pinch of sea salt in it. Place the rice in your hands and form into a triangular shape by cupping your hands into a "V" and applying pressure to mold the rice. The triangle should be firmly packed. With your index finger, poke a hole into the center of the rice and insert the umeboshi plum. Then close the hole by packing the triangle firmly again.

Place a square of the toasted nori on one side of the triangle and the other square on the other side. Pack the rice triangle again so that the nori sticks to it. You may occasionally need to dampen your hands with a very small amount of the salted water to prevent rice and nori from sticking to them. If there are uncovered spots on the triangle you can patch them by sticking small pieces of toasted nori on them until the triangle is completely covered with nori.

Sushi

Homemade sushi (made from brown rice and nonchemicalized ingredients and without raw fish) can be eaten frequently as a snack, at parties, or as a handy lunch item. Many types of sushi can be made, using a variety of ingredients. The following recipe is for a simple vegetable sushi:

nori
cooked brown rice
carrots, cut into strips
scallion leaves
umeboshi plum or paste

Step One: Roast one side of a sheet of nori over a flame until it turns green, and place on a bamboo sushi mat. Wet both hands with water, and spread cooked brown rice evenly on the sheet of nori. Leave about $\frac{1}{2}$ to 1 inch of the top of the nori uncovered with rice, and about $\frac{1}{8}$ to $\frac{1}{4}$ inch of the bottom uncovered.

Step Two: Slice a carrot into lengthwise strips 8- to 10-inches long and about $\frac{1}{4}$ inch thick. Place carrot strips in water with a pinch of sea salt. Boil for 2 to 3 minutes. The carrots should be slightly crisp. Remove and allow to cool. Separate the green-leaf portion of several scallions from the roots, so that each strip is about 8 to 10 inches in length. Place carrot and scallion strips approximately $\frac{1}{2}$ to 1 inch from the bottom of the sheet of nori. Then lightly spread $\frac{1}{6}$ to $\frac{1}{8}$ teaspoon puréed umeboshi along the entire length of the carrot and scallion strips.

Step Three: Roll up the rice and nori, using a sushi mat, pressing the mat firmly against the rice and nori until it is completely rolled into a round log shape. The vegetables should be centered in the roll. If they are not centered, they were most likely placed too far from the bottom edge of the nori and rice.

Step Four: Use a very sharp knife to slice the roll into rounds that are about ½ to 1 inch thick. The knife may need to be moistened after each slice. If this is not done, the knife may not slice properly, and it may cause the nori to tear.

Step Five: Arrange rounds on a platter with the cut side up, showing the rice and vegetables, or pack in a lunch box.

Variations: Substitute strips of pickle, deep-fried *tofu*, cooked *tempeh*, or root or green vegetables inside the sushi.

Soft Rice (*Kayu*)

1 cup brown rice, washed
5 cups water
pinch of sea salt

Place all ingredients in a pressure cooker and cover. Bring to pressure, reduce the flame to medium-low and cook for 50 to 55 minutes. Serve with umeboshi and roasted nori strips or your favorite condiment and scallions.

Variations:

- 1 cup rice and 1-inch strip of kombu (instead of sea salt)
- 1 cup rice and 1 umeboshi plum (instead of sea salt)
- ¾ cup rice and ¼ cup of another grain

Genuine Brown Rice Cream

1 cup brown rice, washed
5 cups water
pinch of sea salt or 1-inch strip kombu

Heat a stainless-steel skillet and dry-roast the rice until golden yellow. Place the roasted rice, water, and sea salt or kombu in a pressure cooker. Cover and bring to pressure. Reduce the flame to medium-low and cook for 1 ½ to 2 hours. Remove from the flame and allow the pressure to come down. Remove the cover.

To boil, place ingredients (use 10 cups water for boiling) in a heavy pot. Cover and simmer for 2 hours or until the liquid is reduced to half the original amount.

Place the soft-cooked rice in a sack made of several layers of cotton cheesecloth or one layer of unbleached cotton muslin. Tie the sack and squeeze out the creamy liquid. Reheat the creamy liquid and serve with or without condiments.

Fried Rice

> **1–2 Tbsp dark sesame oil**
> **½ cup celery, diced**
> **1 cup onion, diced**
> **1 Tbsp scallion roots, minced**
> **½ cup carrot, sliced in thin matchsticks**
> **½ cup burdock, sliced in thin matchsticks**
> **1–2 Tbsp water, if the rice is dry**
> **2 cups cooked brown rice**
> **1 Tbsp parsley or scallion, chopped, for garnish**
> **tamari soy sauce or sea salt**

Place oil in a skillet and heat up. Add the scallion roots and sauté 1 minute. Next, place the onion and celery in the skillet and sauté 1 to 2 minutes. Add the carrot and burdock. Place the rice on top of the vegetables and, if the rice is dry, add water. Cover the skillet and reduce the flame to low.

Simmer for 15 to 20 minutes or until the vegetables are soft and the rice is warm. Just before the vegetables and rice are done, add the tamari soy sauce to taste or a small amount of sea salt for a mild salt taste. Add the chopped parsley or scallions, cover and cook another 2 to 3 minutes. Mix all ingredients together and serve hot.

Variations:

- brown rice, sweet corn, tofu, toasted nori strips
- brown rice and scallions
- brown rice and parsley
- brown rice, onions, carrots, cabbage
- brown rice, tempeh, celery, carrots, parsley
- brown rice, azuki beans, scallions

Brown Rice and Beans

Brown rice and beans can be prepared in several ways:

1. *Boil* the beans with water to cover for 20 minutes. Add to the rice along with the remaining cooking water and sea salt. Cook as for plain brown rice. This method can be used often with azuki beans.

2. *Soak* the beans 6 to 8 hours or overnight. Discard the soaking water, and add the beans to the rice along with water and sea salt. Then pressure-cook as you would plain brown rice.

3. *Dry-roast* the beans. This method is used only with white or black soybeans. Wash the beans, and dry-roast several minutes on a medium flame, stirring constantly. Add the beans to the rice, along with water and sea salt. Pressure-cook as for plain brown rice.

When combining beans with rice, the percentage of beans is usually kept between 10 to 20 percent, with the exception of azuki beans, which can make up as much as 30 percent of the dish. The soaking water from azuki beans can be included as part of the water measurement in cooking. The soaking water from other beans is usually discarded when cooking them with rice.

Sweet Brown Rice

Sweet rice is a more glutenous variety of brown rice. It is rich in protein and is more fatty than regular rice. Sweet rice is used less often than regular brown rice and may be included several times per week. It can be served plain, cooked with the ingredients listed below, or pounded and made into mochi.

Sweet rice is delicious when cooked in the same way as regular brown rice.

Variations:

- 1 cup sweet rice and 1 cup azuki beans (boiled 15 minutes)
- 1 ½ cups sweet rice and ½ cup dried chestnuts (dry-roasted until golden, and soak for 10 minutes)
- 1 ½ cups sweet rice and ½ cup dry-roasted black soybeans
- 2 cups sweet rice and 2-inch strip kombu (instead of sea salt)

Mochi (Pounded Sweet Rice)

Mochi is cooked sweet rice that has been pounded with a wooden pestle for 30 to 40 minutes or more, until it becomes sticky. It is then dried for 2 to 3 days.

Mochi can be purchased pre-packaged in most natural food stores. To serve, cut into small squares and dry-roast in a skillet until slightly browned on both sides, and the mochi puffs up slightly.

Mochi may also be steamed, baked, broiled, pan-fried in oil, deep-fried or added to soups and stews. Mochi may be eaten with a variety of toppings, including tamari soy sauce, warm brown rice syrup, or toasted soybean flour (*kinako*). Mochi can also be dry-roasted or toasted and placed in miso soup.

Recipes for making homemade mochi are included in the cookbooks listed in the bibliography.

Other Grains

Pressure-cooked Barley

> 2 cups barley, soaked 6–8 hours
> 2 ½–3 cups water
> pinch of sea salt per cup of barley

Cook same as for brown rice, using method #2.

Variations: Barley may be boiled, or pressure-cooked with a variety of other grains, beans, and vegetables. Cook same as for plain brown rice. For soft barley cereal, add 4 to 5 cups of water to 1 cup of barley and pressure cook for about 1 to 1 ¼ hours. Serve hot and garnish with chopped scallions, parsley, toasted nori, gomashio, or your favorite condiment.

For barley soup, simply use 6 to 7 cups water per cup of barley, and add several types of sliced ground or root vegetables. Either boil for 1 to 1 ½ hours or pressure-cook as above. Season with sea salt, tamari soy sauce, or puréed barley miso just before the dish is finished cooking. Garnish and serve.

Pressure-cooked Millet and Vegetables

> 2 cups millet, washed

2 ½–3 cups water
1 cup hard winter squash, cut in 1-inch chunks
½ cup carrots, sliced in chunks
¼ cup cabbage, sliced in 1-inch squares
pinch of sea salt per cup of millet

Place all ingredients in a pressure cooker, cover and bring to pressure. Reduce the flame to medium-low and cook for about 15 to 20 minutes. Remove and allow the pressure to come down. Remove the cover and place the millet in a wooden serving bowl. Garnish and serve.

Variations: Dry-roast millet until golden yellow and combine with vegetables and cook as above. Millet may be boiled with vegetables using about 3 cups of boiling water per cup of millet. Cook for 30 to 35 minutes on a medium-low flame. For soft millet cereal cook with 5 cups of water per cup of millet, and either boil for 30 to 35 minutes or pressure-cook for 15 to 20. Millet can also be used in making soups and stews.

Buckwheat (Kasha)

1 cup buckwheat groats, washed
2 cups boiling water
pinch of sea salt

Dry-roast the washed buckwheat for about 5 minutes, stirring constantly. Place the sea salt and buckwheat in boiling water. Cover and reduce the flame to medium-low. Simmer for 20 to 30 minutes or until the buckwheat is soft and all water has been absorbed. Remove and place in a serving bowl, garnish and serve.

Variations:

• Cook buckwheat together with vegetables such as onions, carrots and cabbage; parsley and onions; or sauerkraut, tempeh, cabbage and parsley.

• Buckwheat can also be cooked plain, removed and allowed to cool, and combined with various cooked vegetables to make a light buckwheat salad.

• For a hearty morning cereal, use 4 to 5 cups of boiling water and cook as above, plain or with vegetables.

• Buckwheat can also be used in making a hearty fall or winter soup or a light, refreshing spring or summer soup. For soups, simply use 5 to 6 cups of water, and cook together with vegetables for about 20 to

25 minutes. Season with sea salt or tamari soy sauce, garnish and serve.

Special note: persons with skin conditions or those who have had surgery in the past two years are advised to temporarily avoid buckwheat or products that contain it such as soba noodles.

Wheat and Rye

Wheat and rye are hard grains and require thorough chewing to make them digestible. They are usually mixed in small quantities with brown rice or crushed into flour and used to make bread. Wheat and rye may be soaked 6 to 8 hours or dry-roasted for several minutes in a skillet to make them more digestible and softer when combining them with other grains. However, if you wish to occasionally prepare a plain wheat or rye dish, add 2 cups of water per cup of grain and pressure-cook as you would plain brown rice. Wheat and rye may take several minutes longer to pressure-cook than rice (approximately 60 minutes).

Corn

There are several varieties of soft and hard corn available in natural food markets. Sweet corn is available in many varieties ranging from yellow to white in color. It can be eaten as corn on the cob and because it is perishable is usually eaten in season. Hard corn can be used as a whole grain and because it is dried, can be stored for long periods, making it available in any season. Several types of hard, dried corn are available.

Hard, dried varieties of corn are traditionally cooked with pure wood ashes which help soften the hard shell and add calcium and other minerals to the corn. However if you use wood ashes, be sure that newspapers and other items that contain chemicals have not been burnt in the same ashes.

Whole Corn

> **2 cups whole dried corn, washed, soaked overnight (preferably dent corn)**
> **2 cups pure sifted wood ash, tied in a clean cotton muslin bag or sack**
> **4 cups water**
> **pinch of sea salt**

Place the corn in a pressure cooker. Add the wood ash and two cups of water. Cover and pressure-cook for 1 to 1 ½ hours. Remove from the flame and allow the pressure to come down. Remove the cover and place the corn in a strainer or colander. Rinse all of the wood ashes from the corn. Place the corn into a clean pressure cooker, add sea salt and pressure-cook for 1 more hour. Remove from the flame, allow the pressure to come down and place the cooked corn in a serving dish or use in making soups, vegetable dishes, or salads.

Arepa (Corn Cakes)

Before preparing the arepas, we must prepare a dough, called *masa*. First, cook the corn as above but use 4 cups of corn and 8 to 10 cups of water. Then remove and allow the corn to cool completely. Place the cooked corn in a hand grinder (do not use a blender) and grind to a soft consistency. Knead the ground corn for 10 to 15 minutes by hand. You may add a little water for a doughy consistency. You now have masa or corn dough. This will yield about 1 $\frac{1}{2}$ to 2 pounds of masa.

1 $\frac{1}{2}$ lbs corn dough (masa)
$\frac{1}{4}$ Tsp sea salt
water
dark sesame oil

Crumble the dough and add sea salt. Knead the dough with a small amount of water until it becomes soft. Form the dough into 6 to 8 fist-sized balls. Brush a small amount of dark sesame oil in a cast-iron skillet and heat up. Flatten the balls of dough into round cakes about $\frac{1}{2}$ inch thick, and cook for 2 to 3 minutes on each side, or until a crust forms on the cakes. Next, bake the cakes in a 350°F. oven for about 20 minutes, or until the cakes puff up. The arepas are done when they make a hollow, popping sound when tapped.

Flour Products

Noodles and Pasta

Noodles and pasta are easier to digest than hard, baked flour products. For this reason they can be eaten more frequently. There are many types of noodles and pastas to choose from. There are Japanese noodles such as udon (a whole wheat noodle), soba (buckwheat noodles), somen (a thin whole wheat noodle), as well as others. American made whole wheat pastas include spaghetti, elbows, shells, spirals and various others. Japanese noodles are made with sea salt and therefore it is not necessary to add salt when cooking. American whole wheat pastas do not contain salt, therefore you may add a pinch to aid in the cooking process. In any of the recipes in this section, please feel free to substitute any whole grain noodle or pasta for the one listed.

Fried Udon or Soba

> **6 cups water**
> **1 package udon or soba, 8 oz**
> **1 Tbsp dark sesame oil**
> **1 cup cabbage, shredded**
> **½ cup onions, sliced in thin half-moons**
> **½ cup carrots, sliced in thin matchsticks**
> **¼ cup scallions, sliced**
> **tamari soy sauce**

Place the water in a pot and bring to a boil. Add the udon or soba and stir once or twice to prevent the noodles from sticking. Return to a boil. Reduce the flame to medium-high and cook several minutes until the noodles are the same color inside as outside. If the inside or center of the noodle is white or lighter in color than the outside, cook a little longer. When done, place the noodles in a strainer or colander and rinse thoroughly under cold water to stop the cooking action, and to prevent the noodles from sticking together. Set the noodles aside and allow to drain. They are now ready to use.

Brush dark sesame oil in a skillet and heat up. Add the onions and sauté 1 to 2 minutes. Layer the cabbage and carrots on top of the onions. Place the noodles on top of the vegetables, cover, and cook on a low flame for 5 to 7 minutes until the vegetables are tender and the noodles are hot. Add the scallions and a small amount of tamari soy sauce for a mild salt taste, cover, and continue to cook 1 to 2 minutes until the scallions are done. Mix and place in a serving bowl.

Variations:

- udon or soba and chopped scallions
- udon or soba and chopped parsley
- udon or soba, tofu cubes, carrots, celery, onions
- udon or soba, tempeh slices, onions, celery, cabbage

Udon with Vegetables and Kuzu Sauce

1 package udon (8 oz), cooked
3 shiitake mushrooms, soaked, stems removed, and sliced
½ cup onions, sliced in 1/4-inch-thick wedges
½ cup carrots, sliced on a thin diagonal
¼ cup celery, sliced on a thin diagonal
1 cup broccoli, sliced in small flowerettes
1 cup tofu, cubed, and pan-fried until golden
1 strip kombu, 3 to 4 inches long, soaked
2 ½ cups water
3 Tbsp kuzu, diluted in 3 Tbsp water
1 ½–2 Tbsp tamari soy sauce
grated ginger (optional) for garnish
sliced scallions for garnish

Place the water, shiitake, and kombu in a pot and bring to a boil. Cover and simmer 4 to 5 minutes. Remove the kombu and set aside for future use. Continue to cook the shiitake for another 5 to 7 minutes. Add the onions, carrots, celery, tofu, and broccoli. Cover, reduce the flame to medium, and simmer until the vegetables are tender but still slightly crisp and brightly colored. Reduce the flame to low and add the diluted kuzu, stirring constantly to prevent lumping. When thick, add the tamari soy sauce for a mild salt taste and simmer 2 to 3 minutes. Place the cooked noodles in individual serving bowls and pour the vegetable kuzu sauce over them. Garnish with a dab of fresh grated ginger and a few sliced scallions, and serve hot.

Udon or Soba and Broth

(Please refer to the section on soups for recipe.)

Whole Wheat Sourdough Bread

There are many types of unyeasted whole wheat sourdough breads available in most natural food stores for occasional enjoyment. Whole wheat bread can be eaten plain, with various natural spreads, occasionally toasted, or steamed (which makes it moister and easier to digest). Recipes for making whole wheat sourdough bread at home are presented in the macrobiotic cookbooks listed in the bibliography. Generally, bread is eaten less often than noodles, especially when it is toasted.

Onion, carrot, squash, or sesame butter can be used as spreads on occasion.

Fu (Puffed Wheat Gluten)

Fu is made from the gluten of whole wheat flour, and is naturally rich in protein. It is available pre-packaged in most natural food stores and comes in rounds or thin flat sheets. Fu can be used in soups, vegetable dishes, fried, and in some bean dishes. It is a dried flour product which must be soaked to reconstitute. After soaking for 5 to 10 minutes, simply slice and use. Because it is a moist, more easily digested product, it can be eaten a little more often than hard, baked flour products.

Seitan (Wheat Gluten)

Seitan is made from the gluten of whole wheat flour but unlike fu, it is not dried. It is also high in protein (it is sometimes called "wheat-meat"), and is more chewy than fu. Seitan can be purchased pre-packaged in most natural food stores or can be made at home. Recipes for homemade seitan are included in most macrobiotic cookbooks.

Seitan Stew

(Please refer to the section on soups for recipe.)

Soup

Soups may comprise about 5 to 10 percent of each person's daily food intake. For most people, the average is about one or two cups or bowls of soup per day, depending on individual desires and preferences. Soups can include vegetables, grains, beans, sea vegetables, noodles or other grain products, bean products like tofu, tempeh, or others, or occasionally, fish or seafood. Soups can be moderately seasoned with either miso, tamari soy sauce, sea salt, umeboshi plum or paste, or occasional ginger.

Light miso soup, with vegetables and sea vegetables, is recommended for daily consumption, on average one small bowl or cup per day. *Mugi* (barley) miso is recommended for regular consumption, followed by soybean (*Hatcho*) miso. A second bowl or cup of soup may also be enjoyed, preferably seasoned mildly with tamari soy sauce or sea salt. Other soup varieties include:

- Bean and vegetable soups
- Grain and vegetable soups (brown rice, millet, barley, pearl barley, etc.)

- Puréed squash and other vegetable soups

- *Selecting the highest-quality natural miso and tamari soy sauce:* Miso is a dark purée made from soybeans, unrefined sea salt, and usually fermented barley or rice, all of which have been aged together. After cooking, the ingredients are inoculated with *koji*, a special mold that stimulates fermentation, and the mixture is allowed to age in wooden kegs for usually a year or more. Miso has been a staple in Far Eastern countries for thousands of years, and contains living enzymes that facilitate digestion, strengthen the quality of the blood, and provide a nutritious balance of complex carbohydrates, essential oils, protein, vitamins, and minerals.

There are various types of miso, and their tastes and flavors differ according to the quality of their ingredients, the climate and environment in which they are prepared, the length of time they have aged, and the method of preparation. Barley (mugi) miso is made from fermented barley, soybeans, and sea salt, and is the sweetest and most suitable miso for daily cooking. The highest-quality barley miso is aged naturally for two summers or longer. Miso that has been naturally fermented from whole, round soybeans—without chemically treated ingredients or artificial aging procedures—is recommended for restoring natural immunity. Naturally fermented soybean (Hatcho) miso can also be used as a supplement to barley miso.

Similiarly, natural soy sauce, known in macrobiotics as tamari soy sauce, should also be the highest quality. Soy sauce is traditionally made from organically grown soybeans and wheat, good quality water, and unrefined sea salt, and is fermented naturally for several years in well-aged cedar vats.

Modern commercial soy sauces are a far different product. They are made with defatted soybean meal, chemically grown grains, refined salt, and usually contain *monosodium glutamate* (a flavoring agent), caramel, sugar, or other additives or preservatives. Moreover, commercial varieties are artificially aged in temperature-controlled stainless-steel or epoxy-coated vats to reduce the time required for aging to several months.

Soup Recipes

Basic Vegetable-Miso Soup

  4–5 cups water
  ½ cup wakame, washed, soaked, and sliced

2 cups onions, sliced in thin half-moons
3–4 Tsp puréed barley or soybean (Hatcho) miso
sliced scallions for garnish

Place the water in a pot and bring to a boil. Add the wakame, reduce the flame to medium-low, cover, and simmer for 3 to 4 minutes. Add the onions, cover, and simmer another 2 to 4 minutes until the onions and wakame are tender. Reduce the flame to very low, and add the puréed miso. Simmer another 2 to 3 minutes. Place in individual serving bowls and garnish with a few sliced scallions. Serve hot.

Kombu may be substituted for wakame. Simply soak for 3 to 4 minutes, slice in very thin matchsticks and simmer for 5 to 10 minutes before adding the vegetables; or leave whole, simmer for 3 to 5 minutes, and remove.

Variations:

- carrot, onion, cabbage, and wakame or kombu
- daikon, wakame or kombu
- daikon, shiitake, wakame or kombu
- daikon, celery, wakame or kombu, and parsley garnish
- squash, onion, wakame or kombu
- celery, onion, scallion and toasted nori garnish
- carrot, onion, wakame or kombu, and tofu cubes
- onion, shiitake, kombu, and parsley garnish
- turnip, carrot, wakame or kombu
- wakame, onion, and toasted mochi
- sweet corn, onions, and wakame or kombu

These are only a few of the variety of miso soups that can be created using different combinations of vegetables. Please experiment and create new recipes or refer to cookbooks for recipes.

Miso Soup with Rice

2 cups cooked brown rice
4–5 cups water
¼ cup wakame or kombu, washed, soaked and sliced
1 cup sliced scallions and scallion roots
3 Tsp puréed barley or soybean (Hatcho) miso
sliced scallions for garnish

Place water in a pot and bring to a boil. Add the wakame or kombu, cover and simmer for 3 to 4 minutes. Add the scallion, scallion roots and cooked rice. Cover, reduce the flame to medium-low, and simmer about 10 minutes or so. Reduce the flame to very low, and add the puréed miso. Cover and simmer 2 to 3 minutes. Place in individual serving bowls and garnish with sliced scallions.

Variations:

- cooked millet, celery, onions, squash or carrots
- cooked barley, shiitake mushroom, celery, scallions
- cooked brown rice, daikon, shiitake, scallions

Again, these are only several of the many grain-miso soup recipes that can be created. Please refer to macrobiotic cookbooks for recipe ideas.

Udon or Soba with Tamari Soy Sauce Broth

> 1 **package udon or soba (8 oz), cooked, rinsed, and drained**
> **4–5 cups water, (soaking water from shiitake and kombu may be used in this measurement)**
> **1 strip kombu, 3 inches long, washed, and soaked**
> **2–3 shiitake mushrooms, soaked**
> **2 ½–3 ½ Tbsp tamari soy sauce**
> **¼ cup sliced scallions for garnish**

Place the kombu, shiitake, and water in a pot. Bring to a boil. Cover, and reduce the flame to medium-low. Simmer the kombu for 3 to 5 minutes, then remove, setting it aside for future use in other dishes. Simmer the shiitake for another 5 to 7 minutes, and set aside for future use. Reduce the flame to low, and add the tamari soy sauce. Simmer for 2 to 3 minutes. Place the cooked noodles in individual serving bowls, and ladle the hot tamari broth over them. Garnish with sliced scallions, and serve hot.

Variations: The shiitake mushrooms are an optional item in this recipe. You may use kombu only to prepare the stock. Other vegetables may be added to the broth after removing the kombu and shiitake. Simmer until tender, then season with tamari soy sauce. Fresh tofu, dried tofu, tempeh, seitan, or even fu may also be used for variety. Also, instead of removing the kombu and shiitake mushrooms, they may be sliced very thin and left in the broth to be eaten with the noodles.

Instead of adding noodles, you may prepare a simple clear tamari-broth soup with a variety of sliced, cooked vegetables in it.

Azuki Bean Soup

> 1 cup azuki beans, washed, and soaked 6–8 hours
> 1 strip kombu, 1 inch long, soaked and diced
> 4–5 cups water (the bean soaking water may be used as part of this measurement)
> 1 cup buttercup squash, cubed
> ½ cup onions, sliced
> ¼ cup carrots, sliced in chunks
> ¼ cup celery, sliced in thick diagonals
> ¼–½ Tsp sea salt
> tamari soy sauce (optional)
> sliced scallions or chopped parsley for garnish

Place the kombu in a pot. Add the onions, celery, squash, and carrots. Place the azuki beans on top. Add the water, cover, and bring to a boil. Reduce the flame to medium-low, and simmer until about 80 percent done. Add the sea salt, and continue to simmer until completely soft, which may take another 20 to 25 minutes. You may add several drops of tamari soy sauce just before serving for a slightly different flavor but it is not necessary. Garnish and serve.

Lentil Soup

> 1 cup green lentils, washed
> 1 strip kombu, 4–5 inches long, washed, soaked, and diced
> ½ cup onions, diced
> ½ cup carrots, diced
> ¼ cup celery, diced
> 2 Tbsp burdock, diced
> 1 cup whole wheat elbow pasta, cooked, rinsed, and drained
> ¼ cup chopped parsley
> 4–5 cups water
> ¼–½ Tsp sea salt
> tamari soy sauce to taste (optional)

Place the kombu, onions, celery, carrots, and burdock in the pot. Set the lentils on top. Cook as above. When 80 percent done, add the sea salt and cook another 20 minutes. Add the cooked pasta and the chopped parsley. Cook another 5 minutes or so. For a mild salt taste, you may add a little tamari soy sauce at the same time you add the pasta.

Variations: Vegetables other than those in this recipe may also be used. You may also add 1/4 cup soaked barley to this soup, letting it cook with the lentils from the beginning.

Soybean Stew

> 1 cup white soybeans, washed, and soaked 6–8 hours
> 1 strip kombu, 3–4 inches long, washed, soaked, and diced
> 2 shiitake mushrooms, soaked, stems removed, and diced
> ¼ cup dried daikon, washed, soaked, and sliced
> ¼ cup dried tofu, soaked, and cubed
> ¼ cup celery, diced
> ½ cup carrots, diced
> 2 Tbsp burdock, diced
> 3 Tbsp fresh or dried lotus root, soaked
> ½ cup cooked seitan
> 3 cups water
> grated ginger for garnish
> tamari soy sauce to taste
> sliced scallions for garnish

Place the kombu in a pressure cooker. Add the beans and water. Cover, and bring up to pressure. Reduce the flame to medium-low, and cook for 30 minutes. Remove from the flame and allow the pressure to come down. Remove the cover, and add the shiitake, dried daikon, dried tofu, celery, carrots, burdock, lotus root, and seitan.

Place the cover back on the pressure cooker, and bring up to pressure again. Reduce the flame to medium-low, and simmer another 20 to 25 minutes. Remove from the flame and allow the pressure to come down. Remove the cover and add a small amount of tamari soy sauce for a mild salt taste, and simmer another 3 to 4 minutes. Place in individual serving bowls and garnish with a dab of grated ginger and a few sliced scallions.

Variations: Other vegetables may be used in soybean stew. Ground or root vegetables are most appropriate in this dish. Soaked chick-peas can be used in place of soybeans for a different recipe. Simply soak the chick-peas 6 to 8 hours, pressure-cook 1 to 1 ¼ hours with root vegetables, and season with tamari soy sauce, puréed miso, or sea salt. Garnish and serve.

Millet Squash Soup

> ½ cup millet, washed, and dry-roasted until golden yellow
> 4–5 cups water
> 1 strip kombu, 1 inch long, soaked, and diced
> 1 cup winter squash, cubed
> ½ cup onions, diced
> ¼ cup celery, diced
> ¼ cup dried daikon, soaked and sliced
> ¼–½ Tsp sea salt
> sliced scallions for garnish
> toasted nori strips for garnish

Layer ingredients in a pot in the following order: kombu, celery, onions, dried daikon, squash. Finally, place the millet on top of the vegetables. Add a small pinch of sea salt and enough water to just cover the millet. Cover, and bring to a boil. Reduce the flame to low and simmer until the millet is soft. This may take about 30 minutes. Occasionally, during cooking, you may need to add water, as the millet expands and absorbs water. Add only enough to just cover the millet each time until the millet is done. When done, you may add a little more water for the desired thickness you choose. Add the remaining sea salt at this time. Cover, and continue to cook another 10 minutes or so. Place in individual serving bowls, garnish, and serve.

Variations: Of course other ground or root vegetables may be substituted for those above. Cooked seitan, dried-tofu cubes, or tempeh may also be used in the above recipe for variety. This soup may be seasoned with tamari soy sauce or puréed barley miso for a different flavor, energy, and color.

Other Variations: Instead of using millet, try using soaked brown rice or barley in the above recipe. Cooking time for rice or barley will be slightly longer than for millet (approximately 1 to 1 ¼ hours total). Buckwheat can also be used in making soups, using the above instructions. Dry-roast the buckwheat first before cooking with vegetables.

Brown Rice Stew

(See the section on grains for basic recipe and instructions. To alter for soup, simply add a little more water and seasoning. Sea salt or tamari soy sauce may be used as seasonings instead of puréed miso.)

Barley Soup

(See the section on grains for basic recipe and instructions. To alter for soup, simply add a little more water and seasoning. Sea salt or tamari soy sauce may be used as a seasonings instead of puréed miso.)

Buckwheat Soup

> ½ cup buckwheat, dry-roasted
> 4–5 cups water
> 1 cup onions, diced
> ½ cup celery, diced
> ¼ cup parsley, minced
> pinch of sea salt
> tamari soy sauce

Place the buckwheat in a pot. Add the onions, celery, water and sea salt. Cover, and bring to a boil. Reduce the flame to medium-low and simmer for about 15 to 20 minutes. Season with a small amount of tamari soy sauce for a mild salt taste, and add the minced parsley. Reduce the flame to low and simmer for another 4 to 5 minutes. Serve hot.

Puréed Squash Soup

> 4 cups buttercup squash or Hokkaido pumpkin, washed, skin and seeds removed, and cubed
> 4–5 cups water
> ¼–½ Tsp sea salt
> sliced scallions, or chopped parsley for garnish
> toasted nori strips for garnish

Place the squash in a pot, add a small pinch of sea salt, and the water. Cover, and bring to a boil. Reduce the flame to medium-low, and simmer several minutes, until the squash is soft. Remove the squash, and purée in a hand food mill to a creamy consistency. Place back in the pot, season with sea salt, and continue to cook another 10 minutes or so. Place in serving bowls, garnish, and serve.

Variations: Substitute the following for squash and cook in the same manner as above: carrots, cauliflower, broccoli, or summer squash.

Seitan Vegetable Stew

> 2 cups seitan, cooked
> 1 strip kombu, 3–4 inches long, soaked and cubed
> ½ cup onions, sliced in thick wedges
> 1 cup carrots, sliced in chunks
> ½ cup celery, sliced on a thick diagonal
> 1 cup Brussels sprouts, washed and sliced in half
> ¼ cup burdock, sliced on a diagonal
> ¼ cup leeks, sliced on a thick diagonal
> 4 cups water, or tamari-seasoned cooking water from seitan
> 4 Tbsp kuzu, diluted in 4–5 Tbsp water
> tamari soy sauce
> sliced scallions for garnish

Layer ingredients in the following order: kombu, celery, onions, carrots, Brussels sprouts, leeks, burdock, and seitan. Add the water, and bring to a boil. Cover, and reduce the flame to medium-low. Simmer until the vegetables are soft. Season with a small amount of tamari soy sauce for a mild salt taste, and simmer for several more minutes. Add the diluted kuzu, stirring constantly to prevent lumping. When thick, reduce the flame to low, and simmer for 2 to 3 minutes. Place in individual serving bowls, and garnish with sliced scallions.

Variations: A small amount of soaked barley, rice, or millet may be added at the beginning of cooking for a different flavor and texture, if desired. Other vegetables may be used as well, such as shiitake, white mushrooms, squash, turnips, ruttabaga, cabbage, lotus root, sweet corn, and fresh daikon.

Simple Vegetable Stews

By omitting the seitan in the above recipe, you can prepare a simple vegetable stew. Vegetables may also be sautéed on occasion before cooking for a slightly different, richer flavor. Another variation is to substitute pan-fried, or deep-fried tofu or tempeh for seitan to create variety.

Koi-koku (Carp-Burdock-Miso Soup)

1 small fresh carp
burdock (same in weight as carp), shaved
½–1 cup used bancha twigs, wrapped and tied tightly in a cheesecloth sack
½–1 Tbsp fresh grated ginger
dark sesame oil (optional)
puréed barley miso to taste
water
sliced scallions for garnish

Ask the fish seller to carefully remove the gallbladder and the yellow bitter bone (thyroid) and leave the rest of the fish intact. This includes the head, fins, tail, and scales. Next, ask him to cut the fish into chunks. He may even remove the eyes, if you wish. Wash the carp, and set aside.

Place a small amount of dark sesame oil in a pressure cooker, and heat up. Add the shaved burdock, and sauté for 2 to 3 minutes. Place the cheesecloth sack filled with used bancha twigs on top of the burdock. The used tea twigs will help to soften the hard bones of the carp. Do not use fresh, unused twigs as they will make the soup taste very bitter. Set the carp on top of the burdock and twigs. Add enough water to cover the carp and burdock.

Place the cover on the pressure cooker, and bring up to pressure. Reduce the flame to medium-low and cook for 1 ½ to 2 hours. Remove from the flame, and allow the pressure to come down. Remove the cover, add enough puréed miso for a mild salt taste (½ to 1 teaspoon puréed barley miso per cup of soup), and add the ginger. Reduce the flame to low, and simmer until the bones are soft. Place in serving bowls, and garnish with sliced scallions.

Carp soup is very strong and is best eaten in small volume. One cup at a time, daily, for two or three days is sufficient in most cases. If taken in larger quantities, it may cause cravings for fruits, liquids, sweets, or other strong yin foods.

Carp soup can be stored in a tightly sealed glass jar in the refrigerator for about 5 to 7 days. However, if frozen, it loses freshness and energy.

Variations: For those with restricted oil intakes, water-sauté the burdock instead of using oil. Carp soup may be boiled instead of pressure-cooked, for 4 to 6 hours, until the bones are soft. As liquid evaporates during boiling, add a little more water.

If carp is not available, you may substitute fresh-water trout. Have the insides removed and leave the rest of the trout intact. If burdock is not available, you may substitute carrots, sliced in matchsticks. (Half burdock and half carrots can also be used.) If you use trout, the time needed for pressure-cooking is reduced to 50 to 60 minutes. After seasoning with puréed miso and grated ginger, simmer for several more minutes on a low flame. Garnish and serve hot.

Note: In this dish, a small amount of oil is used for the purpose of softening the bones and high mineral textures of the fish. For persons with serious illness, oil is allowable in this dish.

Fish and Vegetable Soup

> 1–1 ½ lbs white-meat fish (scrod, cod, haddock, sole, etc.)
> 4–5 cups water
> ½ cup onions, sliced in thick wedges
> 1 cup carrots, sliced in chunks
> ¼ cup celery, sliced on a thick diagonal
> ½ cup daikon, quartered and sliced in ¼-inch pieces
> 2 Tbsp burdock, quartered and sliced
> 1 strip kombu, 1–2 inches long, soaked, and diced
> sea salt, tamari soy sauce, or puréed barley miso
> sliced scallions or parsley for garnish

Place the kombu in a pot and add the onions, celery, daikon, carrots, and burdock. Add the water and a small pinch of sea salt. Cover, and bring to a boil. Reduce the flame to medium-low, and simmer until the vegetables are soft and tender. Add the fish, cover, and reduce the flame to low. Simmer 4 to 5 minutes until the fish is done. Season with a small amount of sea salt, tamari soy sauce, or puréed barley miso for a mild salt taste. Simmer 5 to 10 minutes more if using sea salt, or 2 to 3 minutes if using tamari soy sauce or puréed miso. Garnish and serve hot.

You may occasionally add a small amount of grated ginger at the end of cooking for a different flavor. Please feel free to use other ground or root vegetables instead of the ones listed above.

Vegetables

Roughly one-quarter to one-third (25 to 30 percent) of each person's daily intake can include vegetables. Nature provides an incredible variety of local vegetables to choose from. Those recommended for regular use include:

Regular Use:
Acorn squash
Bok choy
Broccoli
Brussels sprouts
Burdock
Butternut squash
Cabbage
Carrots
Carrot tops
Cauliflower
Chinese cabbage
Collard greens
Daikon
Daikon greens
Dandelion roots
Dandelion leaves
Hubbard squash
Hokkaido pumpkin
Jinenjo
Kale
Leeks
Lotus root
Mustard greens
Onion
Parsley
Parsnip
Pumpkin
Radish
Red cabbage
Rutabaga
Scallions
Turnip
Turnip greens
Watercress

Occasional Use:
Celery
Chives
Coltsfoot
Cucumber
Endive

Escarole
Green beans
Green peas
Iceberg lettuce
Jerusalem artichoke
Kohlrabi
Lambs-quarters
Mushrooms
Patty pan squash
Romaine lettuce
Salsify
Shiitake mushroom
Snap beans
Snow peas
Sprouts
Summer squash
Wax beans

Avoid (for Optimum Health)
Artichoke
Bamboo shoots
Beets
Curly dock
Eggplant
Fennel
Ferns
Ginseng
Green/Red pepper
New Zealand spinach
Okra
Plantain
Purslane
Shepherd's purse
Potato
Sorrel
Spinach
Sweet potato
Swiss chard
Tomato
Taro (albi) potato
Yams
Zucchini

Vegetables can be served in soups, or with grains, beans, or sea vegetables. They can also be used in making rice rolls (homemade sushi), served with noodles or pasta, cooked with fish, or served alone. The cooking methods used for vegetables include boiling, steaming, pressing, sautéing (both waterless and with oil), and pickling. A variety of natural seasonings, including miso, tamari soy sauce, sea salt, and brown rice or umeboshi vinegar are recommended. To ensure adequate variety in the selection of vegetables, it is recommended that three to five vegetable side dishes be eaten daily.

• *Selecting the highest-quality vegetables:* In the macrobiotic diet, and especially for persons seeking to restore natural immunity, it is recommended that, whenever possible, vegetables be organic and natural in quality. Canned, frozen, and (in temperate zones) vegetables of tropical origin are best avoided.

Scientific tests show that organic produce contains up to three times more minerals and trace elements than inorganic produce. In one study, supermarket vegetables were found to have as little as 25 percent the mineral content of organic vegetables. For those who are unable to start their own backyard garden, the chief source of vegetables can be the natural food store, co-op, or farmer's market. In many outlets, organic produce is clearly marked and certified by an organic grower's association or state agency which periodically tests soil conditions and monitors cultivation standards.

Vegetable Recipes

The following methods are used often in cooking vegetables:

• *Steaming:* Steaming produces a light, refreshing quality, and can be used daily or often to prepare vegetables. Steaming can be used for most vegetables, and there are two basic methods:

1. *With a steamer basket.* Steamer baskets are available in two styles. One is a stainless-steel, collapsible basket than fits down inside a cooking pot. The other is a bamboo basket which fits on top of a cooking pot. To use these steamers, place about 1/2 inch of water in a pot. Set the stainless-steel steamer down inside the pot, or place the bamboo type on top of the pot. Next slice your vegetables, and place in the steamer. Cover, and bring the water to a boil. Steam until the vegetables are tender. When steaming greens, try to make sure the vegetables are tender but still bright green and slightly crisp. A few drops of tamari soy

sauce can occasionally be sprinkled on the vegetables, at the end of cooking, for a different flavor.

2. *Without a steamer basket.* To steam vegetables without a steamer, place about ¼ to ½ inch of water in a pot and bring to a boil. Place the vegetables in the boiling water, cover, and steam for 2 to 5 minutes depending on the type of vegetables used, or until tender. Again, at the very end of cooking, a few drops of tamari soy sauce may be sprinkled over the vegetables for a different flavor.

Steamed Greens

This particular dish may be eaten daily or often. To prepare, take greens such as turnip, daikon, carrot tops, kale, parsley, watercress, collards, cabbage, Chinese cabbage, radish tops, and so on. Wash and slice the greens, and place in a steamer or in a small amount of boiling water. Cover and steam several minutes until tender but still bright green.

If you are steaming several types of vegetables, it is best to do each separately to ensure even, proper cooking. They may be mixed after cooking. Also, the stems of green vegetables are often harder than the leafy portion and are best steamed separately, or at least chopped very finely before steaming.

It is convenient to use a steamer basket for this method of cooking, and to take about 2 to 3 minutes for steaming, depending upon the quantity and thickness of the vegetables used.

You may save the water from steaming for use as a soup stock, or as a base for a vegetable sauce which can be thickened with kuzu and lightly seasoned with sea salt, tamari soy sauce, or puréed miso. Serve over the vegetables.

• *Boiling* (*Blanched Vegetables*)*:* Lightly boiled vegetables may also be eaten daily or often. The following methods can be used regularly:

Boiled (Blanched) Kale or Other Greens

In Japanese, this style of cooking is called *ohitashi*. Wash the kale, and either leave whole or slice. Place 2 to 3 inches of water in a pot and bring to a boil. Place the kale in the water, cover, and boil 1 to 2 minutes, until deep green but slightly crisp. Remove, drain, and place in a serving bowl.

The kale may be served plain or with a sauce such as kuzu, tamari-ginger, or sesame-umeboshi dressing. You may also garnish with roasted seeds or a little gomashio.

Other green vegetables can also be cooked this way. Boil for a very short time, until the vegetables are tender but still have a crisp texture and a deep, vibrant color. The cooking time depends upon the vegetable. For example, watercress takes only 35 to 40 seconds, while collard greens may take 1 to 2 minutes.

Boiled (Blanched) Salad

This dish can also be served daily or often. Many kinds of boiled salad can be prepared simply by varying the combination of vegetables or the type of dressing served with the salad. Boiled salad can be served with or without dressing. The following is an example of boiled salad:

> **1 cup Chinese cabbage, washed, sliced on a diagonal**
> **1 cup watercress, washed, and left whole**
> **$\frac{1}{4}$ cup carrots, sliced in matchsticks**
> **2 Tbsp celery, sliced on a thin diagonal**
> **water**

Place 2 to 3 inches of water in a pot, and bring to a boil. Place the Chinese cabbage in the pot, cover, and boil for 1 to 2 minutes, or until tender but still a little crisp. Remove, place in a strainer, and allow to drain and cool. Next, place the carrots in the boiling water, cover, and simmer for 1 minute or so. Remove, drain, and allow to cool. Next do the celery, and then the watercress. After draining the watercress, you may slice it in 1-inch lengths. Place all the cooked vegetables in a serving bowl and mix. Serve plain or with a dressing.

Variations:
- Kale, carrots, cabbage, and onions
- celery and carrots
- watercress, Chinese cabbage, and sliced red radish
- daikon, carrots, Chinese cabbage, and turnip greens
- broccoli, carrots, onion, and cabbage

When making boiled salad, it is best to cook each vegetable separately in the same water. Cook the vegetables with the mildest tastes first, such as onions, daikon, or Chinese cabbage. Then do the stronger-tasting ones like celery, burdock, and watercress.

● *Salad Dressing Suggestions:*

1.   Purée 1 umeboshi plum, or 1 teaspoon umeboshi paste, with ½ cup of water in a suribachi. (Chopped parsley, scallions, or roasted sesame seeds may also be blended in for variety.)

2.   Dilute ½ teaspoon barley miso in ½ cup warm water, and add about ½ to 1 teaspoon brown rice vinegar. Mix.

3.   Dilute 1 teaspoon tamari soy sauce with ½ cup water and a small amount of chopped parsley. Mix.

4.   Lightly sprinkle a desired macrobiotic condiment on the salad.

Nishime

Nishime is another method of boiling, and is sometimes referred to as "waterless cooking" because of the low volume of water used. Vegetables are cut in large chunks or rounds, and root or round-shaped vegetables are mostly used. The vegetables are placed in a very small amount of water and cooked on a low flame for 35 to 40 minutes or so. A heavy stainless-steel pot with a heavy cover is recommended for this style of cooking. Pan-fried, deep-fried, or fresh tofu and tempeh may be cooked with the vegetables, as well as dried tofu, seitan, or fu. Nishime can be eaten 2 to 4 times per week on average.

This style of cooking produces a very sweet flavor and soft texture, and because of the slow, peaceful cooking process, imparts relaxing and calming energy.

> 1 strip kombu, washed, soaked, and cut into 1-inch squares
> 1 cup daikon, sliced in 1-inch-thick rounds
> ½ cup carrots, sliced in chunks
> 1 cup buttercup or butternut squash, or Hokkaido pumpkin, sliced in large chunks
> ¼ cup burdock, sliced on a thick diagonal
> ¼ cup fresh lotus root, sliced in ¼-inch-thick rounds
> ¼ cup turnips, sliced in thick chunks
> 1 cup cabbage, sliced in 2-inch-thick chunks
> water
> pinch of sea salt
> tamari soy sauce

Place the kombu on the bottom of the pot and add about ½ inch of water. Layer the vegetables on top of the kombu in the following order: daikon, turnips, squash, carrots, lotus root, burdock, and cabbage. Add a pinch of sea salt, cover, and bring to a boil. Reduce the flame to low and simmer for 30 to 35 minutes or until the vegetables are soft and sweet. Add several drops of tamari soy sauce, cover, and simmer for another 5 minutes or so until almost all remaining liquid is gone. Mix the vegetables to evenly coat them with the sweet cooking liquid that remains. Place in a serving bowl.

Variations:
- carrot, cabbage, burdock, kombu
- carrot, lotus root, burdock, kombu
- daikon, shiitake mushrooms, kombu
- turnip, shiitake mushrooms, kombu
- onions, cabbage, winter squash, kombu
- onions, shiitake, kombu
- daikon and kombu

Root vegetables retain their shape even when cooked for a long period. However, squash may dissolve if it is cooked too long. Therefore, squash may be added after the other vegetables have cooked for a time. The following dish is another example of nishime.

Daikon, Kombu, and Daikon Greens

> **2 cups daikon, sliced in ½-inch-thick rounds**
> **1 strip kombu, 2–3 inches long, soaked, and cubed**
> **1 cup daikon greens, sliced**
> **water**
> **tamari soy sauce**

Place the kombu in a pot and set the daikon rounds on top. Add about ½ to 1 inch of water, cover the pot, and bring to a boil. Reduce the flame to medium-low and simmer for 20 to 30 minutes or until the daikon and kombu are soft and tender. Season with a small amount of tamari soy sauce. Then, place the greens on top of the daikon, cover, and simmer 2 to 3 minutes until the greens become tender but still bright green. Mix and serve.

Variations:
- turnip, turnip greens, kombu
- carrots and carrot tops (chop finely and cook with high steam for about 7 to 10 minutes; then add carrot tops and cook another minute or so)
- dandelion root and greens (cook same as carrots)

Root and green combinations can be included 3 or 4 times per week on average.

Dried Daikon and Kombu

This dish can be eaten approximately 2 to 3 times per week; 1 cup per meal is usually sufficient. This style of cooking is known as *nitsuke*.

> ½ cup dried daikon, rinsed, soaked 10 minutes, and sliced
> 1 strip kombu, 4 inches long, soaked, and sliced in thin matchsticks
> tamari soy sauce
> water

Place the kombu in a heavy skillet or pot, and add the dried daikon. Include enough kombu soaking water to half or three-quarters cover the daikon. Cover, bring to a boil, and reduce the flame to medium-low. Simmer for 30 to 40 minutes until soft and sweet. Add a small amount of tamari soy sauce for a mild taste, cover, and continue to cook several minutes until all liquid is gone.

Variations:
- dried daikon, kombu, shiitake mushroom
- dried daikon, kombu, carrots, and onions

- *Sautéing:* Sautéed vegetables can generally be eaten 2 to 3 times per week, using any of the methods described below. There are several ways in which to sauté vegetables. The following are used most often in macrobiotic cooking:

1. *Oil-sautéing*—For persons in general good health, vegetables may be sautéed in high-quality vegetable oil 2 to 3 times per week on average. With this style of sautéing a few drops of water can sometimes be added for extra moisture and to speed the cooking process. The vegetables may be finely sliced or cut in larger pieces. Leafy greens can be prepared in this way, as can root or ground vegetables.

Oil-sautéed Vegetables

> ½ cup onions, sliced in thin half-moons
> ½ cup carrots, sliced in thin matchsticks
> ½ cup cabbage, shredded

pinch of sea salt or tamari soy sauce
dark sesame oil
water

Brush a small amount of dark sesame oil in a skillet and heat up. Add the onions, and sauté 1 to 2 minutes. Place the carrots in the skillet, and sauté 2 to 3 minutes. Add to cabbage and a pinch of sea salt, and sauté 1 to 2 minutes. Place several drops of water in the skillet, cover, and reduce the flame to medium-low. Simmer 4 to 5 minutes or until tender but still slightly crisp and brightly colored. If you choose to season with tamari soy sauce instead of sea salt, add it at the end of cooking.

2. *Water-sautéing*—This method is especially good for those who wish to limit their intake of oil. Place enough water in a skillet to just cover the bottom, and heat up. Add the vegetables, and sauté as you would if you were using oil. Season either with sea salt or several drops of tamari soy sauce.

Water-sautéed Vegetables

   $\frac{1}{2}$ **cup onion, sliced in thin half-moons**
   $\frac{1}{2}$ **cup carrot, sliced in thin matchsticks**
   $\frac{1}{2}$ **cup Chinese cabbage, sliced on a thin diagonal**
   $\frac{1}{4}$ **cup celery, sliced on a thin diagnal**
   dark sesame oil
   tamari soy sauce
   water

Place enough water in a skillet to just cover the bottom, and heat up. Add the onion, and sauté 1 to 2 minutes. Add the celery, and sauté 1 to 2 minutes. Place the carrots in the skillet, and sauté 2 to 3 minutes. Set the Chinese cabbage on top of the other vegetables. Add a few more drops of water, cover, and reduce the flame to medium-low. Simmer 3 to 4 minutes until tender but still crisp. Add a few drops of tamari soy sauce, cover, and simmer another 1 to 2 minutes. Remove the cover and cook off any remaining liquid.

3. *Kinpira*—This style of cooking combines elements of sautéing and boiling and is similar to braising. It is used mostly for root vegetables. Vegetables are thinly sliced, cut in matchsticks, or in the case of burdock, shaved, and then sautéed for several minutes in a small amount of sesame oil. (Those with restricted oil intakes may water-sautée instead.)

A small amount of water is then added to half-cover the vegetables or lightly cover the bottom of the skillet. The vegetables are then covered with a lid and cooked on a medium-low flame until about 80 percent done. A small amount of tamari soy sauce can be added for a mild salt taste, and the vegetables are covered again and cooked for another several minutes. The cover is then removed and the remaining liquid is cooked away. (This style of cooking is also used for arame or hijiki sea vegetable.)

Carrot and Burdock Kinpira

>**1 cup burdock, shaved**
>**1 cup carrots, sliced in matchsticks**
>**water**
>**tamari soy sauce**
>**dark sesame oil (optional)**

Place a small amount of dark sesame oil in a skillet and heat up. Add the burdock, and sauté for 2 to 3 minutes. Set the carrots on top of the burdock. Do not mix. Add enough water to lightly cover the bottom of the skillet, and bring to a boil. Cover, and reduce the flame to medium-low. Cook several minutes until the vegetables are about 80 percent done. This may take 7 to 10 minutes. Add a few drops of tamari soy sauce, cover, and cook for several more minutes. Remove the cover, and cook until all remaining liquid evaporates.

Variations:
- carrot, burdock, dried tofu
- carrot, burdock, lotus root
- carrot, onion, lotus root
- onions, turnip, lotus root
- carrot, onion, burdock, seitan

These dishes may be eaten 2 to 3 times per week, averaging about ½ to 1 cup per serving.

- *Raw Vegetables:* Persons in general good health may enjoy raw salad several times per week on average. Vegetables such as radish, celery, cabbage, carrot, lettuce, cucumber, and other recommended varieties may be used. The salad dressings presented earlier in this section may be used, or choose from others listed in macrobiotic cookbooks.

● *Pressed Vegetables:* Pressed vegetables (often referred to as "pressed salad") are light and refreshing. They may be eaten daily (about ½ cup per serving) or often. Pressed vegetables are combined with a salty pickling agent such as sea salt or umeboshi vinegar and are pressed for 2 hours or more. When done, the vegetables are lightly pickled instead of raw, and are easier to digest. Pressed salad can be prepared in the following ways:

1. *With a pickle press*—A *pickle press* is a specially made plastic jar (they come in several sizes) with a screw on the lid and a moveable plastic plate that fits inside for applying pressure. They are available at most natural food stores. To prepare pressed salad, slice vegetables very thinly and place in a bowl. Add a small amount of either sea salt, brown rice vinegar, or umeboshi vinegar, and mix well. Put the chopped vegetables in the pickle press, and place the cover on top. Screw the plate down to apply pressure. Let the vegetables sit for 2 to 4 hours before serving. If they are too sslty, rinse them quickly under cold water and squeeze out any excess liquid.

2. *With bowl and plate*—If you do not have a pickle press, you can make one. Simply slice your vegetables as described above, and place in a bowl with one of the above-mentioned pickling agents, and mix well. Place a plate or saucer that is a little smaller than the bowl inside so that it rests on top of the vegetables. Next, fill a large glass jar with water or take a heavy, clean rock and place it on top of the plate for pressure. Let sit for 2 to 4 hours. If too salty when done, simply rinse quickly under cold water and squeeze out any excess liquid.

Pressed Salad

 2 cups lettuce, thinly sliced
 ¼ cup celery, sliced on a thin diagonal
 ½ cup cucumber, sliced in thin rounds
 ¼ cup onion, sliced in very thin rounds
 ¼ cup red radish, sliced in very thin rounds
 2–3 Tbsp umeboshi vinegar

Place all ingredients in a bowl and mix well. Place in a pickle press or bowl, and apply pressure. Let sit for 2 to 4 hours. Remove, and squeeze out excess liquid. If too salty, rinse quickly under cold water, then squeeze out excess liquid.

• *Pickling:*

(Please refer to the section on pickles for specific recipes or suggestions.)

• *Other Methods*: Baking and pressure-cooking tend to make the energy in vegetables more drying or concentrated. These methods are not recommended for regular use in preparing vegetables. A lighter and fresher quality of energy is preferred for regular use.

Beans and Bean Products

Beans and bean products may be eaten daily or often, so that they comprise about 5 to 10 percent of daily intake. The following may be used in cooking:

Regular Use:
Azuki beans
Black soybeans
Chick-peas (garbanzo beans)
Lentils (green)

Navy beans
Pinto beans
Soybeans
Split peas
Whole dried peas

Occasional Use:
Black-eyed peas
Black turtle beans
Great northern beans
Kidney beans
Mung beans

Occasional Use Bean Products:
Dried tofu
Fresh tofu
Natto
Tempeh

Beans and bean products can be cooked in the following ways: with kombu (about 10 percent); with carrots and onions (about 20 percent); with acorn/butternut squash; with chestnuts (about 20 to 30 percent); in soup with vegetables; and with whole grains (about 10 to 15 percent beans).

• *Selecting the highest-quality beans:* Smaller, low-fat varieties of beans, such as those listed in the regular-use column are preferred for daily or frequent use over larger or more fatty beans. Of the varieties of azuki beans available, higher-grade beans—those with a deep red or maroon color and shiny surface—are preferred over those with a dull surface or faded color. High-grade azuki beans are grown in northern Japan on the island of Hokkaido in mineral-rich volcanic soil. They are carefully selected after harvesting so that they generally have a uniform color and shininess. For general daily use, either variety is fine, but for strengthening health and immune ability, the higher-grade beans are recommended.

Bean Recipes

Most beans require soaking for 6 to 8 hours before cooking to make them softer and more digestible. Exceptions to this are green lentils and split peas, which are soft in comparison to other beans and cook more quickly. Beans may be soaked in cold, warm, or hot water. Soaking in cold water gives them a slightly firmer texture. They may require more cooking time than beans soaked in hot water. Warm water makes the beans softer, more easy to digest, and quicker to cook. If you use hot water, beans only need to be soaked for 4 to 6 hours.

With the exception of azuki beans and black soybeans, the water from soaking beans can be discarded. The soaking water from these two beans may be added during cooking.

It is best to cook beans with a small strip of kombu. The minerals in the kombu soften the hard outer shell of the beans, making them more digestible. Kombu also enhances the flavor of beans.

The most frequently recommended methods for cooking bean side dishes are:

1. *Boiling*—Place 1 cup of dried, soaked beans in a pot, add a 3- to 4-inch piece of kombu and 3 $\frac{1}{2}$ to 4 cups of cold water. Bring to a boil, cover, and reduce the flame to medium-low. Simmer until the beans are about 80 percent done. Season with $\frac{1}{4}$ teaspoon sea salt per cup of uncooked beans or the equivalent amount of tamari soy sauce or puréed miso. Cover the pot and simmer until the beans are soft. When done, remove the cover and boil off any excess water until you have the desired consistency.

2. *Shocking Method*—Place a 3- to 4-inch strip of kombu in a pot and set 1 cup of soaked beans on top. Add water (2 $\frac{1}{2}$ cups per cup of beans). Leave the pot uncovered and cook slowly on a low flame until the water comes to a boil. Place a lid down inside the pot so that it rests on the beans. The lid will keep the beans from jumping around. As the beans cook, they will expand in size. Occasionally pour a small amount of water gently down the side of the pot as needed. Continue to cook until the beans are about 80 percent done. At this point, season as above,

leave the cover off, and continue to cook until the beans are soft. Turn up the heat at this point and cook off any excess liquid that remains.

Below are several bean recipes that illustrate these methods:

Azuki Beans with Kombu and Squash

> 1 cup azuki beans, soaked 4–6 hours
> 1 cup hard winter squash, cubed (use acorn, buttercup, butternut squash or Hokkaido pumpkin; carrots or parsnips may be substituted if squash is not available)
> 1 strip kombu, 1–2 inches long, soaked and diced
> water
> sea salt

Place the kombu on the bottom of a pot. Set the squash on top. Place the azuki beans on top of the squash. Add water to just cover the squash. Bring to a boil, cover, and reduce the flame to low. Simmer until about 80 percent done. Season with ¼ teaspoon of sea salt per cup of beans, cover, and continue to cook another 15 to 20 minutes until soft and creamy.

Variations:
- 1 cup azuki beans, ½ cup lotus seeds, kombu
- 1 cup azuki beans, ½ cup dried chestnuts, kombu
- 1 cup azuki beans, ¼ cup soaked wheat berries, kombu
- 1 cup azuki beans, ¼ cup dried apples, 1 tablespoon raisins, kombu
(this dish can be used as a sweet dessert)

Use either of the methods described above to prepare.

Soybean Stew

(Please refer to the section on beans for recipe.)

Soybeans and Hijiki

(Please refer to the section on sea vegetables for recipe.)

Soybeans and Kombu

> 1 cup soybeans, soaked 6–8 hours in 2 ½ cups water

1 strip kombu, 6 inches long, soaked and cubed
2 ½ cups water
tamari soy sauce

Drain off soaking water and place the kombu and soybeans in a pressure cooker. Add fresh water, and boil for 15 minutes, skimming off any skins that float to the surface. Cover the pressure cooker and bring up to pressure. Reduce the flame to medium-low, and cook for approximately 50 minutes. Remove from the flame and allow the pressure to come down. Remove the cover, add a small amount of tamari soy sauce, and simmer uncovered for another 5 to 10 minutes. Remove, garnish and serve.

Variations:
• soybeans, kombu, onions, and carrots
• soybeans, kombu, carrots, lotus root, burdock, seitan, celery, shiitake mushrooms, and dried daikon (thicken at the end of cooking with a small amount of diluted kuzu)

• *Black Soybeans:*   Black soybeans are washed and soaked in a slightly different way than other beans because of their soft skins. To wash, first dampen a clean kitchen towel. Place the beans in the towel and cover completely. Roll the bean-filled towel back and forth several times to rub off dust and soil. Place the beans in a bowl, dampen the towel again, and repeat. This can be done 2 to 3 times until the beans are clean.

After washing the beans, place them in a bowl. Add about 3 cups of water for each cup of beans, and ¼ teaspoon of sea salt. Soak the beans 6 to 8 hours or overnight. Place the beans in a pot, together with the salt-seasoned soaking water, and bring to a boil. Do not cover the beans. Reduce the flame to medium-low, and simmer until the beans are about 90 percent done, which may take about 2 to 3 hours. During cooking you may need to add water occasionally but add only enough to just cover the beans each time.

As the beans cook, a gray foam will rise to the surface. Skim off and discard. Repeat until the foam no longer appears. When the beans are about 90 percent done, add several drops of tamari soy sauce. Do not mix with a spoon. You may however, gently shake the pot up and down 2 to 3 times to mix the beans and coat them with bean juice, which will make the skins a very shiny black color. Continue cooking until no liquid remains. Total cooking time varies from 3 to 3 ½ hours.

Chick-peas and Vegetables

> 1 cup chick-peas, soaked 6–8 hours or overnight
> 1 cup carrots, sliced in chunks
> ½ cup celery, sliced on a thick diagonal
> 1 strip kombu, 1–2 inches long, soaked and diced
> water
> sea salt or puréed barley miso

Place the kombu, celery, carrots, and chick-peas in a pot, and add water to just cover. Prepare using either of the methods described above. When 80 percent done, season with tamari soy sauce, sea salt, or puréed barley miso. If boiling, chick-peas may take 3 to 4 hours.

Green Lentils with Onions and Kombu

> 1 cup green lentils
> 1 cup onions, sliced in thick wedges or diced
> 1 strip kombu, 2 inches long, soaked, and diced
> sea salt
> water
> chopped parsley garnish

Place the kombu in a pot, and set the onions on top. Add the lentils. Add enough water to just cover the lentils. Bring to a boil, reduce the flame to medium-low, and cover. Simmer about 35 minutes or until about 80 percent done. Occasionally, during cooking you may need to add small amounts of water as the beans expand and absorb liquid. Each time add just enough water to cover the lentils. When the lentils are almost done, season with approximately 1/4 teaspoon of sea salt per cup of beans. Cover and simmer another 10 to 15 minutes.

Variations:
- lentils, onions, carrots, celery, kombu
- lentils, onions, carrots, burdock, celery, kombu and parsley

Bean Product Recipes

Dried Tofu with Kombu and Carrots

> ½ cup dried tofu, soaked, and cubed or sliced in rectangles
> 1 cup carrots, sliced in thick matchsticks

1 strip kombu, 2–3 inches long, soaked, and sliced in very thin matchsticks
water
tamari soy sauce

Place the kombu in a pot. Add the dried tofu and carrots. Add enough water to just cover the dried tofu, and bring to a boil. Reduce the flame to medium-low, cover, and simmer about 25 to 30 minutes or until the kombu is soft. Add several drops of tamari soy sauce, cover, and continue to cook for 3 to 5 minutes. Remove the cover, and simmer until excess liquid is gone.

Scrambled Tofu

1 cake fresh tofu, 1 1b, drained
½ cup onions, diced
½ cup carrots, sliced in matchsticks
¼ cup burdock, sliced in matchsticks
¼ cup celery, sliced on a thin diagonal
dark sesame oil
tamari soy sauce
chopped scallion garnish

Brush a small amount of dark sesame oil in the bottom of a skillet, and heat up. Add the onions, and sauté 1 to 2 minutes. Next add the celery, and sauté 1 to 2 minutes. Set the carrots and burdock on top of the celery and onions. Crumble the tofu and spread on top of the vegetables. Cover, and bring to a boil. Reduce the flame to medium-low, and simmer until the tofu is soft and fluffy and the vegetables are tender. Add a small amount of chopped scallions and several drops of tamari soy sauce. Cover and simmer another 2 to 3 minutes.

Variations:
- sweet corn, onions, and parsley or scallions
- green beans, carrots, and onions
- carrots, onions, and toasted nori squares
- season with a small amount of umeboshi vinegar instead of tamari soy sauce
- season with a pinch of sea salt instead of tamari soy sauce or umeboshi vinegar
- water-sauté the vegetables instead of using oil

Tempeh with Sauerkraut and Cabbage

1 cup tempeh, cubed
1 cup green cabbage, shredded
¼ cup sauerkraut, chopped
small amount of sauerkraut juice
tamari soy sause

Heat a skillet and add the tempeh cubes. Place a drop of tamari soy sauce on each cube, and brown slightly. Add the sauerkraut and cabbage. Add enough sauerkraut juice or plain water to half-cover the tempeh. Bring to a boil, cover, and reduce the flame to low. Simmer about 20 to 25 minutes. Remove the cover and cook off any remaining liquid.

Variations:
- tempeh and leeks
- tempeh, scallions, and ginger juice
- tempeh and onions, with parsley garnish
- season with tamari soy sauce or a little umeboshi paste or plum instead of sauerkraut juice

- *Natto:* Natto, or lightly fermented whole soybeans, is usually combined with a little tamari soy sauce and chopped scallions, mixed, and eaten together with cooked brown rice or other grains, or on top of noodles. Natto can also be added to a very simple wakame-onion miso soup, or daikon-wakame miso soup on occasion. Recipes for using natto are presented in macrobiotic cookbooks as are instructions for making it at home.

Sea Vegetables

Sea vegetables may be used daily in cooking. Side dishes can be made with arame or hijiki and included several times per week. Wakame and kombu can be used daily in miso and other soups, in vegetable and bean dishes, or as condiments. Toasted nori is also recommended for daily or regular use, while agar-agar can be used from time to time in making a natural jelled dessert known as *kanten*. Below is a list of sea vegetables used in macrobiotic cooking.

Regular Use (almost daily):
Arame

Occasional or Optional Use:
Agar-agar

Regular Use (almost daily):	*Occasional or Optional Use:*
Hijiki	Dulse
Kombu	Irish moss
Wakame	Mekabu
Toasted nori	Sea palm
	Other traditionally used sea vegetables

● *Selecting the highest-quality natural sea vegetables:* Sea vegetables are rich in minerals, and help clean the blood. Sea vegetables that are naturally processed according to traditional methods are preferred, and these are the varieties available in natural food stores.

Recent scientific studies have upheld many of the traditional beliefs associating sea vegetables with a variety of health benefits. In 1984, medical researchers at Harvard University reported that a diet containing 5 percent kombu significantly delayed the inducement of breast cancer in experimental animals. Extrapolating these results to human subjects, the investigators concluded, "Seaweed may be an important factor in explaining the low rates of certain cancers in Japan." Japanese women, whose diet normally includes about 3 to 5 percent sea vegetables, have from three to nine times less breast-cancer incidence than American women, for whom sea vegetables are not a part of their usual diet.

Sea Vegetable Recipes

Arame with Carrots and Onions

> **1 oz dried arame, rinsed, drained, and allowed to sit 3–5 minutes**
> **¹⁄₂ cup onions, sliced in thin half-moons**
> **¹⁄₂ cup carrots, sliced in matchsticks**
> **dark sesame oil**
> **water**
> **tamari soy sauce**

Lightly brush dark sesame oil in a skillet and heat up. Place the onions in the skillet and sauté 1 to 2 minutes. Place the sliced carrots on top of the onions. Slice the arame and set on top of the carrots. Do not mix. Add enough water to just cover the vegetables but not the arame, and a very small amount of tamari soy sauce. Bring to a boil, reduce the flame to medium-low, and cover. Simmer for about 25 to 40 minutes. Lightly season with a few drops of tamari for a mild salt taste. Cover and cook another 5 to 7 minutes. Remove the cover, and continue to cook until almost all liquid is gone. Mix and cook off remaining liquid. Garnish and serve.

Variations:
- arame, onions and lotus root
- arame, onions, carrots, and tempeh (plain or fried)
- arame and roasted sesame seed garnish
- arame and dried daikon
- arame, onions, and sweet corn
- water-sauté the vegetables
- sauté arame first then add vegetables and cook

Hijiki with Onions and Lotus Root

Depending on the texture or hardness of the hijiki, the cooking time may vary. Softer varieties of hijiki may only need to be cooked 30 to 40 minutes until soft, while harder varieties may require as much as 1 hour cooking time. Please adjust the cooking time depending on the variety of hijiki that is available to you.

> 1 oz hijiki, washed, soaked 3–5 minutes, and sliced
> ½ cup onions, sliced in thin half-moons
> ½ cup fresh lotus root, washed, halved, and thinly sliced
> dark sesame oil
> water
> tamari soy sauce

Lightly brush dark sesame oil in a skillet and heat. Add the onions and sauté 1 to 2 minutes. Add the lotus root and sauté 1 to 2 minutes. Place the hijiki on top of the vegetables. Add enough water to cover the vegetables but not the hijiki. Bring to a boil, cover, and reduce the flame to medium-low. Simmer for 30 to 45 minutes depending on the texture or hardness of the hijiki. Season with a few drops of tamari soy sauce for a mild salt taste, cover, and continue to cook another 10 to 15 minutes. Remove the cover, mix, and simmer until all remaining liquid is gone. Garnish and serve.

Variations:
- hijiki, onions, and carrots
- hijiki, onions, carrots, and tempeh (plain or fried)
- hijiki, onions, carrots, and fried tofu

- hijiki and roasted or soaked yellow soybeans
- hijiki and dried daikon
- hijiki, onions, carrots, and dried tofu
- water-sauté the vegetables
- sauté hijiki first, then add vegetables

Boiled Kombu with Carrots and Burdock

2 strips kombu, 6 inches long, soaked, and cubed
1 cup burdock, sliced on thick diagonals
1 ½ cups carrot, sliced in chunks
water
tamari soy sauce

Place the kombu in the bottom of a pot. Add the burdock and carrots. Add enough water to half-cover the vegetables. Bring to a boil, cover, and reduce the flame to medium-low. Simmer for 30 to 35 minutes or until the kombu and vegetables are soft and tender. Season with a few drops of tamari soy sauce, cover, and simmer another 5 to 10 minutes. Remove the cover and cook off all remaining liquid. Mix and serve.

Variations:
- kombu, carrots, and onions
- kombu, carrots, and dried tofu
- kombu, carrots, daikon, and fried tofu
- kombu and matchstick pieces of ginger
- kombu and dried daikon
- kombu, dried daikon, and shiitake mushrooms

Wakame, Onions and Carrots

1 oz dried wakame, washed, soaked, and sliced
½ cup onions, sliced in thick wedges
½ cup carrots, sliced in chunks
water
tamari soy sauce

Place the onions, carrots, and wakame in a pot. Add enough water to half-cover the vegetables. Bring to a boil, cover, and reduce the flame to medium-low. Simmer 25 to 30 minutes or until the vegetables are soft. Add a few drops of tamari soy sauce for a mild salt taste. Cover and simmer another 10 to 15 minutes.

Variations:
- wakame, onions, carrots, and parsnips
- wakame, onions, and parsnips

• *Toasted Nori:* Nori, a light, thin sea vegetable that usually comes in dried sheets, does not require washing or soaking, but to increase its digestibility, it can be dry-roasted. Take a sheet of nori from the package, and hold it so that the smooth, shiny side faces upward. Turn the flame on your stove to medium, and hold the nori about 6 inches above it. Slowly rotate or move the nori above the flame until it changes from purplish brown to green. You may cut it into strips or squares for use as a garnish on soups, stews, noodles or grains, or simply break off small pieces and eat as a snack. Toasted nori can also be used in making rice balls and sushi by wrapping cooked rice and other ingredients inside it. Please see the section on grains for recipes.

Condiments

A variety of condiments may be used, some daily and others occasionally. Small amounts may be used on grains, soups, vegetables, beans, and other dishes. Condiments allow everyone to freely adjust the taste and nutritional value of foods, and stimulate and contribute to better appetite and digestion. The most frequently used varieties include:

Main Condiments:
Gomashio (a half-crushed mixture of roasted sesame seeds and roasted sea salt)
Sea-vegetable powder
Sea-vegetable powder with roasted sesame seeds
Tekka (selected root vegetables sautéed with dark sesame oil and seasoned with soybean, or Hatcho, miso)
Umeboshi plum (pickled plums)

Other Condiments:
Cooked miso with scallions or onions
Nori condiment (nori cooked with tamari soy sauce)
Roasted sesame seeds
Shiso-leaf powder
Shio kombu (kombu cooked with tamari soy sauce)
Green-nori flakes

Brown rice vinegar (used mostly as a seasoning)
Umeboshi plum and raw scallions or onions
Umeboshi vinegar (used mostly as a seasoning)
Other traditionally used condiments (not highly stimulating ones)

• *Selecting the highest-quality natural condiments:* In macrobiotic cooking, condiments and garnishes provide nutritional and energetic balance to the meal. Among regular condiments, gomashio, or sesame salt, is especially nutritious. It contains a high amount of calcium, iron, and other nutrients and is an excellent way to obtain polyunsaturated vegetable oil in whole form. Also, because they are roasted, the sesame seeds in gomashio are easier to digest. The roasted salt with which they are combined provides a harmonious balance to the oil in the seeds.

The proportion of sesame seeds to sea salt can range from 10 to 1 to 18 to 1, depending on individual condition and need. The best quality sesame seeds for use in gomashio are natural black sesame seeds. Be careful when choosing seeds, however, because some black seeds are dyed. To distinguish dyed seeds from natural black seeds, put them in warm water. The artificial coloring in the dyed seeds will gradually dissolve and the water will turn black.

To further test the quality of sesame seeds, place them in water. The most yang, nutritious seeds slowly sink to the bottom. The more yin or damaged seeds float to the top. Black sesame seeds that slowly sink are the best quality for use and have the maximum effectiveness in strengthening natural immunity.

Tekka is a traditional condiment made from minced burdock, carrots, lotus root, Hatcho miso, and dark sesame oil. These ingredients are cooked down, over many hours, into a concentrated black powder. Toward the end of cooking, the mixture is seasoned with ginger. Tekka is recommended for regular use. Since it provides a very strong, concentrated form of energy, this condiment can be used in small amounts sprinkled on grains, noodles, or vegetables. It can be purchased ready-made, in natural food stores.

Umeboshi plums are also recommended for regular use. The plums grow in the warmer, southern and middle regions of Japan and are related to the apricot. Traditionally fermented with sea salt and pickled with shiso leaves, umeboshi plums have a tangy flavor, combining a sour and salty taste. They are a very balanced food, give a strong centering energy, and have a wide range of uses. Once again, the quality of modern, commercially prepared umeboshi plums is different from the quality of the past. Their aging is artifically speeded up, and synthetic colorings are often added to give them the deep red color that naturally comes from aging.

Even though umeboshi plums in natural food stores are generally good quality, their taste and energy differ widely. Those that have aged the longest are less tart and salty and give stronger energy, and are especially recommended. If it were possible to obtain them, umeboshi plums that have aged for more than five years would be ideal. The plums become almost transparent, and are very strong in their effects, so that only a tiny piece is enough to balance grains or other foods.

Condiment Recipes

Gomashio (Sesame Salt)

> 1 cup black sesame seeds, washed, and drained
> 1 Tbsp sea salt

Place the sea salt in a hot skillet and dry-roast several minutes over a medium flame until it becomes shiny. Remove and grind to a fine powder in a suribachi. Next, place the damp sesame seeds in a heated skillet and dry-roast over a medium-low flame, stirring them constantly with a wooden rice paddle. Shake the skillet back and forth occasionally to evenly roast. When the seeds give off a nutty fragrance, and begin popping, take a seed and crush it between your thumb and ring finger. It if crushes easily, the seeds are done. If not, roast them a little longer.

When the seeds are done, place them in the suribachi and slowly grind together with the sea salt. Continue grinding until the seeds are about half crushed. Allow to cool and store in a tightly sealed glass container. Use moderately on grains, noodles, or vegetable dishes.

Variation: Use tan instead of black sesame seeds.

Sea-vegetable Powders

Take several pieces of kombu, wakame, or dulse and place them, unwashed, on a baking sheet. Roast in a 350°F oven for approximately 15 to 20 minutes, or until crispy and dark but not burnt, or place in a dry skillet and roast until crispy and dark. Remove and break the roasted sea vegetable into small pieces over a suribachi. Crush into a fine powder. Allow to cool and store in a tightly sealed glass container. Sprinkle lightly on grains, noodles or vegetable dishes.

Sea-vegetable and Roasted Sesame-seed Powders

Roast one of the above sea vegetables as explained. After roasting, grind into a fine powder in a suribachi. Dry-roast washed and drained tan sesame seeds as you would if making gomashio. When done, place the roasted seeds in the suribachi and grind with the sea-vegetable powder until the seeds are about 50 percent crushed. Allow to cool and store in a tightly sealed glass container. Use as you would gomashio or roasted sea-vegetable powders. The average proportion of seeds to powdered sea vegetable can be about 60 percent to 40 percent.

Tekka

Since it traditionally takes about sixteen hours to prepare, tekka is usually bought ready-made at a natural food store. If you wish to prepare your own tekka, the recipe can be found in macrobiotic cookbooks.

Nori Condiment

5 sheets nori, unroasted
water
tamari soy sauce

Tear the nori into small squares and place in a saucepan. Add water to just cover. Bring to a boil, cover, and reduce the flame to low. Simmer until the nori becomes a smooth, thick paste. Season with several drops of tamari soy sauce for a mild salt taste and continue to cook until all liquid is gone. Allow to cool and store in the refrigerator, in a tightly sealed glass container. Eat with grains, noodles, or vegetable dishes. A small amount of freshly grated ginger may be added at the end of cooking for a special flavor.

Variation: On occasion, a few drops of barley malt, brown rice syrup, or *mirin* (the fermented liquid of sweet rice) may be added at the end of cooking for a sweeter taste.

Pickles

A small amount of naturally made vegetable pickles can be eaten daily or often as a supplement to main dishes. Pickles stimulate appetite and help digestion. Some varieties—such as pickled daikon, or *takuan*—can be bought prepackaged in natural food stores. Others—such as quick pickles—can be prepared at home. Certain varieties take just a few hours to prepare, while others require more time.

A wide variety of pickles are fine for regular use, including salt, salt brine, bran, miso, tamari soy sauce, umeboshi vinegar, and others. Natural sauerkraut may also be used in small volume on an occasional basis. Below are the varieties of pickles recommended for use:

Regular Use:
Rice-bran pickles
Brine pickles
Miso bean pickles
Miso pickles
Pressed pickles
Sauerkraut
Tamari soy sauce pickles
Takuan pickles
Amazaké pickles

Avoid (for Optimum Health):
Dill pickles
Herb pickles
Garlic pickles
Spiced pickles
Vinegar pickles (commercial apple cider vinegar or wine vinegar pickles)

Vegetables Used Often in Making Pickles:
Burdock root
Broccoli
Cabbage
Carrots
Cauliflower
Chinese cabbage
Cucumbers
Daikon
Leeks
Lotus root
Mustard greens
Olives
Onions
Pumpkin
Radishes, red and white
Red cabbage
Scallions
Squash
Turnips

• *Selecting the highest-quality natural pickles:* The best pickles are made from natural ingredients, such as fresh organic vegetables, high-quality natural sea salt, and naturally fermented miso, tamari soy sauce, umeboshi, and vinegars. Pickles processed with strong spices, sugar, artificial vinegar, or chemicals are best avoided for maximum health. Spicy pickles, for example, are often eaten to balance the consumption of meat and other animal foods. However, in temperate climates, the intake of strong spices or artificial vinegar creates imbalance with the surrounding environment and can weaken natural immune power.

Pickle Recipes

Umeboshi-Vegetable Pickles

Place 7 to 8 umeboshi plums in a glass jar and add 2 quarts of water. Shake well and allow to sit several hours until the water becomes pink. Place a variety of thinly sliced vegetables (red radish, daikon, carrot, onion, cauliflower flowerettes, broccoli flowerettes, red onion, cabbage, etc.) in the water. Cover the jar with clean, cotton cheesecloth and place in a cool place for 3 to 5 days. When done, remove and serve. If too salty, rinse quickly under cold water before serving.

Quick Tamari Soy Sauce-Vegetable Pickles

Slice a variety of root or ground vegetables into thin slices and place in a glass jar. Cover with a mixture of ½ water and ½ tamari soy sauce. Shake and cover the jar with clean, cotton cheesecloth. Allow to sit in a cool place for 2 to 3 hours. Remove and serve, or, if too salty, rinse quickly and serve.

Longer Tamari Soy Sauce-Vegetable Pickles

Prepare as above only allow the vegetables to pickle in the tamari-water solution for 3 to 5 days. Remove, rinse and serve.

Brine Pickles

Boil 3 to 4 cups of water together with 1 teaspoon of sea salt until the salt is completely dissolved. Allow to cool completely. Place a 3-inch piece of kombu in a jar and pour the cool salt brine over it. Place thin slices of root or ground vegetables such as carrots, daikon, radishes, onions, broccoli, cauliflower, and cucumber, in the water. Cover the jar with clean, cotton cheesecloth and let sit in a slightly cool and dark place (not the refrigerator) for 3 days. These pickles are best stored in the refrigerator.

Other Pickles

A variety of pre-packaged pickles can be purchased at most natural food stores, including daikon-rice-bran pickles, takuan pickles, ginger pickles, and sauerkraut. If the pickles taste too salty, simply rinse or soak for ½ hour before eating.

Supplementary Foods ───────────────────────

A variety of supplementary foods can be enjoyed occasionally in the Standard Macrobiotic Diet. Some items can be eaten several times per week, and others—such as seasonings and beverages—are used daily but in smaller amounts than the foods listed above. Supplementary foods include:

White-meat Fish

For variety, enjoyment, and nourishment, fish and seafood may be enjoyed on occasion by those in ordinary good health. The frequency of eating fish and seafood varies according to climate, age, sex, and personal needs, and can range from once in a while to more regularly, the standard being about once or twice per week in a temperate climate.

The kinds of fish and seafood recommended are those with less fat and cholesterol and those that are most easily digested, especially low-fat, white-meat varieties. As a separate side dish, fresh fish is usually prepared in a small to moderate amount as a supplement to whole grains and vegetables, which still comprise the major volume of the meal. Fish may also be served in soups or stews and cooked with other foods. The varieties of white-meat fish recommended for occasional consumption include the following examples:

Ocean Varieties:
Cod
Flounder
Haddock
Halibut
Herring
Ocean trout
Perch
Scrod
Shad
Smelt
Sole
Other varieties of white-meat
   ocean fish

Fresh-water Varieties:
Bass
Carp
Catfish
Pike
Trout
Whitefish
Other varieties of white-meat,
   fresh-water fish

Dried Fish:
Bonito flakes (dried bonita,
   freshly shredded)
Chirimen iriko (very small
   dried fish)
Dried white-meat fish

Note: Shellfish such as lobster, crabmeat, and shrimp are best limited or avoided for optimum health as they are high in cholesterol.

• *Selecting the highest-quality fish and seafood:* In the past, fish was one of the most uncontaminated and least processed foods. However, in modern times, its quality has been greatly affected by pollution, and seafood has been subjected to many potentially harmful industrial processing techniques. Finding a reliable source of truly fresh and uncontaminated fish is very important for people who wish to include this supplementary food in their diet. As a general rule, seawater species are less polluted than fresh-water varieties. Among deep-water species, moreover, white-meat fish are less fatty and oily than red-meat and blue-skinned varieties. Store-bought fish and seafood should be obtained as fresh as possible. Avoid frozen, smoked, canned, prestuffed, prebreaded, concentrated, or otherwise commercially processed varieties. However, fish or seafood that has been dried, pickled, or naturally processed without artificial preservatives may occasionally be used.

When selecting fresh fish, things to look for include good color, smooth skin, clear eyes (rather than cloudy), good odor (a fishy smell shows decay), clean and intact gills, and resiliency when poked.

In the kitchen, fish and seafood should be stored, cleaned, and cut separately from vegetables, fruit, and other plant foods, even though they may later be cooked together. Using a separate knife and cutting board for this purpose prevents the heavier animal-quality vibrations, odor, and taste from interfering with the lighter energy of vegetable foods.

Also, fish and seafood are best served with garnishes that help offset the effects caused by their proteins and fats. A small side dish or serving of grated daikon or grated radish, with a few drops of tamari soy sauce and a touch of grated ginger helps neutralize these effects.

Fish Recipes

Koi-koku (Carp-Burdock-Miso Soup)

(Please refer to the section on soups for recipe.)

Trout-Carrot Miso Soup

(Please refer to the section on soups for recipe.)

Fish Soup or Stew

(Please refer to the section on soups for recipe.)

Broiled or Grilled White-meat Fish

To broil or grill fish, marinate in a mixture of equal parts water and tamari soy sauce and a few drops or fresh ginger juice for 1 hour, or simply sprinkle with freshly squeezed lemon juice and a few drops of tamari soy sauce. Broil or grill until tender and flaky. Remove and serve with a garnish and grated daikon.

Steamed or Boiled White-meat Fish

Marinate as above or place plain fish in a steamer basket or saucepan. Steam or boil until tender and flaky. Remove and serve with a garnish and grated daikon.

Baked White-meat Fish

Marinate as above and bake as is or stuff the fish fillets with thinly sliced vegetables, cover, and bake at 450° to 475°F for 20 minutes or until soft and tender. Serve with a garnish and grated daikon.

Variation: Bake with a thin layer of puréed miso covering the fish.

Fruit

In general, fruit can be enjoyed on occasion by those in normal good health. Frequency of consumption varies according to climate, season, age, level of activity, and personal need and health considerations. The average is about two to four times per week.

However, for those who wish to rebuild natural immune ability, it is recommended that fruit be eaten only when craved. In this circumstance, the first preference would be dried fruit that is soaked and then cooked with a pinch of sea salt. The second choice is a small volume of fresh fruit that is cooked with a pinch of sea salt. Fresh fruits are ideally consumed in the season in which they are grown, and are least preferable for the restoration of natural immunity. If fresh fruit is craved however, it is recommened that it be eaten in small amounts with a pinch of sea salt sprinkled on it.

Among fruits, locally grown or temperate-climate varieties are preferred, especially for persons living in these regions. As much as possible, it is best to avoid consumption of tropical fruit, especially for persons wishing to recover natural immunity. Below, the varieties of fruit that can be eaten in a temperate climate are presented according to season of availability or optimum season for use:

Spring:
Plums
Cherries
Strawberries
Dried fruit

Summer:
Apricots
Blueberries
Blackberries
Cantaloupes
Cherries
Dried fruit
Grapes
Peaches
Raisins
Raspberries
Strawberries
Tangerines
Watermelon

Autumn:
Apples
Pears
Grapes
Dried fruit
Raisins

Winter:
Pears
Raisins
Dried fruit

Dried Fruit (Unsulphured):
Apples
Apricots
Peaches
Pears
Raisins
Cherries
Plums
Prunes

Avoid in a Temperate Climate:
Banana
Dates
Figs
Pineapple
Other tropical fruits

• *Selecting the highest-quality natural fruit:* Obtaining good-quality fruit is essential because of the exceptionally poor quality of most commercially available supplies. Whenever possible, organically grown fruit should be obtained. Organic or more naturally grown fruit will generally be slightly smaller in size, duller in appearance, and contain more blemishes and evidence of nibbling by small insects than commercially grown fruit. However, it will generally have a more symmetrical shape, fresher aroma, and sweeter taste than the other kind.

Cooked Fruit Recipes

Stewed Fruit with Kuzu

> 2 cups apple juice or water (or half and half)
> 1 cup sliced apples or pears
> 1 Tbsp raisins
> pinch of sea salt
> 3 heaping Tsp kuzu

Place the raisins, apple juice or water, and pinch of sea salt in a pot and bring to a boil. Reduce the flame to medium-low, cover, and simmer until the apples are soft. Turn the flame down low. Dilute the kuzu in a small amount of water and pour it into the apple mixture, stirring constantly to prevent lumping. When thick, simmer 1 minute. Remove and serve.

Variations:
- use other northern varieties of fruit
- use ½ cup dried fruit, soaked and sliced

Amazaké Pudding

> 1 pint amazaké
> 1 cup apples or pears
> 3 Tsp kuzu, diluted

Place the apples and amazaké in a saucepan and bring to a boil. Reduce the flame to medium-low, and simmer until the fruit is soft. Reduce the flame to low, add the diluted kuzu, stirring constantly to prevent lumping. Simmer 1 minute or so until thick. Remove and serve.

Variations:
- use other northern varieties of fruit
- use ½ cup dried fruit, soaked, and sliced
- omit fruit entirely and prepare plain
- add 1 teaspoon of prepared, instant grain coffee to the amazaké

Baked Apples

Wash the apples, core, and place in a baking dish with a little water.

Cover and bake at 350° to 375°F for about 30 minutes or until soft. Remove and serve.

Applesauce

Wash, peel if waxed, core, and slice the apples. Place in a pot with a pinch of sea salt. Add enough water to just lightly cover the bottom of the pot. Cover and bring to a boil. Reduce the flame to medium-low and simmer until the apples are soft. Purée in a hand food mill. Serve.

Dried Chestnuts and Dried Apples

> 1 cup dried chestnuts
> ½ cup dried apples, soaked, and sliced
> 2 ½ cups water
> pinch of sea salt

Wash the chestnuts and dry-roast in a skillet, over a low flame, for several minutes. Remove and place in a pressure cooker. Add the water and allow the chestnuts to soak for about 10 minutes. Add the dried apples and pinch of sea salt. Place the cover on the pressure cooker and bring up to pressure. Reduce the flame to medium-low and simmer for about 40 minutes. Remove the cooker from the stove and allow the pressure to come down. Take the cover off and serve.

Azuki Beans, Chestnuts, and Raisins

> ½ cup azuki beans, soaked 6–8 hours
> ½ cup dried chestnuts, dry-roasted and soaked 10 minutes
> 2 Tbsp raisins
> 2 ½ cups water
> 1 strip kombu, 2–3 inches long, soaked and diced
> ¼ Tsp sea salt

Place the kombu, azuki beans, chestnuts, raisins and water in a pot. Cover and bring to a boil. Reduce the flame to medium-low, and simmer for about 2 to 2 ½ hours. As the beans are cooking, you may need to add a small amount of water from time to time. When the beans are about 80 percent done, season with sea salt, cover and simmer for another 15 minutes or until soft.

Kanten

> **4 cups water**
> **2 cups dried apples, soaked and sliced**
> **agar-agar flakes (follow package instructions for proper amount of liquid)**
> **pinch of sea salt**

Place the water, sea salt, dried apples and kanten (agar-agar) flakes in a pot. Bring to a boil, reduce the flame to low, cover, and simmer until the apples are soft. Remove and pour the apples and liquid into a dish. Refrigerate or place in a cool place until jelled. Kanten is usually ready to serve in 45 to 60 minutes. Slice or spoon into serving dishes.

Nuts ───────────────────────────

Nuts can be eaten from time to time as snacks and garnishes. It is best to keep their consumption occasional and to eat them in small amounts. Nuts that are roasted and lightly salted (with natural sea salt) or a small amount of tamari soy sauce are preferred. Among the many types of nuts, non-tropical varieties that are lower in fat are recommended. Below are several varieties of nuts for use:

Occasional Use:	*Nuts to Avoid (Tropical*
Almonds	*Varieties) for Optimum*
Peanuts	*Health:*
Walnuts	Brazil nuts
Peacans	Cashews
	Hazel nuts
	Macadamia nuts
	Pistachio nuts

• *Selecting the highest-quality nuts (see discussion of seeds below):*

Roasted Nut Recipes

Roasted Nuts

Nuts can be roasted in two basic ways:

• *In the oven*—Place the nuts on a baking sheet and bake in a 350°F oven until slightly brown. When they are almost done, add a few drops of tamari soy sauce and mix to evenly coat. Bake another 2 to 3 minutes.

• *In a skillet*—Place a skillet on the stove and heat up. Add the nuts and reduce the flame to low. Stir constantly to evenly roast and prevent burning. Roast until a light golden brown, sprinkle a few drops of tamari soy sauce on them and roast for another minute or two. Remove and serve.

Variation: Dry-roasted sea salt that has been ground to a fine powder in a suribachi may also be lightly sprinkled on roasted nuts instead of tamari soy sauce.

Seeds

A variety of seeds may be eaten from time to time as snacks. They can be lightly roasted with or without salt. Varieties of seeds include:

Pumpkin seeds
Sesame seeds
Sunflower seeds
Other traditionally consumed seeds

• *Selecting the highest-quality natural nuts and seeds:* Whenever possible, choose seeds and nuts that have been grown organically. Most of the commercially grown nuts in the United States are produced with artificial fertilizers and subjected to intensive spraying with insecticides and fungicides. Moreover, after harvest, many commercially sold nuts are treated with a further round of chemicals in order to retard spoilage and extend their shelf life.

Good-quality seeds and nuts should be firm, not rubbery. If shelled, their surfaces should generally be smooth and regular, with a minimum of scratches, chips, or cracks. They should not be too hard or dried out, and an off-smell or discoloration is usually an indication of rancidity.

Roasted Seed Recipes

Roasted Pumpkin or Squash Seeds

Rinse the seeds under cold water and drain. Heat a skillet and place the damp seeds in it. Dry-roast, stirring constantly until the seeds become golden brown and begin to puff up slightly and pop. Plain roasted, unseasoned pumpkin or squash seeds are preferred. On occasion, you may season mildly with a few drops of tamari soy sauce, mix, and roast for another several seconds until the tamari soy sauce on the seeds dries. Remove and place in a serving bowl.

Snacks

A variety of natural, high-quality snacks can be eaten from time to time. They can be made from grains, beans, nuts or seeds, sea vegetables, and temperate-climate fruits. The following foods can be used as snacks:

Leftovers
Noodles
Popcorn (homemade and unbuttered)
Puffed whole cereal grains
Rice balls
Rice cakes
Seeds
Homemade sushi (without sugar, seasoning, or MSG)
Mochi
Steamed sourdough bread

• *Selecting the highest-quality natural snacks:* For optimum health, it is important to select the highest-quality natural snacks, while avoiding items made with refined sweeteners, honey, carob, tropical fruits, or poor-quality oils. Snacks made from foods within the Standard Macrobiotic Diet are preferred, and many of these can be prepared at home. Those that are easiest to digest, such as rice balls, homemade sushi, mochi, and noodles are preferred for regular use. Hard, baked flour products, such as crackers, cookies, and muffins can interfere with digestion and cause stagnation in the body.

Snack Recipes

Steamed Sourdough Bread

Slice several pieces of whole wheat sourdough or any other unyeasted whole grain bread. Place about ½ inch of water in a pot. Insert a steamer basket and place the sliced bread in the steamer. Cover and bring the water to a boil. Reduce the flame to medium, and steam 4 to 5 minutes or until the bread is soft and warm. Remove and serve as is, with naturally processed and salted sesame butter, miso-tahini spread, or other appropriate spreads.

Miso-Tahini Spread

2–3 Tbsp organic sesame tahini
barley miso
1–2 Tbsp chopped scallions
water

Place the tahini in a small saucepan. Add a small amount of barley miso (mugi miso) for a mild salt taste, together with the chopped scallions. Add several drops of water and mix well. Place on a medium flame and simmer 2 to 3 minutes until the scallions are cooked, mixing constantly to evenly cook and to prevent burning. Remove and serve on steamed bread, rice cakes, or other appropriate snacks.

Variations:
- substitute organic sesame butter for tahini
- add chopped onions or parsley instead of scallions

Sweets

The naturally sweet flavor of cooked vegetables is preferred for optimum health. One or several of the vegetables listed below can be included in dishes on a daily basis:

Cabbage
Carrots
Daikon
Onions
Parsnips
Pumpkin
Squash

In addition, a small amount of concentrated sweeteners made from whole cereal grains may be included when craved. Dried chestnuts, which also impart a sweet flavor may also be included on occasion, along with occasional consumption of hot apple juice or cider. Additional sweeteners include:

Amazaké
Barley malt
Brown rice syrup
Chestnuts (cooked)
Hot apple cider (with a pinch of sea salt)
Hot apple juice (with a pinch of sea salt)
Mirin

• *Selecting the highest-quality natural sweeteners:* The sweet flavor in macrobiotic cooking comes primarily from the complex carbohydrates in whole grains, beans, and fresh vegetables. Carbohydrates are generally known as sugars, but in speaking of sugar we should specify the variety. Single sugars, or *monosaccharides* are found in fruit and honey and include *glucose* and *fructose.* Double sugars or *disaccharides* are found in cane sugar and milk and include *sucrose* and *lactose.* Complex sugars or *polysaccharides* are found in grains, beans, and vegetables. In the normal digestive process, complex sugars are decomposed gradually and at a nearly even rate by various enzymes in the mouth, stomach, pancreas, and intestines. Complex sugars enter the bloodstream slowly after being broken down into smaller saccharide units. During the process, the pH of the blood maintains a normally healthy, slightly alkaline quality.

In contrast, single and double sugars (together known as simple sugars) are metabolized quickly, causing the blood to become over-acidic. To compensate, stored minerals, including calcium, are mobilized for the so-called buffer action necessary to maintain the normal weak alkaline quality of the blood. This chemical process produces excessive carbon dioxide and water which are normally eliminated through breathing and urination. Moreover, the pancreas secretes insulin which allows excess sugar in the blood to be removed and enter the cells of the body. This produces a burst of energy as the glucose (the end product of all sugar metabolism) is oxidized. Carbon dioxide and water are given off as waste products.

Much of the sugar that enters the bloodstream is originally stored in the liver in the form of *glycogen* until needed, when it is again changed into glucose. When the amount of glycogen exceeds the liver's storage capacity of about 50 grams, it is released into the bloodstream in the form of *fatty acid.* This fatty acid is stored first in the more inactive places of the body, such as the buttocks, thighs, and midsection. Then, if cane sugar, fruit sugar, dairy sugar, and other simple sugars are eaten in excessive amounts, fatty acid is continuously attracted to organs with more dense, or compact structures such as the heart, liver, and kidneys, which gradually become filled with fat and mucus.

As these accumulations penetrate the inner tissues, the normal functioning of the organs begins to weaken. In some cases, blockage—as in atherosclerosis—can occur. The buildup of fat can also lead to the formation of cysts, tumors, and eventually cancer. Still another form of degeneration may occur when the body's internal supply of minerals is mobilized to offset the effects of simple-sugar consumption. For example, calcium from the teeth and bones may be depleted to balance the excessive intake of candy, soft drinks, and sugary desserts.

In order to prevent these degenerative effects, it is important to minimize or limit the consumption of refined carbohydrates, especially simple sugars, as well as naturally occurring lactose and fructose in dairy foods and fruits, and to derive the sweetness of complex carbohydrate primarily in the form of grains, beans, bean products, and fresh vegetables.

Sweet Recipes

Amazaké

Amazaké can be used in making desserts and puddings or may simply be heated in a saucepan and used as an occasional beverage.

Barley Malt or Brown Rice Syrup

These sweeteners may be used occasionally in making desserts, added in small amounts to soft-cooked breakfast cereals, or added to bancha tea for an additional sweet flavor.

Chestnuts

(Please refer to the sections on grains, beans, and desserts for recipes.)

Seasonings

A variety of naturally processed seasonings are fine for regular use. Unrefined sea salt is used regularly in cooking whole grains, beans, and many vegetables. Tamari soy sauce, miso, and umeboshi plums, which have been salted and pickled, are also used frequently. In general, however, the use of seasonings is best kept moderate. Rather than using them to add a salty flavor to your dishes, it is better to use them to bring forth the natural light sweetness of the whole grains, vegetables, beans, sea vegetables and other ingredients you are cooking with. The use of salt is a highly individual matter, and is based on factors such as age, sex, activity, and the climate in which we are living. Please consult the other publications listed in the bibliography for recommendations.

The following seasonings are used most often in macrobiotic cooking:

Regular Use:
Miso, especially barley (mugi)
   and soybean (Hatcho)
Tamari soy sauce
Unrefined white sea salt

Occasional Use:
Ginger
Horseradish
Mirin

Rice vineger
Umeboshi vinegar
Umeboshi plum or paste
Sesame oil (dark)

Avoid (for Optimum Health):
All commercial seasonings
All stimulating and aromatic
   spices and herbs
All irradiated spices and herbs

• *Selecting the highest-quality natural seasonings:* Salt is essential to life. The quality of salt, the amount consumed, and the way salt is used in cooking are paramount questions in the life of an individual, family, community, and culture. In proper volume, good-quality, unrefined natural sea salt, containing trace minerals and elements, contributes to smooth metabolism, steady energy and vitality, and a clear, focused mind. Too little salt or no salt at all can lead to anemia, lack of vitality, stagnated blood, and loss of direction in life. Too much salt can produce another type of anemia, hyperactivity, rigid thinking, aggressive behavior, and excessive retention of fluids, leading to kidney troubles and other physical, mental, and emotional disorders.

The poor quality of overly refined table salt is one of the major factors in the deteriorating health in modern society. Compared to the macrobiotic way of eating, the usual modern diet contains about three to four times the amount of sodium. In addition to the large amount of refined salt used in frozen, canned, and convenience foods, and salt added to foods at the table, sodium is consumed in large volume in animal foods, including meat, eggs, poultry, and dairy products. Excessive sodium from these sources, as well as the consumption of refined salt, is a major factor in some forms of cardiovascular disease and other degenerative conditions.

General guidelines for using sea salt, miso, tamari soy sauce, umeboshi plums and other natural seasonings are presented in the recipes in this chapter, as well as in macrobiotic cookbooks.

Beverages

A variety of natural beverages can be included for daily, regular, or occasional consumption. The frequency and amount of beverage intake vary according to the individual's personal condition and needs as well as the climate, season, and other environmental factors. Generally, it is advisable to drink comfortably and when thirsty and to avoid icy cold drinks. The following beverages are used most often in the practice of macrobiotics:

Regular Use:
Bancha twig tea (*Kukicha*)
Bancha stem tea
Roasted barley tea
Roasted brown rice tea
Natural spring water (suitable
  for daily use)
High-quality natural well
  water

Occasional Use:
Grain coffee (100% roasted
  cereal grains)
Sweet vegetable broth
Dandelion tea
Kombu tea
Umeboshi tea
Mu tea
Freshly squeezed carrot juice
  (if desired, about 2 cups per
  week)

Infrequent Use:
Green leaf tea
Green magma
Vegetable juice
Northern climate fruit juice
Beer (natural quality)
Saké (natural quality)
Wine (natural quality)

Avoid (for Optimum Health):
Distilled water
Coffee
Cold or iced drinks
Hard liquor
Aromatic herbal teas
Mineral water and all bubbling
  waters
Chemically colored tea
Stimulant beverages
Sugared drinks
Tap water
Artificial, chemically treated
  beverages
Tropical fruit juices

• *Selecting the highest-quality beverages:* A source of good-quality water is essential for daily cooking and drinking. Natural spring water or deep well water that is moving and alive (charged with natural energy from the environment) is best. Municipal tap water often contains chemical additives such as the disinfectant chlorine, as well as pesticide residues, detergents, nitrates, and heavy metals such as lead. There are several mechanical methods used to filter tap water of impurities, but these are less desirable than natural spring water that comes up from the earth before it is bottled, or clear well water drawn from an underground vein. However, spring and well water should be tested to see if they are suitable for daily use.

The natural mineral content of spring or well water varies considerably. Usually hard water containing more minerals is preferred for drinking, while soft water containing less minerals is used primarily for washing. Bottled spring waters differ widely in quality, and changing brands may improve the energy and taste of foods and beverages. Spring water may often be ordered in large 5-gallon containers and be delivered directly to the house or be purchased at the natural food store in 2 ½-gallon or 1-gallon containers.

Bancha tea is the most frequently consumed beverage in most macrobiotic households. It is picked in midsummer from the large and mature leaves, stems, and twigs of the tea bush. These are called respectively bancha leaf tea, bancha stem tea, and bancha twig tea. Traditionally picked by hand in the high mountains, the bancha leaves, stems, and twigs are roasted and cooled up to four separate times in large iron cauldrons. This procedure, as well as the late harvest when the caffeine has naturally receded from the tea bush, makes for a tea containing virtually no caffeine or tannin, especially in the stem and twig parts. Also, unlike other teas which are acidic, bancha is slightly alkaline and thus has a soothing, beneficial effect on digestion, blood quality, and the mind. Bancha twig tea is also known as *kukicha*, from the Japanese words for "twig tea."

Beverage Recipes

Bancha Twig Tea (Kukicha)

Place 1 tablespoon of bancha twigs in 1 quart of water and bring to a boil. Reduce the flame to low. Simmer 1 to 3 minutes for a mild taste or up to 15 minutes for a stronger tea. Drink while hot.

Bancha Stem Tea

This tea is made entirely of twigs and contains no leaves. It is prepared in the same manner as kukicha but requires a slightly longer cooking time.

Roasted Grain Tea

Dry-roast about ½ cup of washed barley or brown rice in a skillet until golden yellow, stirring constantly to prevent burning. Place the roasted grain in a quart of water and bring to a boil. Reduce the flame to low and simmer for about 15 to 20 minutes. Drink while hot.

Roasted Barley Tea

You may purchase pre-packaged, unhulled, roasted barley tea in most natural food stores. Place 1 tablespoon of roasted barley in a quart of water and bring to a boil. Reduce the flame to low and simmer 1 to 3 minutes for a mild tea or up to 10 minutes for a stronger-flavored beverage. Drink while hot or at room temperature in hotter weather.

Sweet Vegetable Broth

> ½ **cup carrots, diced**
> ½ **cup onions, diced**
> ½ **cup winter squash, sliced very thin**
> ½ **cup green cabbage, sliced very thin**
> **2 quarts water**

Place all ingredients in a pot, cover, and bring to a boil. Reduce the flame to low, and simmer for 10 to 15 minutes. Remove from flame and strain the sweet broth through a fine-meshed strainer. Drink 1 cup or 2 cups per day. Store in a glass jar in the refrigerator and heat up as needed. Save the cooked vegetables from making the broth and use in soups.

Conclusion

These recipes are recommended for everyone who wishes to maintain healthy natural immune ability. However, many other recipes have been traditionally used in different cultures, and are suitable in the climates or regions in which they developed. Traditional recipes and natural methods of food processing can also be adapted and used from time to time. Additional recipes common in macrobiotic cooking are also presented in the following cookbooks which are recommended for further study:

1. *Aveline Kushi's Complete Guide to Macrobiotic Cooking*, by Aveline Kushi with Alex Jack, Warner Books, 1985.

2. *The Changing Seasons Macrobiotic Cookbook*, by Aveline Kushi and Wendy Esko, Avery Publishing Group, 1985.

3. *Aveline Kushi's Introducing Macrobiotic Cooking*, by Wendy Esko, Japan Publications, 1987.

4. *Macrobiotic Cooking for Everyone*, by Edward and Wendy Esko, Japan Publications, 1980.

5. *How to Cook with Miso*, by Aveline Kushi, Japan Publications, 1979.

6. *The Macrobiotic Cancer Prevention Cookbook*, by Aveline Kushi with Wendy Esko, Avery Publishing Group, 1988.

7. *The Macrobiotic Food and Cooking Series*, by Aveline Kushi, Japan Publications, (assorted titles).

8. *The Quick and Natural Macrobiotic Cookbook*, by Aveline Kushi and Wendy Esko, Contemporary Books, 1989.

2. Home Care for AIDS-related Symptoms

A variety of special dishes, drinks, and preparations can be included as a part of home care for persons experiencing symptoms related to immune deficiency. When properly applied, these traditional dishes, drinks, and natural applications are completely safe, and can be included as a part of a naturally balanced diet and way of life. These special preparations can be made at home, in the kitchen, using a variety of commonly available foods.

The foods, drinks, and other forms of home care listed below are presented for educational purposes and are not substitutes for qualified medical care. Anyone with a serious condition is advised to contact their physician at the earliest opportunity. Moreover, do not hesitate to get in touch with a qualified macrobiotic teacher or center for guidance on the appropriate use of these natural preparations.

• *Strengthening Natural Immunity:* The following natural preparations can be of help in strengthening natural immune function:

1. *Baked Kombu Powder*
Preparation: Take several pieces of dried, unwashed kombu and break into small pieces. Place in a dry skillet. Roast on a medium flame, stirring occasionally until crisp, but not burnt, for about 15 to 20 minutes. Remove and place in a suribachi. (As an alternative, you may place the kombu on a baking sheet. Bake at 350°F for approximately 10 to 15 minutes or until dark and crisp but not burnt or black. Remove and place the baked kombu in a suribachi.) Grind to a fine powder.

Use: Sprinkle one or two teaspoons of kombu powder on grains, vegetables, or other foods daily for a period of 2 to 3 weeks. Kombu powder can also be occasionally used to prepare tea. To make kombu-powder tea, place one or two teaspoons in a cup and pour boiling water over it. Stir and drink hot.

2. *Roasted Barley Tea* (*Mugi-cha*)—Prepackaged roasted barley for making tea may be purchased at most natural food stores. Barley can also be roasted at home.

Preparation: Instructions for preparing barley tea are presented in the beverage section of the *Macrobiotic Food and Recipe Suggestions.*

Use: Barley tea can be enjoyed daily or often along with other recommended beverages.

Variation: A small piece of natural licorice may occasionally be added to barley tea while simmering for a slightly different flavor and to further strengthen natural immunity.

3. *Mu Tea*—Depending on which variety you select, this special beverage is made from a combination of either 9 or 16 herbs. This strong, sweet-tasting tea has been traditionally used to restore strength and vitality to the entire body, including the immune system. Mu #9 includes herbs such as peony root, Japanese parsley root, hoelen, cinnamon, licorice, peach kernels, gingerroot, rhemannia, and a small amount of ginseng. Ginseng is an extremely contractive root that is normally avoided in macrobiotic cooking. However, it is used in very small amounts in mu tea and is balanced by the other ingredients. Mu tea may be purchased in most natural food stores.

Preparation: Directions for preparing mu tea are included on the package.

Use: Either variety of mu tea (#9 or #16) may be enjoyed three or four times per week along with other recommended beverages.

• *Fatigue:* The following dishes and drinks can be helpful in recovering from fatigue:

1. *Carp-and-Burdock-Miso Soup (Koi-koku)*
Preparation: Instructions for preparing this traditional dish are presented in the soup section of the *Macrobiotic Food and Recipe Suggestions.*

Use: Carp soup is very strong and is best eaten in small volume. One cup daily, for two to five days is sufficient in most cases. If taken in larger quantities, it may cause cravings for fruits, sweets, or other-strong yin foods. Carp soup can be stored in the refrigerator in a tightly sealed glass jar for about five days. However, frozen carp soup loses freshness as well as power to restore energy and strength.

2. *Fresh-water Trout and Carrot Miso Soup*—This variation can be substituted when carp or burdock root are not available.
Preparation: Instructions for preparing this soup are presented in the soup section of the *Macrobiotic Food and Recipe Suggestions.*

Use: This soup can be used in place of carp and burdock miso soup as recommended above.

3. *Ranshio* (*Raw Fertile Egg and Tamari Soy Sauce*)—This strongly contracting drink is made with a fresh fertile egg.

Preparation: Crack an organic fertilized egg in half. Place the whole egg—white and yolk—in a cup. Half-fill one of the empty shell halves with tamari soy sauce. Pour the tamari into the cup with the raw egg. Stir and drink slowly.

Use: Because of its strong contractive properties, this drink should be taken no more than once a day for two days only.

4. *Ume Extract*—A small amount of this concentrate, made from umeboshi plums, can be used to restore vitality and recover from fatigue. Ume extract comes in a small jar and is available from most natural food stores.

Preparation: Dip the tip of a chopstick into ume extract so that a small dab sticks to the end of it. Place the dab of extract in a cup and pour boiling water over it. Stir to dilute and drink hot. You may also eat the dab of extract rather than diluting it in water, if you do not mind the strong sour taste.

Use: Ume extract may be taken two to three times per week for several weeks.

• *Fever:* The following preparations can be of use in helping a fever to naturally discharge:

1. *Ojiya* (*Soft Miso Rice*)—Ojiya may be prepared in a number of ways, using brown rice in combination with vegetables or sea vegetables. The most commonly included ingredients are:

1 cup brown rice
½ cup daikon, sliced
sliced scallions for garnish
1 sheet toasted nori, cut in strips or squares
½ Tsp puréed barley miso per cup of cooked rice
5 cups water

Preparation: Place the rice, daikon, and water in a pressure cooker. Cover, bring up to pressure, and reduce the flame to medium-low. Cook the rice for 50 minutes. Remove from the flame and allow the pressure to come down. Remove the cover, and place the cooker, uncovered, on a very low flame.

Add the puréed miso and mix in. Simmer for 2 to 3 minutes without boiling. Place the rice in a serving bowl and garnish with a few sliced scallions and several strips or squares of toasted nori. Eat while hot.

Use: Ojiya may be enjoyed every day for several days or longer during a fever. It may also be included as a regular dish several times per week.

2. *Ume-Sho-Kuzu—Kuzu* (or *kudzu* as it is known in the southern United States where it is found in abundance) grows wild in the mountains of Japan and has very deep roots. It is traditionally harvested and processed by hand into a white chalk-like substance. It is often used in macrobiotic cooking as a thickener in sauces, stews, and desserts. Its health properties include strengthening the digestive organs. This traditional preparation combines the effects of umeboshi and kuzu. It can be used to strengthen the intestines and digestive system as a whole and restore active energy lost during fever.

Preparation: Dilute a heaping teaspoon of kuzu powder in 2 teaspoons water. Add another cup of water and mix well. Then, separate the meat of an umeboshi plum from the seed, and add it. Bring the water to a boil, stirring constantly to prevent lumping. Reduce the flame to medium-low and simmer until thick and translucent. Near the end, add ½ to 1 teaspoon of tamari soy sauce and simmer for several seconds more. For a lighter preparation that may help induce sweating, add a small amount of grated ginger at the end. Pour into a bowl and drink hot.

Use: One or two bowls may be taken per day for two to three days during fever.

3. *Grated Daikon Tea*—Daikon, or white radish, is an indispensable part of traditional Far Eastern cuisine and is now grown in America. The smaller, thinner daikon, shaped somewhat like a carrot, grows more quickly than the larger varieties and has a strong, sharp taste. The big, juicy varieties grow up to several feet in length and are sweeter to the taste.

Tea made from grated raw daikon was traditionally used to help reduce fever by inducing sweating. *Please note, however, that this tea is not recommended for someone with a weakened condition or for small children.* Two varieties of grated daikon tea can be prepared:

● **Daikon Tea 1**

Preparation: Grate 1 to 2 tablespoons of fresh daikon and place in a tea cup. Add ¼ to ½ teaspoon of fresh grated ginger, and a tablespoon of tamari soy sauce. Pour weak, hot bancha tea or boiling water over the ingredients. Stir and drink hot.

Use: Take one cup daily for 2 to 3 days. It is best not to take this tea for more than 3 days in a row. Again, persons in a weakened condition are advised to use another tea in place of this one.

• **Daikon Tea 2**—This variation of daikon tea can be used to induce urination and calm and relax the body.

Preparation: Grate a small amount of daikon and place it in a piece of cotton cheesecloth. Squeeze 2 tablespoons of juice through the cheesecloth and mix it with about 6 tablespoons of water. Place in a saucepan and add a pinch of sea salt. Bring to a boil, reduce the flame to low, and simmer for about a minute. Drink hot.

Use: Take one cup daily for 2 to 3 days. It is better not to use this tea for more than 3 days in a row unless otherwise indicated. Again, it is best if those with a weakened condition do not use this tea.

4. *Dried Daikon Tea*—This tea can be used to help reduce fever in a person who is unable to use raw grated daikon.

Preparation: Place ¼ cup of dried daikon in a saucepan and add 2 cups of water. Bring to a boil, reduce the flame to low, and cover. Simmer for about 10 minutes. Drink hot.

Use: Take one cup daily for 2 to 3 days. Daikon tea is best not taken for more than 3 days in a row unless otherwise indicated.

• *Diarrhea:* Ume-sho-kuzu, introduced above, can also help strengthen the digestive tract and restore bowel function to normal.

Preparation: See above.

Use: Persons with acute diarrhea may take 1 or 2 cups daily for 2 to 3 days. Those with chronic diarrhea may take 1 cup daily for up to 5 days, or until the condition stabilizes.

Note: The use of ginger is optional. Persons in a weakened condition may omit it in this recipe.

• *Coughing:* The following teas, made from freshly grated or powdered lotus root, can be helpful in easing respiratory congestion and coughing:

1. *Fresh Lotus Root Tea*—In Far Eastern countries, lotus root has been known for centuries as being effective in easing respiratory problems, including coughs and congestion. The root of the lotus flower plant grows underwater in segmented lengths, is light brown in color,

and contains hollow chambers. It can be regularly included in a variety of dishes—such as with other root vegetables or with sea vegetables—or can be used to prepare tea or external plasters. It is available at many natural food and Oriental food markets.

Preparation: Take a 4-inch piece of lotus root and after washing, grate it on a flat grater. Place in a piece of cheesecloth and squeeze all of the liquid into a measuring cup. Add an equal amount of water to the lotus root juice and place it in a saucepan. Add a small pinch of sea salt and bring to a boil. Reduce the flame to low and simmer for 3 to 5 minutes. Drink hot.

Use: Drink 1 to 2 cups per day for several days.

2.   *Powdered Lotus Root Tea*—Prepackaged, powdered lotus root tea is available in most natural food stores. It can be used when fresh lotus root cannot be located. Directions for preparation are printed on the package. Powdered lotus root tea can be used as you would tea made from the freshly ground root.

Special Note: Persons experiencing respiratory problems resulting from immune deficiency are advised to completely avoid cigarette smoking.

● *Pneumonia:*   The following preparations can be helpful in lowering the high fever that frequently accompanies acute pnuemonia.

1.   *Carp Plaster*—Carp is a very yin, slow moving fish. It can be more effective than an ice pack in lowering the high fever and neutralizing other excessive factors associated with pneumonia.

Preparation and Use: If you can obtain a live carp, after killing it, extract a small quantity of its blood for use as a special drink. Place about 1 teaspoon of the carp's blood into a small cup and drink it. If a live carp cannot be obtained, this step can be omitted.

Wrap the carp in a towel and crush it with a hammer in the way you would crush a block of ice. Then, apply the towel to the chest, and check your temperature every half hour, since it often drops quickly once the carp pack is applied. Remove the pack once the temperature reaches 97°F. This may take from ½ to 1 hour or longer in some cases. It may even be necessary to apply a fresh carp pack until the temperature drops and breathing becomes easier.

Variation: If carp cannot be located, cold or iced ground beef can be applied directly to the chest for the amount of time indicated above. Since ground beef contains plenty of fat, it can be helpful in reducing fever, although it is less effective than carp plaster.

• *Hypoglycemia:*   Cravings for sweets are often due to low blood sugar, or *hypoglycemia.* This condition is widespread today; as many as 60 percent of American adults may experience it to one degree or another. A person with this condition often has strong cravings for sweets, together with mood swings that include depression and anxiety. These symptoms often become acute in the afternoon or evening.

A main cause of hypoglycemia is the chronic overintake of foods such as chicken, cheese, eggs, and shellfish. These items can make the pancreas hard and tight and interfere with the secretion of *glucagon,* or anti-insulin, the pancreatic hormone that causes blood sugar to rise. Insulin, an opposite hormone, lowers blood sugar. Avoiding these foods and eating more complex carbohydrates, such as those in whole grains, beans, vegetables, and sea vegetables, helps solve the problem. Many of these foods have a naturally sweet flavor, and this taste can be emphasized in daily cooking. At the same time, the following drink can be helpful in relieving hypoglycemia and restoring normal functioning to the pancreas:

1.   *Sweet Vegetable Drink*—This special drink is made from naturally sweet vegetables. It relaxes the pancreas and provides naturally occurring complex carbohydrates which stabilize the level of blood sugar.

Preparation: Instructions for preparing this drink are presented in the beverage section of the *Macrobiotic Food and Recipe Suggestions.*

Use: One or two cups can be taken daily or several times per week depending on the severity of the sweet cravings. Sweet vegetable drink may be taken indefinitely until the symptoms of hypoglycemia begin to diminish. To serve, heat in a saucepan until warm or allow it to sit until it reaches room temperature.

3. Way of Life Suggestions

Together with eating well, there are a number of practices that we recommend for a healthier and more natural life. Practices such as keeping physically active and using natural cooking utensils, fabrics, and materials in the home are especially recommended. In the past, people lived more closely to nature and ate a more wholesome, natural diet. With each generation, we have gotten further and further from our roots in nature and have experienced a corresponding rise in chronic illnesses. The suggestions presented below complement a balanced, natural diet and can help one enjoy more satisfying and harmonious living.

1. *Hot Towel Body-scrub*—Every morning and every night, scrub the body with a hot, damp towel until the circulation becomes active. When a complete body-scrub is not possible, at least do the hands, feet, fingers, and toes.

Daily body-scrubbing activates circulation, releases stagnation, and helps break down fats deposited under the skin. After many years of consuming cheese and other dairy products, chicken, meat, eggs, and other animal foods, many people develop a layer of hard fat just below the skin. This condition occurs in thin people as well as in the overweight and produces hard, dry skin and often the reduced capacity to sweat.

The skin is one of the body's major organs of elimination. When the pores and sweat glands become constricted and blocked with fatty deposits, toxic excess that is normally discharged through the skin can start to accumulate. This can lead to the buildup of toxins throughout the body, creating a medium for the eventual weakening of natural immunity. It is therefore important to avoid the foods that cause these fats to develop and to practice daily body-scrubbing to open the pores and allow excess to come out.

Body-scrubbing can be done before or after a bath or shower. All that is needed is a sink with hot water and a medium-sized cotton towel. Turn the hot water on. Hold the towel at either end and place the center part under the stream of hot water. Wring out the towel, and while it is still hot and steamy, begin to scrub with it. Do a section of the body at a time, for example, beginning with the hands and fingers, and working up the arms to the shoulders, neck, and face, and then downward to the chest, upper back, abdomen, lower back buttocks, legs, feet, and toes. Scrub until the skin turns slightly red or until each part becomes warm. Reheat the towel by running it under the hot water after doing each section or as soon as it starts to cool.

A hot towel body-scrub is ideal once or twice a day. When done in the morning, it vitalizes and energizes. When done in the evening, it relaxes and refreshes and makes sleep more comfortable. The total body-scrub takes about ten minutes to do.

2. *Ginger Body-scrub*—A special body-scrub can also be done with hot ginger water. Ginger body-scrubs work like plain hot towels to stimulate circulation, dissolve stagnation, and energize certain areas of the body. Freshly grated ginger makes the heat even more stimulating and penetrating.

To prepare the ginger body-scrub, you will need a medium-sized piece of fresh ginger root (available at most natural food or Oriental markets), a flat metal grater, some cheesecloth, a medium-sized cotton towel, and a medium- to large-sized pot with a lid.

Grate the ginger root on the metal grater and place a golfball-sized amount in a double layer of cheesecloth. Tie the cheesecloth at the top to form a sack. Then, place a gallon of water in a pot and bring it up to, but not over, the boiling point. Turn the flame down to low just before the water starts to boil.

Next, hold the sack over the pot and squeeze as much of the ginger juice as you can into the water. Then drop the sack into the pot. Make sure the water does not boil, as this will weaken the effect of the ginger. Place the lid on the pot and let the ginger sack simmer in the water for about 5 minutes. Then, fold the towel several times lengthwise, so that it becomes long and thin. Hold it from both ends and dip the center into the hot ginger water. Wring it out tightly, and if it is too hot to place on the skin, shake it slightly. Begin scrubbing as described above. As the towel cools, reheat it by dipping it in the hot ginger water.

Many people find plain hot water body-scrubbing more convenient during the week, and use the ginger body-scrub on weekends when more time is available. One pot of hot ginger water can be used for two body-scrubs. Simply reheat the water before use (do not bring to a boil).

3. *Chewing and Eating*—Chew very well, until each mouthful becomes liquid. Eat as calmly and peacefully as possible. You may eat as much food as you need or desire, provided chewing is thorough and pro-

portions are correct. Try not to eat before bedtime, preferably three hours, except in unusual circumstances. Snacks are best eaten in moderate amounts, and not to the extent that they replace regular meals. Try to eat regularly, two or three meals a day is preferred, and refrain from over-eating.

4. *Exercise and Activity*—Keep as active as possible. Daily activities such as cooking and cleaning are excellent forms of exercise. If desired, one may also try systematic exercises such as yoga, martial arts, aerobics, and sports, but not to the point of exhaustion. Walking is an ideal form of activity, and it is recommended to go outdoors every day, regardless of weather. A half-hour walk per day is recommended.

5. *Clothing, Accessories, and Body Care*—Try not to wear synthetic clothing or woolen articles directly against the skin. Wear cotton instead. Keep jewelry and accessories as simple, graceful, and natural as possible. Bedding materials that come in contact with the body, such as sheets or pillowcases, are also best when made of cotton. Use natural cosmetics, soaps, shampoos, and other body-care products. Brush the teeth with natural preparations or sea salt. Avoid taking long hot baths or showers, including saunas, steam baths, or whirlpools, as these cause the body to lose minerals.

6. *Stoves and Other Appliances*—Electric and microwave cooking are best avoided for maximum health. Those with these cooking stoves are advised to convert to gas at the earliest opportunity. Try to minimize time spent in front of the television. Color television in particular emits unnatural radiation that can be physically draining. Turn the television off during mealtimes. Heating pads, electric blankets, portable radios with earphones, and other electric devices can disrupt the body's natural flow of energy. They are not recommended for regular use.

7. *Attitude and Mental Outlook*—Sing a happy song every day. Cultivate positive and ambitious wishes toward life. Try to live each day happily without being worried about health. Greet everyone and everything with gratitude, particularly offering thanks before and after each meal. Be grateful to parents, family members, ancestors, other people and society, and to nature and the universe. Develop the spirit of mutual assistance toward brotherhood and sisterhood extended to society at large.

8. *Sexual Activity*—Regulate sexual behavior by avoiding multiple partners. To prevent the spread of AIDS, "safe" sexual practices are recommended. Individuals with AIDS may also consider whether to continue sexual activity or to refrain, according to their discretion.

9. *Daily Living*—Shift to a more orderly life-style from chaotic living. Try to get to bed before midnight and to get up early in the morning. Maintain an orderly environment, avoiding disorderly, dark, and depressing surroundings.

10. *Home Environment*—Cleanliness and proper sanitation are very important. Keep the home clean and orderly. Make the kitchen, bathroom, bedrooms, and living rooms shiny clean. Keep the atmosphere of the home bright and cheerful. Put many green plants in the living room, bedroom, and throughout the house to freshen and enrich the air. Do not let the air in any part of the house become stagnant. Open the windows to allow fresh air to circulate when necessary.

11. *Social Occasions*—Avoid events or gatherings that disturb natural harmony and peacefulness, or are in any way chaotic. It is essential to completely avoid alcohol or drugs at social events or other occasions regardless of how others are behaving. Regulate life-style so that it is not stressful.

4

Personal Experiences

Mark Mead

Frank—Kaposi's Sarcoma
New York City, June 1987 ──────────────

Mark: Let's start with your reason for getting into macrobiotics.

Frank: Well, I was sick with a stomach ailment for well over a year from 1984 through part of 1985. It came to a head in early 1985 and the medical community couldn't really put their finger on it although it seemed like a parasitic infection. After visiting a number of doctors who were medicating it improperly, I finally saw an AIDS specialist who said that (a) I definitely had a parasitic infection, and (b) I also had ARC as far as he could tell, because my immune parameters were all depressed.

Mark: Do you remember what the numbers were?

Frank: The number of T helpers was 200 and the ratio of T4 to T8's was 0.6. That was in 1984. In the early part of 1985 the ratio fluctuated between 0.6 and 0.8, and the T-helper number varied between 250 and about 450, but rarely every going above 400. So it was consistently below normal. What they didn't see in my case was a downhill trend of the T-cells. And they stayed pretty stable—the lowest reading, the 200 count, was the very first I had, and it hasn't been that low since early 1984. So my doctor thought that for all that time I was probably carrying a parasite that compromised my immune system, but he felt the numbers were low enough to warrant an ARC diagnosis. The other mitigating circumstance was that I had no constitutional symptoms really—no weight loss, no night sweats, and only a few fevers that were so low-grade they weren't even considered ARC fevers. But, at the time, he was one of the AIDS specialists in the city. This was before a virus was discovered, before Rock Hudson got sick.

Mark: This was just before the epidemic struck.

Frank: Just before. As a matter of fact, the month he diagnosed me he put me on disability. He really said it's time to make my will. He had me horrified. The month I started getting government checks, the Rock Hudson story broke and I was convinced that this was going to be it. Interestingly enough, although this expert scared me, he also scared me into taking my condition seriously. He also treated the parasites much more effectively than any other doctor had, with massive amounts of medicine. He also told me about macrobiotics which was, you know, little known at that time.

Mark: Can you mention the doctor's name?

Frank: Sure. Dr. Roger Enlow. He used to be the director of Gay Lesbian Health concerns for the city. Anyway, he simply said to me, you really shouldn't be eating dairy products, you shouldn't be eating red meat. It was clear to him that my stomach was very irritated. For two months I had been taking incredible doses of anti-parasite medicine. I was literally having hallucinations. I was peeing brown. I was dizzy. I couldn't taste anything. The medicine left me so ravaged that I wasn't quite sure that I had even gotten well. And I couldn't eat. Stupid me, though, I was still going to have a burger, still going out to eat. It was the parasites, they ruled me. I never thought that I had any control over anything. And he said to me, I want you to cut out meat and dairy. You might look into a vegetarian diet for a couple of months just to see how you react. So I said fine. He said he had met a man named Larry Kushi, who turned out to be Michio's son, at a scientific convention. He found Larry and his diet interesting. Whatever it was, the seed had been planted. All he did was mention the word "macrobiotics." I had two friends down the street who were following the current fad of macrobiotic eating. Very trendy. They had yin and yang charts in the kitchen, they were pressure-cooking whole grains, and one friend said, "Oh great, this is what I've been waiting for you to do. If you'll just give me two weeks, I'll cook for you. I'll take you out to restaurants, and answer any questions you have. Let's go book shopping. I want to be your guide." So I agreed. I ate at macrobiotic restaurants a lot at first. I bought a pressure cooker, I started burning my first few pots of rice, steaming some vegetables, working my way through basic books. Didn't go near seaweed or beans —I left that up to the restaurant and my friend.

Mark: What was the first book you read?

Frank: The first edition of *The Book of Macrobiotics*. And the next book was *Macrobiotic Cooking for Everybody* by Edward and Wendy Esko. And I ate at uptown Souen.

Mark: Did you take any cooking classes?

Frank: Eventually I did.

Mark: So you began officially when?

Frank: August 1985.

Mark: That was when your friends introduced you?

Frank: Right. I took it a lot more seriously than they did. As a matter of fact, within three or four months of my beginning macrobiotics, they dropped the whole thing. Now, I see them coming out of Dunkin Donuts in the neighborhood all the time. And both of them have health concerns too. At that point I gave up a lot of foods—dairy, meat, sugar, caffeine, junk, and preservatives. I went clean, although I hadn't quite balanced it all out yet. Then I went to meetings of the HEAL group every single week, and met people who were macrobiotic including cooks, so I gave myself a social network. I had a community support group. I also went to the macrobiotic center's support group. They used to have a lot of pot luck dinners. So I found myself almost every night of the week with something macrobiotic or holistic to do. And the important thing was that I found people to do it all with. I wasn't isolated. I signed up in early 1986 for both levels of cooking classes in a row with Karen Jones and loved them. It was great.

Mark: This was at the Center?

Frank: Yes. When they were uptown. And it felt really good because I knew I had a real awareness of what the foods were. It was so practical. I could go home and do this stuff. I felt terrific and went to about ten different lectures that year at the Center. Murray Snyder, Steve Gagne, Bill Tara, Denny Waxman—all fine teachers. I did a lot of other healing things like the Louise Hay workshops, the AIDS mastery. A lot of macrobiotic concepts were implicitly there.

Mark: Can you give some examples?

Frank: There's a big front and back to AIDS, and a front and back to your own diagnosis. And also the idea of discharge, especially discharge of emotions. One thing I don't think was ever clearly brought out in macrobiotics is that a lot of the emotional stuff we deal with is a form of discharge.

Mark: Actually that's a major premise of macrobiotics.

Frank: It's a really important one. Yes. I guess I really was exposed to it but more in terms of discharge as headaches, diarrhea, and all that other stuff. Discharge can also be two days of extreme depression followed by mood swing. These workshops were about getting anger out, getting love out, and finding where you might have some blockages. I found it compatible with macrobiotic awareness; I found it macrobiotic. And then of course the newspaper you read becomes macrobiotic, the *New York Times* becomes macrobiotic. You read about this happening on this side of the world, and you think, "Ah well, we'll pay for that later" or "We're paying for that now." You put it in context, in an orderly perspective.

Mark: And you see more order now in the way things are happening?

Frank: Oh, absolutely. It wasn't that I didn't have any insight before, I just didn't have the bigger view on life. What I like about macrobiotics is the global sense of everything—the world perspective, the big picture on everything. And that really helped me get out of my little egocentric, dualistic world view. So now when I read the paper it's different. The world is making more sense.

Mark: How has your attitude changed toward your life, toward your friends, toward your family, and people in general, work, problems, and so forth?

Frank: From the beginning I felt a little more self-assured, more self-confident. But the very first thing was that I began to look a lot better. I used to be very fat. My peak weight about five years ago was 230 pounds. I was really big.

Mark: How much do you weigh now?

Frank: Now, about 155, and I feel great. I mean, I fluctuate some, but I was never thin, never trim. And I had terrible acne, on and off. And now my skin's a lot clearer and my eyes shine. Even the shape of my face has changed. I used to be real chubby and droopy. My appearance changed and then my energy level changed. That all happened within four or five months.

Mark: Your friends must have been amazed.

Frank: I think no one recognizes me from my college days. But not only did my complexion change. Within four or five months my blood numbers shot way up. In January of 1984 my T-cells were 200. In January of 1986 they were about 1,000. The ratio in January of 1984 was 0.6 and the ratio in January of 1986 was 1.75. I felt that I was basically cured. I didn't use the word "cure" but I knew something was happening right. And all of the blood parameters got into shape by January of 1986. However, within four or five months into 1986 they were somewhat down, but nowhere near where they were before.

Mark: Can you attribute that to anything?

Frank: Not really. I tried to look at it diet-wise. Also, there are natural lymphocyte cycles. It's a tricky thing, dealing with those tests because of that. Dr. Enlow was testing my T-cells weekly, because he thought I was a real interesting case.

Mark: For how long?

Frank: For four or five months.

Mark: At the beginning of macrobiotics?

Frank: No, this was even before the initial medication. He was very concerned to see what the medicine was going to do to the blood, so he tracked me before, during, and after the medicine. At a certain point he discontinued it because he was stopping his work with AIDS. He referred me to the doctor that I see now, who has much respect for what I'm doing. He's not necessarily pro macrobiotics, but he's very encouraging with anything one does with conviction and good sense. I think when he first saw me over a year ago, he was skeptical about what I was doing. And now he wouldn't think of trying to change what I'm doing. For example, he used to occasionally suggest my getting involved with some drug research program, just to keep some form of help. And now he just lets me be.

I have had to exercise my patient rights with medical specialists who wanted to dominate my course of healing. The minute I got that kind of arrogance I was out the door. Once I literally got up and took off the examination gown. This guy was examining me and wanted to do a bone marrow biopsy. So he walked in after knowing me ten minutes, with a huge needle and was going to go in my back. And he said, we need to do a biopsy. You'll be uncomfortable for . . .

Mark: How long was the needle?

Frank: It was a huge syringe. The needle has to go to your bone marrow in the middle of your hip. So it's got to be long, not a tiny little injection needle.

Mark: So what happened?

Frank: So I looked at the needle and I said, "Wait a minute, what are you doing?" And he replied, "Well, we need to check your bone marrow, and then we might have to do a spinal if it's necessary. We need to see if . . ." I said, "Wait a minute. Hold on! I really don't think this is necessary." As it turns out, it wasn't necessary. There was a simple blood test that could have told them basically the same thing. And I let someone else do the blood test.

Mark: What do you see in store for you in terms of macrobiotics?

Frank: Well, people often say to me, "When are you going to be done?" So, how long I have to do this is a big question for them. You know, it's the old medical tact. It's like how long is this prescription— three weeks or a month or a decade? And people ask me, "If you're finally cured of AIDS, will you start eating normal again?" I try to tell them they're totally missing the point, that's not what this is about. For me the food is just ground level, the fundamental part. The food is something I simply have to do now. What's next? I really have to say—and people don't believe me when I say it—I have really not missed ice cream, liquor, marijuana, coffee and so on. I'll confess to occasionally missing coffee but I have roasted bancha tea and I'm fine. Certainly not once have I missed meat.

I took to the food like a fish to water. It was just splendid. Every day there's something new to deal with, a new way to rethink something. And I'm reminded that it's not a process that particularly stops. It's not supposed to stop. You don't ever particularly arrive at your whole being. I mean, some people might like to think that they do but I don't quite know how fully they plan on living.

Mark: In other words, you see life as a process rather than as achieving an ultimate goal?

Frank: An ultimate goal or a series of goals. You get out of school and then you begin to live life through continuous movement every single day. The other component is healing AIDS in particular. I don't know if I'd ever feel out of the woods even if a "cure" is found or an antiviral drug is developed. People say to me, "So you're on a maintenance mode. You're kind of treading water, or you're hedging your bet or you're doing this for the time being. This is like a survival thing for you." And I answer, "Well, yes. Except that I've never looked, felt, worked, or thought, better than since I've been on macrobiotics." But they don't want to hear about this transformation I'm experiencing. They want to hear that there's a gun to my head saying "You must eat tofu, brown rice, seaweed." This is because they can't get beyond that point themselves. Then there's the issue of living in New York. When I travel, sometimes it's very difficult to eat well, but I always manage to eat macrobiotically. Even if it's just a matter of eating fish, rice, and vegetables.

Mark: Do you travel a lot?

Frank: Last year I did a lot on business. I had a job that took me to towns all over. I was copywriting for a marketing company. I would fly to Denver, Cincinnati, Chicago, Boston, but very often in suburbs of these cities. So it wasn't like I could go to a restaurant. I'd wind up eating in hotel restaurants a lot with businessmen who were having steak and salad and martinis. I was proud of my boss for not being humiliated by the fact that I would take out rice balls. The executives would be a little stunned. But my boss was into writers having a funky image, especially from New York.

One time, I was in Baltimore at one of the finest hotels and I said to the waiter, well I'm on a special diet. I can't eat certain foods. Could you just steam some vegetables and fish? I was real low key about it. And I don't think any of the other businessmen even noticed. Ten minutes later, out from the kitchen comes the head chef, the stereotype French chef. He's got a big hat on, and he says, "Who is on this special diet? I want to hear." He was fascinated by people who chose special diets. So I said, "Well, I'm on a vegetarian health food diet." He had heard of macrobiotics and he said to me, "You tell me how you like your food cooked. What can I use? What can I bring you?" And he gave me this incredible plate of brown rice, which he had in his kitchen, which he boiled, fish cooked very plainly with a little bit of sesame oil, a big plate of vegetables—all without butter. The businessmen almost died because I got royal treatment from this chef who had a great deal of respect for people who ate natural food.

Mark: He already knew macrobiotics?

Frank: He'd heard of macrobiotics, and knew what it was. This chef just loved the topic of food and diets. And the businessmen all took notice. My game was revealed.

Mark: How have you fared living and trying to heal in New York?

Frank: I think that New York is such a stress-ridden environment . . . it is also a very polluted environment. The people I associate with all agree the macrobiotics is the only way to eat healthfully within New York City. The first two or three years that I lived here I was real big on delis, quick eating—Burger King, anything. I went literally from junk food to macrobiotics. It was a huge transformation. I'm very conscious of all the garbage, noise, air, chemicals and filth, and how it affects people.

Mark: How long have you lived here?

Frank: Five years. I was born in Brooklyn and grew up on Long Island. Now I live in Manhattan.

Mark: It's a negative environment yet you can still live well?

Frank: Yes. For that I must thank macrobiotics. The other thing about macrobiotics is that it keeps you very clear-headed. There were times when I'd be in my little apartment, standing in the middle of the room literally turning one way, then turning the other, totally confused, unfocused, and stressed out. But now, I really have a lot more gratitude, and I'm a lot more centered. More grounded, more clear. And that's exceptionally important at a time when it seems like things are going crazy. Illness demands so much, you know.

Mark: What's your living situation?

Frank: I live in a studio by myself.

Mark: Do you have social support?

Frank: A lot. Through my community involvement, through my AIDS work and my writing. So that keeps me in touch. It's real important.

Mark: What's been the response of people at HEAL or the other groups in the city?

Frank: Well, HEAL started out very macrobiotic in the beginning. Because one of the people who started HEAL was macrobiotic. Now with so many macrobiotic restaurants open, and with the new New York Center, macrobiotics has grown incredibly here. Whether or not these people are really doing macrobiotics or just stopping into a restaurant a couple of times week is another matter. If they're not doing the actual practice then I don't think they're going to have powerful healing benefits. Very often I'll hear about people who have died and realize that I saw them in the last few months of their life eating desserts at macrobiotic restaurants. So for some of them it's only a last ditch effort. But we are seeing a lot more people who want to do it preventively before they get sick. These people really desire health and well-being.

Mark: That's what you're trying to promote?

Frank: Yes. Once I got out of bed and started doing things for myself I began going to community meetings and got support there. The next logical step for me was to start leading meetings and getting the word out. I couldn't do macrobiotics in a vacuum. And I couldn't do this work, or any of the AIDS community work, without expanding, constantly getting bigger. So, literally, a year ago we couldn't get the *New York Native* to print anything on macrobiotics. Then came that article I wrote in July of 1986, and in December of 1986 they ran a summary for the year called "A Summary of Major Breakthroughs." My article was considered one of the breakthroughs.

Mark: As a freelance writer, do you see improvement in the coverage of alternative therapies?

Frank: "Quack cures" is a convenient label often given by closed-minded people toward things they are ignorant of, or prefer not to know about because of blind devotion to the sacred cow called modern medicine. Curiously enough, the coverage of macrobiotics by medical publications—notably an article that appeared in the April 1986 *Medical World News*—has had far more positive things to say about the New York study. The fact is, no one knows where the ultimate solution to AIDS will come from. We're all still in the experimental stage and nothing has been definitively proven on the medical side either. One thing needs to be more forcibly voiced: that the macrobiotic approach precludes virtually all of the side effects that people experience on conventional antiviral drugs. The diet may not affect the virus immediately, but I'm confident that by restoring and potentiating the immune system, macrobiotics will some day be demonstrated clinically effective against AIDS. Time will tell, but we've got to maintain open minds. After all, we're not just talking about the common cold anymore.

Mark: Could you say a bit more about the orientation of medical research?

Frank: Memorial Sloane Kettering Institute is doing a study on shiitake mushrooms. But of course what do they try to do? They want to be able to extract the active chemical ingredient, the *lentanin*, from the shiitake and mass-produce it as a so-called drug. Strange as it sounds, only then will people buy it. It doesn't matter to me as long as people some day get the point: natural substances really works! Perhaps AIDS will help break down some of the walls of allopathic medicine and get people to start thinking about taking care of themselves. In this vein, just today there was another article in the *New York Times* talking about healthy HIV carriers and why they seem to remain without symptoms a long time, perhaps indefinitely. This is an extremely vital area of study, especially since statistics would seem to indicate that, combining the current mortality and transmission rates, half of all New York gay men will be dead within five years.

Mark: What is the current rate of infection in New York and how do you see the AIDS scene changing in the coming years?

Frank: The current rate of infection, new infection, for gay men is down below 1 percent. So gay men have gotten the message. But the rate of infection for IV drug users is skyrocketing. And these people are not worried at all. They're going to be a much tougher nut to crack than homosexuals. Gay men are generally concerned, active citizens and well-educated money earners. And we don't like to die. A lot of gay men have been oversexed, but a lot of people working with AIDS have said that junkies are inherently self-destructive and don't think twice before sticking the deadly needle into their arm. The gay thing is starting to taper off—not just the rate of infection, but the rate of illness as well. Gay people have started taking the bull by the horns. We have thirty or forty people coming to the HEAL meetings now. Last year we couldn't get eight people to sit in a room for two hours. Now these meetings go on for three hours. And participants leave excited about the things they can do for themselves. And macrobiotics, whole foods nutrition, is step one. Macrobiotics is kind of "it" for us. I'm not going to take any chances or be foolish in my way of living. The time to heal, the time to live, is now.

Gary—Kaposi's Sarcoma
New York City, June 1987 ——————————————————————

Mark: Gary, what was your reason for getting into macrobiotics, and how were you introduced to it?

Gary: Well, when I was first diagnosed two-and-a-half years ago, I decided right away that I had to do something. I couldn't just roll up and die so I started looking into all the different possibilities around. I went to several doctors to ask their advice. Some wanted me to go on chemotherapy right away; some wanted to conduct all sorts of tests. One doctor told me not to do anything. He said you have Kaposi's sarcoma

(KS), so you have time to decide what you want to do. Don't rush into anything. I felt uncomfortable with him, but I did like what he had to say. This was January 1985.

Mark: What kind of symptoms did you have?

Gary: KS. I had five spots and they took a biopsy. One of my closest friends who I've known since fourth grade—I'm now forty years old— sent me an article that she saw in the *New York Native* about macrobiotics and AIDS. I read it and decided to look into it. At a HEAL meeting I met some people that had been doing macrobiotics for two or two-and-a-half years at the time, and they were perfectly healthy and happy. At that point I just couldn't believe anybody would live over a year with AIDS. That these people had lived that long meant there had to be something to it. So I decided that this was the route I was going to go. Within a week I started eating macrobiotically. I started going to a macrobiotic restaurant in New York called Souen. I didn't know how to cook this way so I was eating once a day and lost a lot of weight—14 pounds in three weeks. It really startled everybody. And I didn't like the way it felt myself. It's funny now, people look at me and say "Oh, you're macrobiotic? You don't look it." You're not really skinny or anything, and people to this day just can't believe it. But I am.

Mark: Did you see a counselor?

Gary: I wanted to see Michio Kushi so I had to wait until he came down from Boston. I was quite anxious at the time and wanted to get started right away. I began reading books and going to lectures and I started hanging around with several people who had some experience with macrobiotics.

Mark: What were the names of some of the books you read?

Gary: *You Are All Sanpaku*, and a couple of macrobiotic cookbooks. At the time there weren't as many good books as there are now. Michio wrote a wonderful book about a year or so later. It was basically all you wanted to know about macrobiotics, called *The Macrobiotic Way*. Superb book. I must have read about ten books. Then I went to some lectures and classes.

Mark: When you saw Michio what was your impression of what he said to you?

Gary: I had a good feeling about him. He had a genuine smile, he put me at ease. I just was very trusting of him, and I still am. He said not to worry and I trusted him. This is one thing about macrobiotics; I feel that it has given me a positive way of thinking and that I am doing something positive for myself. And it's a hope.

I don't feel it's a cure, although you read about all these different cancer stories and cures that happen, but I don't know about AIDS. Macrobiotics gives me hope at least that I'll be strong and that I'll stay healthy. Meanwhile, hopefully, they will find a cure. Maybe it will be from macrobiotics, I don't know. It would be nice if it was. I recently went through a crisis period where I had to do something about my health—something drastic because I was having a problem with edema. The KS interferes with the flow of fluids in your body and they start to build up and swell. I tried for about six months through macrobiotics to see what I could do. Finally I went to some doctors and researched it. Then I went to the radiation experts to see what they had to say. What it finally boiled down to was a mild form of chemotherapy, which is what I'm on now. I feel that you can do macrobiotics and chemotherapy together—especially if it's a dire necessity.

Mark: Have you done any of the supplementary therapies like acupuncture, herbs, or homeopathy?

Gary: No, I haven't.

Mark: How about exercise or visualization?

Gary: Well, I do some visualization and I still continue to work out, but not the way I used to. It's less weight-oriented and more of a stretching routine.

Mark: How about aerobics?

Gary: Well, I bicycle for about twenty minutes a day, which is plenty of aerobics.

Mark: What about social support?

Garry: I'm very lucky that way. I haven't lost any friends because of what I'm doing. I don't go out as often with them as far as eating out, but I do see them. They're all pretty supportive, and they do meet me at macrobiotic restaurants sometimes. They understand. If they're having a party they always try to have something there for me.

My lover, who is perfectly healthy, has learned to cook. It's nice that we can share this together and that I don't have to do the cooking all the time. It takes a big burden off when somebody else is there supporting you, because I prefer to eat at home—even though we do eat out about once a week.

Mark: Have you had any blood measures done?

Gary: Yes. It's interesting too, because when I was first diagnosed my white-blood count was down to around 1.9 and the last one I had a few weeks ago, it was up to 5.8. So it's quite an increase in my white-blood cells. It's gone up dramatically. And my immune system is in pretty good shape, although I still have a reversed T-cell ratio. I feel very good about the macrobiotic approach. I feel it definitely has helped me.

Mark: You said that you felt that macrobiotics has given you a more positive attitude. Were you more negative before?

Gary: Well, when I was diagnosed I had been living with someone for nine years, and I broke up with him. Things just didn't seem the same so I wasn't very happy. This was about a year before I was diagnosed. I was feeling pretty low. It's funny though. It's almost like the diagnosis gave me a reason to live. It gave me something to hook onto right away, something to get me going to a positive mode. Today I'm a much more positive, happy person. Things are quite different now. Despite my health situation I enjoy my life to the fullest. I do a lot more things than I ever did before. I really enjoy my life a lot more now.

Mark: How about your family? Do you communicate with them?

Gary: Yes. My mother, who lives in Florida, thinks it's nice that I'm doing this.

Mark: Does she know why you're doing it.

Gary: Oh yes. She knows why I'm doing it. She's happy that I'm on this now. And my sister's supportive too. She's willing to cook, although she cooks very simply. She'll cook some brown rice and steam some vegetables and to me that's very boring. I want to eat something really exciting, something a bit more delectable.

Mark: Tell me what's happening with your chemotherapy. How are you reacting to it? How do the doctors think you'll react to it?

Gary: My doctor feels I'm responding quite quickly. He doesn't know what to make of it because he pooh-poohs the macrobiotic diet. When he was away for two weeks I had another doctor who was quite interested in it and I sent her a copy of my diet. She was quite impressed. For instance, she couldn't believe how low my cholesterol level was. She eats pretty healthy herself and when she saw the numbers on it she just was astounded.

Mark: What is most meaningful to you about the macrobiotic approach? Any lessons that you've gotten along the way that you feel are personally significant?

Gary: I think I've become a lot more flexible in my life. I'm appreciating things more. To know simply where my next meal is coming from and to be able to cook dynamically and just go with the flow. Because I was very yang in certain ways—very tight in my thinking, I've become a lot more understanding of people. And I think that's one of the keys for me. I'm a lot more easygoing now than I was.

Mark: What were you like when you started five years ago?

Gary: Well, I wasn't really a wild and crazy guy. I was basically living a married life. I was with somebody for nine years. Then we split up and I went a little wild, which was the wrong time to go wild. But I ate fairy well. I can't say it was a healthy diet when I think about what I ate, but I didn't eat that much red meat but did eat a lot of fish and vegetables. Then again, I also ate a lot of sugar. Lots of dairy and cheese too, but mostly sugar—ice cream and cake, lots of cake.

Mark: Did you use drugs?

Gary: Marijuana and some cocaine. No amphetamines. They always got me nervous. Sugar and marijuana were my big yin. And I had lots of rich desserts.

Mark: Are you eating in the standard macrobiotic way?

Gary: · Well, I have miso soup every day. My tendency is to have a more yang diet anyway, so maybe that balances out the radiation. I can't say that using extremes is a good idea but maybe it balances out better.

Mark: Do you find difficulty trying to make life-style adjustments in the New York environment?

Gary: Well I have more of a desire for peace. I don't like chaotic situations. I'm more aware of it now. And I feel a lot calmer. I guess the diet really calms you. I hate to use the word "centers" but it's true. I feel a lot more centered. I just feel more even tempered. I don't have mood swings now. I guess it's the lack of chocholate chip cookies or something but basically it's an even keel. But we all have emotions and they come out when they should.

Mark: How are you coping with your old sweet tooth?

Gary: The funny thing with desserts is I have more of a problem in the summer time. I'm more prone to want desserts in the summer. Since I've been on the diet, desserts have always been a nemesis for me. But, I've managed to keep it under control most of the time. It's the summer time that I really seem to get a little looser. Exercise counteracts it to some extent, of course. In the summer, I don't know what it is in me, but I just want to have more desserts, more yin.

Mark: Where do you think you got AIDS from?

Gary: It's hard to say. It's basically a weakening of the immune system which gets you susceptible to the virus. I'm sure it had to do with me being depressed. I'm sure what I ate had something to do with it as far as being in a weakened physical and spiritual condition. But that's a difficult question. It's hard to say.

Mark: I was talking about transmission.

Gary: My ex-lover has AIDS, so I could have gotten it from him. But also when I left, for about a year, I had been fooling around more than I ever had in my life which was a long time to be fooling around. Except that they don't know how long the incubation period is. It could be five to eight years. So it didn't necessarily happen then.

Mark: You were monogamous.

Gary: Yes. And I liked it that way, at least in retrospect. But then all hell broke loose. I have some dark ideas of when it could have happened but I don't really know for sure, and what does it matter now? I have to remind myself continually that the past is a dream. Today my ex-lover was questioned on television and they asked him, "Do you think you got AIDS from your lover, from taking care of him and everything?" He replied that he didn't know, and they seemed disappointed. I think it's sad that people are so obsessed with the past, with how the virus got transmitted. We have to start focusing on the present. We have to reflect on our quality of life and we have to create joy here and now.

Paul—Kaposi's Sarcoma ──────────────

Mark: What was your reason for starting macrobiotics and how did you get into it?

Paul: I had always been interested in nutrition and had read various books on health although I didn't know about macrobiotics. Then, when I was diagnosed as having Kaposi's sarcoma three years ago, I was upset. The doctor told me that I had between six and eighteen months to live, and I reacted the way people do. I asked all kinds of questions about what could or couldn't be done for me. As it turned out, it didn't seem like they could do much and the things they were going to do were going to hurt me. I was going to be sick, I was going to go through different things as part of the treatment. That didn't appeal to me, so I went to a fortune-teller that I go to every once in a while when something important happens to me. I wanted to know how long I had to live, so I asked her if she saw me in the hospital within the coming year. Even though I had told her I had been given the diagnosis of incurable cancer beforehand, she said "Gee, I know that I should see this, but I don't. I don't see you in the hospital, or even sick." As we were going on she mentioned the name Michio Kushi in her meditation. She said she had worked with John Lennon and Yoko Ono and that's how she had heard of him. She thought he was in Boston, and that he would be very good for me. Soon after that I went to see Michio and he told me not to worry. He made some life-style recommendations and said that my prospects were good. I felt wonderful when I left his place.

Mark: Did you have any signs of AIDS?

Paul: Yes. When I went to the hospital, my throat felt weird. I looked in my mouth one day and saw two things the size of grapes that were like blood blisters stuck on the inside of my throat. They were protruding like grapes, one on either side, and were very foreign looking. I'd never seen anything like them. One of them broke just before a big dinner party I was having. I said to my neighbors, "When the guests come just go ahead with the dinner party. I'm going to the emergency room." And I ran to the hospital. They had never seen anything like it. They took a biopsy and I suggested to them what it might be because we were all worried about it at that time. And they said that they didn't think so. So three days later the doctor called to say that she was very sorry to tell me that it was Kaposi's sarcoma, which meant I had AIDS. I went to the hospital and wanted to cooperate and do all the things they wanted me to do. But then I just had this urge and went to the fortune-teller, then to Kushi. When I got home from Kushis I called my neighbor up and said, "Come over and bring shopping bags." I emptied my refrigerator and all my cabinets. The next day I went out and filled the cupboards with seaweed, beans, grains, utensils, pots, and everything. I phoned to have a macrobiotic cook come over the day after that. He showed me five, six meals each day he was there. That's how I began the diet. Eric Stapelman was the cook. He's excellent. It worked out well because I'm a quick learner and in a short period of time I learned a lot of different dishes and was able to move quickly into the diet. All along, however, I never felt sick. And I never really had any other symptoms or anything.

The only thing that was really wrong with my life up to that point was that I had a heavy-duty negative attitude, which was quite destructive. I was always struggling with it, but never knew how to control it. It was a very negative attitude about myself and others. I also had strange ups and downs during the day, mood changes that I couldn't explain. From very ecstatic to very depressed, often within minutes. My vision of things was incorrect and unclear, which makes one's life more difficult. It was absolutely unbelievable that in a very short period of time, weeks or maybe a month, I began to see myself and others differently. My perception of reality changed. Because I wasn't tortured any longer by those ups and downs, I was more at ease and began to develop better relationships with people. I made more friends. Before that I had always isolated myself, which is where arrogance came in. Arrogance isolates you and makes you more brittle, less flexible, and more unhappy.

Mark: What does arrogance mean to you?

Paul: Arrogance probably stems from an inability to love oneself and others so that you develop an attitude about yourself that reinforces the fact that there's something wrong with you. You may act like you're better than somebody else but in actuality, it's to turn people away. Then, when they give you a negative reaction you say, "Ah, of course I deserve that because I'm no good. And they're no good either because look at how they're treating me." Very subtly through expressions or mannerisms or whatever, you're giving off that vibe. I've had people tell me afterward that they thought I was a certain way—detached or disconnected. I didn't want to have any close friends. There's a certain rigidity there that's all tied in with the negativity and with the lack of ability to understand one's humanness. All that changed very quickly after I started macrobiotics.

Mark: Was that through any kind of spiritual study that you were doing at the same time? Were you meditating?

Paul: No, and I still don't. That's the one thing I have yet to come to. My spiritual life is not great at this point.

Mark: So mainly it was through diet?

Paul: Yes. Before that I had done lot of sweets, tons of fresh juice every day, tons of fruit and some regular sugar. I would generally avoid sugar, but, there was some of that too. I drank fresh orange juice every day and apple juice every day, thinking I was doing myself a favor, mind you, because there are some people who believe that juice is good for health.

Mark: Did you have any problems with colds or allergies? Were you susceptible to sickness or were you healthy?

Paul: Throughout my life I had nothing terribly serious. I had some colds and allergies but nothing dramatic. I had hepatitis and gonorrhea numerous times. I had to take a lot of antibiotics which is one of the things that weakened me. Heavy-duty antibiotics all the time.

Mark: How about drugs?

Paul: Drugs? No. I have to say no. Although I did smoke maybe three joints a year for a while. I never drank alcohol. So that was also a plus for me. You know the only thing I do, really, is get a lot of sunshine. I'm not supposed to do it but I love the sun. So that's another thing.

So anyway, the more I ate well, the more my vision changed, the more confidence I had, the more I liked myself, the more comfortable I was with myself and others. The whole thing developed. The only difficult part about what's happened in the three years since I've been macrobiotic and supposedly with AIDS is that I still get sick now and then maybe four times a year. It's difficult for me to decide if this is just discharging or if it is AIDS-related, because I have very strange things happen to me, very unusual sinus infections that can come on very strong, but then they go. Or coughing up lots of phlegm, tons of it.

Mark: What was your dairy consumption like before?

Paul: Heavy duty, every day at all meals.

Mark: And flour products too?

Paul: Some, but I would say it was more heavy dairy. I didn't eat much bread.

Mark: So the mucus still comes up?

Paul: Yes, it still comes up and sometimes I get what appears to be a flu for twenty-four hours to three days. I'll get fever and my body just goes crazy. But then it will be over and I'll feel wonderful. I'm told that this is a discharge, but I wonder. In my mind I'm still not sure, although I feel great afterward. It's over with almost as quickly as it comes. It happens about every three months, almost like clockwork. I don't know what it is but as soon as I get over it, I feel good, I have all kinds of energy.

Mark: Does it appear as the seasons are changing?

Paul: It could be. It does happen like that, but the seasons in New York are strange. It's hard to decide when one begins and when one ends. The last real big one I had was in November, Thanksgiving. Then I had another one just six months later.

Mark: Did you see any other macrobiotic teacher besides Michio Kushi?

Paul: No, though I keep in touch, of course, with Shizuko Yamamoto, Dr. Martha Cottrell, and Neil Stapelman.

Mark: Do you get massage?

Paul: A little massage, but not much. Maybe about three times with Shizuko Yamamoto during the three years. It doesn't do anything for me.

Mark: Do you have any blood measures taken at all?

Paul: I'm part of the program. I missed the last two because I was out of town so I don't know what's happening. The last I heard, of course, was that everything was getting better—not that it was that bad with me to start out. I wasn't one of the ones in really sad shape. The last time I went, everybody's had gotten better, mine included. They were trying to trace it to the change in season or whatever. And I haven't been since then.

Mark: How about exercise?

Paul: I enjoy exercising. I swim three times a week, I ride a bicycle. I row, I stretch every day. If I don't, I feel lousy. But I've always been like that. If I feel tired or crummy I exercise and I feel great. Somehow it picks me up.

One of the things I don't like about this diet, however, is that I gotten to be so thin, and I'm not comfortable that way. I don't wear shorts any more and I'm uncomfortable in a bathing suit. I'm self-conscious of the fact that I'm so thin.

Mark: Have you tried acupuncture, herbs, or anything?

Paul: I haven't.

Mark: What do you think are the greatest difficulties for you right now in continuing with macrobiotics? For example, do you have cravings?

Paul: Yes. I have cravings for macrobiotic desserts, which I have anyway. I don't deprive myself of that but I get yelled at, and they tell me that that's the reason why I have these problems every four months.

Mark: How often do you have desserts?

Paul: Oh, I probably have them five times a week—sometimes three in a row. No maple syrup and no fruit, I'm basically a baked-goods person. I like muffins, carrot cake and stuff like that. I can't really understand how if I do everything down to the last detail, that desserts are going to cause problems. I love them so much.

Mark: Do you feel your desire for desserts is somehow related to something else in your life, like eating too much salt, stress, or emotional tension?

Paul: I figure it may have to do with relationships. It's a little difficult in my position to start up a relationship with somebody, because what do you do when you meet someone interested in you? Do you tell them right off the bat? I don't. Nothing has really developed to the point where I've had to make that decision, but it's in the back of my mind how someone might feel if they knew they were getting involved with someone in my situation. The idea of that kind of romantic relationship is out of my life right now, and I miss it. Maybe it doesn't necessarily have to be but that's how I feel about it. That might be part of the need for yin. And just that I really enjoy it. And I don't feel like depriving myself. It's kind of simple. I feel like I can handle it.

Mark: Do you or did you take vitamins?

Paul: Yes. I did take vitamins for about a year. But I didn't find that they did much good. The important thing is I have such a wonderfully positive attitude now, which is just amazing for me—the energy I feel, the positive direction. Part of that is macrobiotics, I'm sure, the food change. But also when you're confronted with what's supposed to be a deadly ailment, you either are going to have a joy for living or you're going to die. So I decided to have the joy for living and appreciate things more. For the first time in my life when I was confronted with this life-or-death thing I actually chose to be positive and put all the wonderful energy that I had put into negative living into positive living. I have a lot of energy to focus and the people around me responded. It has worked out well. Mental attitude is very important. You can eat all the good food you want, and if you don't have the right mental attitude it's not going to do you very much good. It's probably 60:40, I would say.

Mark: What's your work and how does that affect your healing process?

Paul: My work is, fortunately, fairly stress-free. I'm an artist. I paint. There are no deadlines or anything. And that of course is a big plus because when I have gotten into stressful positions outside of work I see that it has a very negative effect. So I can understand how someone that has this illness, plus a heavy stress situation, is in a really tough position. Some of the stress of course you create yourself. Without realizing it, some people are more comfortable in a stressful position, so if they don't have it they'll make sure they find it somehow. But I don't need such stimulation.

Mark: Can you give any advice for people who have difficulty making the transition to macrobiotics?

Paul: For a junk food fanatic, I don't have much to say because of the way we're bombarded with ideas of what's good and what isn't good for us. Everybody agrees on certain things, however, and macrobiotics really just goes a step further than what everybody says. It works well for me.

I love vegetables, I love rice. It wasn't difficult for me to eat these things. I think they're wonderful. I work with some people that eat all the worst things. And they look at the food I'm eating. If I'm bringing my lunch to work and I'm having carrots, broccoli, rice and whatever, they look at it like it's the strangest food they ever saw. And sometimes I say to myself, am I crazy or what? Isn't this what food is? Isn't this real food? And yet they're looking at these common vegetables, like they are off the wall.

Mark: Do you feel that your social support is pretty good in regard to being on the macrobiotic diet?

Paul: Yes, although none of my friends are macrobiotic. They all smoke and drink and do other things, but when they're with me they know that that's what they're going to be doing. If they're coming to dinner with me, we're going to a macrobiotic restaurant. They all do it. Nobody complains, so in a sense I have that support. If I visit my family, they don't cook for me but I can eat whatever I want and nobody's criticizing me. I get teased a lot, but not to a point I can't handle. I feel sorry for them; they're ignorant of what they are doing to themselves.

Mark: Does your family know you have a condition?

Paul: Yes, I have two sisters. Had I known what was going to happen with me, I wouldn't have told them. I probably wouldn't have told anyone. But they knew that I have a problem with my throat and so when I found out what it was, I told them. So my family learned for the first time about my homosexuality, and they got the whole scoop. I really thought I was going to die shortly. I wouldn't have troubled anybody with that if I had known how well I was going to be doing.

Mark: You don't have any regrets now?

Paul: No. It's OK now because it actually brought my family and me closer together. Now I don't have to be as mysterious about how I live and what I'm all about.

Mark: In the early stages you did some body work, right?

Paul: I did some body rubs with body brushes and things, but mostly did aerobic exercise, which really helps eliminate a lot of things and gets your blood moving and oxygen going, and opens the pores.

Mark: What's your ancestry?

Paul: Italian.

Mark: Are you going back to Italy some time?

Paul: I was born here. I do like Italy and I understand they have some great macrobiotic centers, but I haven't been there for about eight years. I was in England last year. I was afraid to go because its the furthest I've gone since starting macrobiotics. But it was wonderful.

I was in London. They have a macrobiotic center there which is incredible. They have excellent food made there every day of the week. I had all of my meals there because I was in a hotel. We had to work, and I was on a busy schedule. They had delicious meals and at least five different desserts every day. None of them had sweetener in them. They were all delicious.

Mark: What was the occasion? Was this a vacation?

Paul: No, I also do some interior design work and I was with somebody buying furniture there. It was a hectic schedule because there were shows at night and we had to see shows during the day. I ate in the limo and the car a lot of times, but at least I ate the right kind of food. I was enjoying it so much that the stress wasn't there.

Mark: Thanks Paul.

Paul: My pleasure.

Rudy—Kaposi's Sarcoma
New York City, August 1987 ━━━━━━━━━━━━━━━━━

Mark: What circumstance brought you to macrobiotics?

Rudy: It all began with imbalanced living. My life-style prior to macrobiotics involved working many, many hours, and using drugs, caffeine, sugar and fast foods as a support system to keep me going. I believed then that this was the only way I could live and be successful as a fashion designer here in New York. Just before beginning macrobiotics, I was in India for a year and that experience prepared me on the level of vegetarianism and spirituality. Before going to India, I had my own fashion design business, which was going quite well for a while. It was primarily women's evening attire made here in New York and sold everywhere in the world, but mostly here in the States. Then my business closed. When it fell apart, I felt like a failure and tried to blame everybody and everything outside of myself.

When the AIDS epidemic swept New York, I began to reflect more deeply. I saw that I had been living a very fast life-style which had taken its toll on my health. This prompted me to begin looking for things to protect myself from AIDS. In finding macrobiotics I immediately regarded it as a preventative, a protective way of leading my life. I don't think I could ever have survived this whole ordeal without the support of macrobiotics. It enabled me to survive the crisis and to recover from whatever discrepancies were in my health. So looking back on my pre-macrobiotic days and the collapse of my business, I now see that it afforded a way out of my self-destructive pattern of living.

Mark: What signs or symptoms made you reorient your life toward macrobiotics?

Rudy: Five years ago I noticed swollen lymph glands underneath my jaw, underneath my arm, and in my groin. Purplish lesions began appearing on my left leg, and I began losing weight rapidly. The doctors suggested having one of the lesions removed and analyzed, but I refused to do that. It's interesting that I responded in that way because I had always been a proponent of modern medicine, always ready for the "quick fix." But when this occasion arose I suddenly felt that I was divinely protected. Something went "click" in my mind and I simply said, "No." One day a dear friend of mine told me, "Your lymph nodes are your sentinels against illness," and I realized that I would be giving up one of my biological guardians. It seemed utterly ludicrous to give up something that might actually, paradoxically, play some role in resolving the disease, so I canned the idea. As far as I'm concerned I was fortunate to have followed my intuition at the time. Otherwise I would've probably embraced modern medicine altogether and run the full gamut of unnecessary, untested AIDS treatments.

Mark: What course did you take after rejecting the conventional approach?

Rudy: A little over four years ago I changed my diet to something I thought was healthy. This included dairy products, in which I indulged all too often. I would eat "healthy" ice cream like honey carob, and lots of so-called natural cheese. I would eat lots of fish and chicken too, and practically no red meat. But I always felt that if I ever fell into a grinder, I would come out hamburger and Swiss cheese. This whimsical health kick went on for about one year before I began living the macrobiotic way. During that time AIDS had become a frightening spectacle in the public eye.

Mark: What was the general viewpoint then in New York among medical professionals, the homosexual community, and the general public concerning AIDS? How were they addressing the crisis?

Rudy: Most saw it then as a death sentence and most still do. Many feel the situation is hopeless. Others are hoping for a technological miracle from science. The majority think the only way to go is to use the new experimental drugs or to follow the protocols that are suggested by the medical establishment. So it takes great courage and faith, I think, to take the road less traveled by, to take the softer path of natural healing.

The media and some of the medical profession really think that the orthodox medical mode is what everybody should be doing. Anyone that chooses to practice something other than that is labeled charlatan or quack doctor, and their patients are considered fools or ignoramuses. We should all be given the opportunity, the latitude, the space, to choose how we want to live and how we want to die, and to choose how we want to recover. No one should be forced into any one particular mode. I feel that we should be granted the freedom of choice. The media in particular needs to respect that.

Mark: Do you think macrobiotics has the answer?

Rudy: Four years ago when I became macrobiotic I thought it was the answer. The answer for everybody. And now I feel that macrobiotics is the answer for some people. I still think its transformational in people's lives. And based on the way our society looks upon success or failure, if you happen to die and you're macrobiotic, in some quarters of our society that looks like failure. To me, however, that doesn't look like failure at all anymore. I think that when you die, and you've been macrobiotic, it's not your failure, or macrobiotics' failure, it's just the way you chose to pass from this realm into the next. I think the quality of that individual's death is totally transforming at a different plane—you could call it spiritual. It really has transformed the passing so it's not connected to all the garbage that would have been connected to it. In this sense, at the level of living well and dying well, macrobiotics is profoundly transformational. It's beautiful.

Mark: So it affords the opportunity to die peacefully and with awareness?

Rudy: Yes. Based on my experience with friends dying, I think you die in a more spiritual mode and are not so disconnected or hopeless. You don't feel your life has been in vain or your life has been wasted. For many the dying becomes a moment of deep, heartfelt appreciation and recognition of truth.

Mark: The idea of "failure" usually carries a lot of connotations. You can look at it in terms of the healing process per se, or you can look at it in more personal terms—that you failed as a person or that you failed your parents or society.

Rudy: Or failed macrobiotics. I have a friend who once thought he was a macrobiotic failure. It was interesting because I saw it from a totally different point of view, and told him, "I really think that you would have been much sicker and unhappier otherwise." It all depends upon the question of self-worth: Is your cup half full or is it half empty? It's all in the perspective you take on your life, your self. It's interesting when you hear conversations with other people who are also in the healing process; you form your own picture of what and how they are doing. Sometimes you think they're doing really well and you're not doing too well. And then you start asking intimate questions and you find out that they're really not doing as well as you're doing, so it's really startling.

Someone once said to me, "Don't ever be jealous of what someone else has, because if you get it you may not find you want it." We may be jealous or envious of somebody's wealth, or social position, but when you really stop to assess the unhappiness they might have as a result of that, you really take a second look. It's a real waste of our energies to get stuck in someone else's trip, especially when you see someone who obviously has "everything"—fame, wealth, success, or whatever—and suddenly they die of AIDS. Of what real value was all that stuff in their life? They're leaving this planet without having gained any insight into why they were here. It seems like a really wasted trip. I'm only saying that about certain people I've observed.

Mark: Are there some common characteristics of people you knew who died, like a consistent pattern of perspective and attitude?

Rudy: Well, it was interesting for me to find out today that Oscar was diagnosed five years ago. I was diagnosed a little more than five years ago, and it took me a year to find macrobiotics. I searched out different paths, I went to psychics, I began eating differently, dropped drugs and heavy stuff. But it took me a year before becoming macrobiotic. So there's this strong parallel between Oscar and I, getting to macrobiotics early in the process and we're both still here after five years. Other people have come and gone. And macrobiotics does prolong people's lives. Most people go to extremes like AZT and all the other experimental drugs, yet still they die, often unhappily. That's their choice and that's the way they say they're buying time. The way we used to look at buying time was, you know, stop the dead reaper from coming to get us. My prayer is that more people will buy time to recreate and enhance the quality of their lives so that when they do leave it, they're leaving at a much higher spiritual level. It's all part of the process of healing.

Mark: So you're suggesting that quality at that time is what's important, not quantity. Because when you're talking about buying, buying implies quantity.

Rudy: Yes, and from our ordinary frame of reference, "buying" is such a materialistic point of view that we have in our society. We're always buying things. It's as if our identity really depends on what we acquire in life, rather than on what's inside us. It's a little terrifying to people when they see you going off to pray and meditate, if you're actively involved in spiritually evolving. It's as if you're going off in orbit, losing touch with the world.

Mark: The other day Oscar mentioned that, for him, there isn't enough time. Rather than buying time or borrowing time for yourself, he said we have just this life to live now, so let's do it. Very bold and honest.

Rudy: Yes. If you look at it from the point of view of this being our only existence. If we're including all the other incarnations we may have had, and if we're including the possibility of coming back, then there's unlimited time. And we've already learned these lessons and have forgotten . . . some of us. Even if this is only one of your many lives on this planet, you still have to work on it this time. That's the nitty-gritty truth of the matter. Then there's also what I call cellular memory. That cosmic cellular memory of all life experience is the fundamental foundation of who we are, physically, spiritually, however we want to put it out on whatever plane.

It's interesting for me too because I was raised as a Roman Catholic. Actually, I raised myself as a Roman Catholic, because I don't believe in that theory that your parents raise you, society raises you. You raise you. And we use our parents as an excuse, we use our religion as an excuse, we use society as an excuse. But in reality, we have raised ourselves, because some of us are totally different from the rest of the people who were raised in our society, in our environment, and in our families. So we cannot blame others. Those things are all influencing us, but it's only one of the influences we allow to attach to ourselves to create who we are. This gets back to our taking responsibility for who we created.

My relationship with God is going through so many transitions right now because the Roman Catholic Church's position on homosexuality alone is mind-boggling. The Church has come right out and declared homosexuality a sin. They said you men are sinners. We can look at it from their point of view, and it really looks like there's a pretty good case for that right now. Some of us want to remain within the framework of the Roman Catholic Church and also still live in society, remain homosexual and macrobiotic, and still be able to chant, meditate, work with crystals, do aerobics or whatever you do to make yourself the person you want to be or whatever you want to experience. It becomes very difficult to try to live in a society where an institution you believe in says that you're invalidated. It's shocking. And then to have a Cardinal come out and say that homosexuals cannot convene on the premises of any Roman Catholic place.

I bring this up because I think it's part of the condition that keeps AIDS in place and makes homosexuals really feel like second-rate citizens on certain levels. Homosexuals found out that they were "different" and they pushed that differentness to the extreme and made themselves overtly feminized or, in the 70s, overtly masculinized when they took the opposite extreme and became macho. So it's like we're moving in two opposite extremes trying to create balance. To have a society that condones how homosexuals do their hair, design their homes and clothes, dance the ballets and do all the things they associate with homosexuals. They condone all of that, but when there's the possibility of those people teaching or influencing their children, society gets crazy. It's an opportunity for all of society to "come of AIDS." We used to say "come of age." Now it's about getting in touch with AIDS and getting in touch with our relationships and our world. It's the heterosexual's relationship with the homosexual, the drug addict, the prostitute or whatever we consider abnormal in our society. And God knows AIDS is the ultimate abnormality—to see people stricken and in four days disappear, it's amazing to me how other people go through all the things they have to go through to die. All the rejection and malice. At the same time I really know that God is beyond formalized religion on the face of this earth.

Mark: Do you think there is a typical homosexual life-style? Is there a typical gay diet?

Rudy: I think that when you're coming from a level of society that says you're different, you really want to do as many different things as possible. You're predisposed to being different. Many homosexuals are considered to be in the vanguard of everything. Take the discotheques; the most outrageous discotheques were first run by homosexuals. Now I'm not trying to say that heterosexuals don't have creative ability. Don't misunderstand me, I'm not one of those snobs who think that only gays know where it's at. But they do have a way of doing things that are considered outside of the mainstream, like not working 9 to 5.

So part of their whole idea is that if they're so different, they're going to try and do as many extreme things as possible within that framework of our society and they want to experience life fully in many different directions. So they sparked the "sexual revolution."

But back to the diet situation. I think when you're living in the "fast lane," you're living outside the norm of society, you want to find out what is the latest movie, the latest piece of clothing, the latest place to dance, the latest drug, the latest music, the newest ballet, play, or whatever, and the best restaurants. You have breakfast, lunch and dinner, and dessert comes with each one of them. You can also have meat, conceivably, with every one of your meals. You eat hamburgers, and other fast foods, and then go out to really glorious, decadent, festival-type meals almost every night if you happen to be on a fat expense account. Or if you make enough money, you lead this excessive, excessive life. And you're drinking the finest wines, the best liquors, and doing the best drugs. So, talk about creativity being produced by yin.

And you are not limiting your sexuality in any way.

Mark: So for you, in that respect, sexuality and promiscuity were yinnizing?

Rudy: Yinnizing? Well sure, in a sense. I think it's part of sexual liberation. It was our right, an extension of our freedom to be. And on certain levels I still think it's everyone's right if that's what they choose. That's their way of choosing to live and die. I still question if AIDS really comes from sexual practices, from the exchange of body fluids. I read all that stuff in the newspaper and just don't completely buy it.

Mark: How do we prepare ourselves for our dearest friends' death? How do they prepare themselves for dying?

Rudy: I always denied their death before. I always thought they had within themselves the capacity to overcome it. I still believe that but I'm also starting to deal with the reality that some people are going to die. So I don't have to be so devastated by their deaths, whenever it occurs. And I think it's really necessary for us to have a mourning period. It's valid to have that time, sending out your white light, your respect, your love, and let them go.

Mark: Let's talk more in terms of people relating to somebody who has AIDS. What kind of advice could we give people who are lovers or intimate friends of people who have AIDS?

Rudy: You know, one of the big burdens of being a support for a partner in this crisis is that you keep on making allowances for that person and that person's illness, and I wonder if that whole attitude of tough love needs to be instituted here.

Mark: What do you mean by tough love?

Rudy: If somebody's really dumping on you, you just tell him off and say "enough of this crap!" I mean, I've watched things like this occur. What this brings forward is a whole new level of bonding between two people, and also it's doing it at a very abstract level in society; it's doing it in an area that's considered beyond the norm. But, all the same things exist in the homosexual life-style that exist in the so-called heterosexual life-style. There are relationships that have been completely monogamous, going on for ten, twenty, thirty, forty years together, and there have been other people who have had open, non-committal relationships where they've had many different kinds of relationships.

We're all seeking balance, and I think that those of us who have chosen to be homosexuals are also looking for balance within our lives, even within our sexual balance. I think one of the things you learn from confronting the possibility of dying is that when you're standing at the precipice of death you make a decision whether you want to live or die. And that decision doesn't include somebody else. It takes a long time for you to even get around to the possibility of whether you want to let somebody into your life. I led a whole life where I could never be alone. I thought I could never exist being alone. When I finally did become macrobiotic, and I finally began living alone, I was much less driven to be attached or to have somebody move in with me. I thought, where are they going to put their clothes, where are they going to put their belong-ings, and am I ready to do that? I know that when you absolutely fall in love, all those questions just go right down the tubes and everything gets worked out. I think promiscuity reflects the desire to find connection, to find love. That sounds pretty extreme but I think having physical contact with somebody is at least going beyond the impartial handshake. And it's interesting to note that promiscuity was just as rampant in the heterosexual "young society" up until recently when people got this AIDS scare.

Mark: When you got into macrobiotics did your friends look at you differently?

Rudy: Well, actually, a very dear friend of mine, Gabriele Knecht became macrobiotic four years ago. We both decided the same weekend. She decided to become macrobiotic and so did I. I was already eating Uncle Ben's brown rice and steaming vegetables and saying, "If, this is going to make me well I'll do it for the rest of my life, but I didn't like it." So that's how we began, and other friends came along for the ride. What followed was my typical judgmental thing—"If you didn't like what I like, buzz off."

Mark: Did they put that out too?

Rudy: Well no, my friends would come along, and they'd eat, but I didn't feel supported by their coming along with me to eat. It felt like they were begrudging me eating this dinner, and I really got to the point where I had to surround myself with only macrobiotic people for my own protection.

Mark: At the AIDS conference in Paris, there was a doctor who lectured on the psychology of AIDS. He said macrobiotic diets, visual imagery, and other holistic practices often bring people to the realization that their life is in their own control and often gives people the sense of being the type of person they've always wanted to be.

Rudy: Well, I believe there's a whole transformation that occurs as a direct result of change in your diet. It's interesting for me to hear someone else's point of view and what their journey included, like when Oscar said that when he read the book he understood it and he could change his condition. It's very interesting, because when I read I kept saying "No, no, no, no. This is all crazy, these people are all nuts." And then, I'd start saying, "Yes, no, yes, no," and suddenly I heard it go click in my mind. I saw that by applying these principles anybody could recover from anything. And it had to do with something beyond just the food. It had to do with the fact that you believe in universal order.

Mark: You seem much more willing to say "recover" than "cure."

Rudy: Those words "cure" and "recovery" are all part of medical dogma in this country and the way we have been thinking about living and dying prior to our discovery of macrobiotics as an alternative or as a recovery tool, whatever you want to call it. I think what's important is how well you live. How alive you truly are.

Mark: In a sense, with the term "recovery," we are recovering a part of ourselves, we're recovering our youthful nature, the vibrancy that we had as kids, our spirit.

Rudy: Beyond calling it spirit in the religious sense, there are people whose spirit or personality has always been dead. They have no spirit of aliveness at all.

Mark: Is that the critical difference in healing fully or successfully?

Rudy: I think the critical difference is that you must believe that you have within yourself the power to do this. And there may be days when you doubt it. But basically it's whether we feel empowered. I think that the majority of people have decided to die. The decision may be a conscious flash in their mind, like maybe one zillionth of a second: "I want to die. I can't handle this any more. Now, how am I going to die without committing suicide? How am I going to die that's socially acceptable? Well, maybe I can get a really serious disease and all society can feel sorry for me and I can become one more of the martyrs." Somebody recently said that gays have decided to become martyrs to AIDS, which is an interesting way of looking at it.

You have to go through all of these crazy attitudes. And you have to really believe or have faith or be enlightened enough to get through it until you become a more spiritualized person.

Mark: Another reason that cure is inappropriate it is that cure, as opposed to recovery, implies coming from the outside. Recovery is something you realize from within.

Rudy: I think what's implicit is that cure is being done for you. Like those miraculous cures in Lourdes: you go there, get in the water, and you believe that's the way to channel the energy and you can do that. It's interesting that I have not heard of anyone with AIDS who has gone to Lourdes. And I used to say years ago, that if I ever became seriously ill I would go to Lourdes. And coming from my point of view in those days, I would have gone to Lourdes and I might have had a cure. You see? I gave up that aspect of my own belief. And other people have not given that up. People go there all the time and are cured.

Mark: How can we strengthen our faith?

Rudy: I think if you have people around that support you and you're lucky enough to have somebody you're bonded with closely, it's easier. I had a situation with a roommate who did not eat the food I ate.

I was so determined that I was not going to be influenced by his food that it did not affect me. In the beginning, when he used to eat that food in front of me and I had already eaten, I'd want to eat what he was eating too. But then I made a decision very clearly that I no longer wanted to eat that way and got very clear that all that food was supporting growth of those lesions, the cancer and the illness already in my body. You've got to be the stupidest person in the universe to eat stuff that supports your illness. I mean, that's sheer stupidity.

Alan—Pneumocystis Carinii Pneumonia, Toxoplasmosis, Cryptococcus Meningitis, Candidiasis, and Kaposi's Sarcoma
New York City, August 1987 ——————————————

Mark: Let's begin with how you got into macrobiotics and how you heard about it.

Alan: My introduction to macrobiotics was part of an evolving process of personal health care. I had always thought of myself as eating well. Then about four years ago I went to a woman who did colonics, and she said to me, "Why don't you stop eating flesh?" Well, she impressed me so much that I ended up getting rid of meat right then and there. After that I was basically vegetarian with a bit of chicken and lots of seafood. Then the AIDS epidemic started, and one thing led to another. I kept reading and hearing that there were decent results through macrobiotics. At that point I had not been diagnosed yet, but friends began coming down with the disease and dying. Other friends who were macrobiotic invited me to go to dinner with them at Souen restaurant, and that was my first introduction to macrobiotic eating. I wasn't really crazy about it, and in the first six or seven months, I ate tempura fish and vegetables every time we went to Souen. The food seemed OK to me, since before that I had my own herb-and-spice garden and cooked with mild spices and lots of flair.

Eventually, however, I contracted pneumonia and was hospitalized. My friend Jerry suggested that I get into macrobiotics as soon as I got out of the hospital, but I was totally oblivious to his suggestion. In the first place, I didn't understand that I was sick. In spite of seeing so many people with the problem, I just didn't think it could happen to me. And even when I became seriously ill, I refused to believe it.

Mark: When did you first recognize that you weren't well?

Alan: I spent a vacation in Paris in September 1985 with my friend

Gerry. We'd been in Spain a couple of weeks and pushed hard because we had a lot of things to do. All of a sudden, I came down with this dreadful cold. It was really quite debilitating and I'd never had anything like that before. When I got back to New York, I went to see my doctor. He just said that it was a bad cold, but started monitoring my white-blood cells and other blood measures because he had many patients who either had AIDS or were worried about getting AIDS. He never told me that my T-cells were down or anything like that. He just monitored me and didn't inform me of the results. But anyway, I never really recovered from that cold—it lingered on. And then I went on another trip to Puerto Rico for two weeks. As soon as I got home, the cold was back again. This went on and off, all the while getting progressively worse. We have a country place in the mountains in upstate New York, and I used to walk up and down the site all the time.

Mark: You walked up and down the hill for exercise?

Alan: Yes. It's so beautiful there. We have seventy acres at the side of the mountain. So we'd start at the bottom—we had no road or anything at that time—and we would walk up. Eventually it got to the point where I had trouble getting all the way up without stopping. And then it got to the point where I had to rest halfway up. Then I'd rest four or five times, and finally I couldn't make it up there at all. I developed a bad cough which kept getting worse, with lots of phlegm, until finally I had to go to the hospital. I just couldn't breathe smoothly or deeply, because of constant coughing and tons of phlegm. It was scary because I felt I was going to choke to death. Finally I ended up in the hospital. I never quite accepted their telling me what my problem was. I'd seen so many people around me, but I never related with their conditions. I thought I was just fine because I'd been healthy all my life, never really sick very often.

Mark: Had you always been physically active?

Alan: Very active. I used to be a ballet dancer. I've done all kinds of things, and I'm not the kind of person who sits still. So when I was in the hospital, my friend Gerry suggested that I read a book called *The Macrobiotic Way* by Michio Kushi. I had already eaten some of the food; I didn't know if it was going to please me, but there were many good reports of people who had tried macrobiotics as a prophylactic and for people who were just diagnosed and didn't want to leave the planet. They figured it was best to eat foods that were very clean and in harmonious balance. So I immediately arranged to meet with a macrobiotic teacher. He wasn't apathetic, though not very empathetic either. He seemed like he had obviously heard my story before.

But as a result of that visit, I started the macrobiotic way with my friend and hired a girl named Lindsey from the New York Macrobiotic Center, who came to my house and redid my kitchen, and got rid of all my aluminum and teflon pots and pans. I threw all my spices out. Everything from before went into the garbage. Lindsey was wonderful; she's truly macrobiotic, very warm, giving, and thoughtful of other people. She started teaching me how to cook. I didn't really want anyone to cook for me because I do believe that you must heal yourself. Nobody else can do it for you. So I started cooking and taking cooking classes and studying the macrobiotic way.

Then, since I wasn't satisfied with the initial visit to a teacher I decided to see Michio Kushi. Michio wanted me to take the seminar, "The Macrobiotic Way," before seeing him. It turned out that I couldn't take it before going to Europe, but I did manage to see Michio anyway before leaving. I was very frightened when going to see Michio because I had seen so many die. In one month, six or eight friends went. While I was in the hospital, I lost a very dear friend of mine, a young boy who was in there only three days and died. I was trying not to deny it, but I was really frightened. So when I walked into Michio's room I said, "Before we start, I must ask just one question, because it's something I haven't asked anyone yet: How long am I going to live?" And Michio sat back in the chair, looking at me pensively, and started to smile. "You'll live as long as you want. If you don't want to live here and now, you'll pass on to the next place, but if you want to stay here, you'll be alright," he said.

"But you'll have to be very good for at least three years. If you make it through three years, you're going to be OK."

That was one thing that really boosted me. Michio was totally warm and empathetic. He taught me the real meaning of what macrobiotics is. He's the greatest example of human kindness and understanding I've ever seen. He knew that I was very upset when I walked into the room, but he didn't get mushy and say, "Oh, you poor thing." Instead, he related to me with a wonderful sense of humor, and it's a very realistic sense of humor. I felt so peaceful and grateful for life, and everytime I've met Michio since, he seems to instill in me those same feelings. I've taken his spiritual seminar and a few other things. As far as I can see, he's got the answers. By the way, I got rid of the pneumocystis in ten days. The doctors couldn't believe how quickly I recovered from it. And that was before I turned fully macrobiotic. I had always eaten in a fairly healthy way, including lots of raw vegetables and spices.

Mark: Is there anything in particular that could have contributed to your condition?

Alan: Well, in my case I don't think that my diet contributed much to AIDS. On the other hand, I had abused myself terribly throughout life by taking a lot of drugs and alcohol. That did much damage, I'm sure, especially the alcohol. And what those things didn't do to me my stressful life did. I had a business which I'm getting rid of now, and I think that could have finished me off had I continued. I'm just very fortunate to be sitting here now.

Mark: Do you believe your sexuality had anything to do with your illness?

Alan: No. I'm one of the few people who doesn't believe that. You see, I was basically monogamous. I think it was mainly the drugs. I did a lot of one drug called MDA, which is an amphetamine and hallucinogen. Potent stuff, indeed! You could just feel this drug throw you against the wall, and then splat! You'd be tired for three days, totally exhausted. We did it every weekend for about three years. I mean, I spent a lot of money on that junk. And then there was the cocaine. Both of those are real sex drugs too. Both give you a big high then a big low. If I could turn back the clock and change anything, I would never have taken those drugs. They're very deceptive. They make you feel euphoric, and, once the dependency starts, you defend them. And the stress is also part of the picture, as I said. I see the drugs on one side and the stress on the other. I don't want to use the terms yin and yang. Let's just say the drugs seem to balance the stress. They attract one another and wear you out horrendously. Again, I really do not think my food intake had much to do with my condition, as it was really pretty clean. But definitely my wine intake contributed.

Mark: What about all the mucus you talked about? Where do you think all that came from?

Alan: Well, that probably came from all the bread, cheese, and oil, but it was just a discharge. What I didn't tell you was that I straightened out four years ago. I've been drug-free now for five years. I used to smoke four packs a day. I was also a very heavy drinker. I drank three to four bottles of wine every day. And if I'd gone on. . . .

Mark: You drank three to four bottles every day?

Alan: Yes, I was a real boozer. But one morning I woke up and said, "I'm never going to drink again." From then on I never touched it and, amazingly, never had any withdrawal problems. It's because I knew I had to do it; it was the only way to get to a more stable level of living. I had been losing myself in the drugs and wine for years. I was very unhappy in business from the very beginning and should never have been doing the drugs and booze. You see, I take things too personally—it's just part of my make-up. When my business began, it took off and did very well for several years. But then it started to stagnate. It wasn't up to par, and I started taking it personally, as a personal failure. I began criticizing my partner. We couldn't get our act together, and I started drinking more and taking more drugs. Of course, it was very "in" to be a druggy in those days, all throughout the seventies. I think also that the tetracycline and all the other drugs I took were really the central cause. Those and stress.

Mark: What did you take the tetracycline for and how often?

Alan: Well, I took it for gonorrhea mainly. Though I only had gonorrhea two or three times, there was one time that they couldn't get any results with the tetracycline because it was a very strong, antibiotic-resistant strain of gonococcal bacteria. That was a very rough time, but finally I got over it. On the other hand, perhaps I never really did get over those things. Perhaps they just kept getting piled up one on top of the other, lowering my resistance constantly. If I had not done the drugs, I don't think I would've contracted AIDS.

Mark: Did you eat much meat and cheese before you started being semi-vegetarian?

Alan: No, not very much. Prior to five years ago, I'd have meat maybe once or twice a week, but never more than that. However, I did like olives and fresh vegetables, and we'd have chicken once a week, usually poached. I'm of European background and was raised in Europe. Europeans aren't generally reared on a lot of meat. We had pasta, potatoes, and minestrone, always fresh soups, and always a garden salad. Not much whole grains, though we did have polenta (cornmeal) on occasion. Everything was fresh, including the meat. Rarely would they go out and buy a piece of meat. They made their own sausages, so it was never packaged.

Mark: Where were you raised? What's your family like?

Alan: France and Italy, and later on, Detroit, Michigan. But my family are northern Italian. This was the family that raised me from the time I was a year old. At that time, my mother and father divorced, and she then married a northern Italian. I went with her until I was twelve years old, when she was killed in a car accident. So it left me with no real blood parents. I still have a father, but I never see him. I mean, I don't have any family ties at all. The people that I care about very much are my family, which is mainly my friend Gerry and the people I work with.

Mark: Do you feel pretty secure and connected with people?

Alan: I'm OK with people, although often I find myself wishing people liked me more. I'm really not very secure in general, and I'm working toward being more secure. It's going to be a lot of work. I've been living with the same person, Gerry, for twenty-four years, and I've only recently become secure with him. The insecurity seems to come mainly from my childhood experience of having the things I really loved taken away from me, like my mother, who was my only real parent since age one. And my father was out of the picture too. All those losses pulled the rug out from me and left me insecure. It's still the same way with me in business and in everything else. I'm always ready to say, "Oh, this person doesn't like me." Not realizing that the person really does like me. I think I'm evolving very nicely now since getting into macrobiotics.

To me, macrobiotics is much more than just food, and that's why I went to the spiritual seminar. At that time, I had another serious illness and was hospitalized with cryptococcal meningitis. About two or three days there, I was almost dead. My vision went awry and I got extremely sick. That was this year, around Christmas time. The meningitis had flared up and I had also contracted toxoplasmosis. As if that wasn't enough, X-rays showed that four masses had developed in my brain. They had so disfigured my brain that it was all shifted to the right. My nerves were pinched, and I was seeing triple. It was a hell of a sick time.

Mark: Were you in terrible pain?

Alan: Horrible pain. Headaches that made me want to jump out the window. So finally I went to the hospital and stayed until my condition stabilized. Along with Michio, Dr. Cottrell was helpful and has continued to be very supportive, very sensitive and compassionate. She is, for me, another great example of macrobiotic spirit, much the way I'd like to be.

One of the oddest things that happened in the hospital was that, for some strange reason, I could not be in the presence of macrobiotic food. The smell of it alone would make me start vomiting, and I could not eat any of it for thirty-two days. I was on a zero diet. I couldn't keep anything down. And they let me out of the hospital throwing up; they didn't care. Two weeks later, I went back for another test and found out I had gotten worse. They put me back in for another two weeks. Once again, the smell of steamed vegetables was so awful to me that I couldn't even have them in my room.

Mark: Do you think that your aversion to food may have somehow been induced by the drugs you received in the hospital?

Alan: Yes, it was definitely a reaction brought on by the drugs. It had to have been. I mean, how could I have eaten the food for six months without any problem and then all of a sudden, after being hospitalized, not even stand the smell of it? I had been given heavy doses of drugs.

From the onset of that hospital visit I was given at least twenty-two different medications a day—for toxoplasmosis, meningitis, candidiasis, and so on, and drugs to keep up my blood levels.

Mark: How long did you take the medications? Did you lose a lot of weight then?

Alan: I took the drugs for seven weeks total—three weeks in the hospital the first time, two weeks out, then two weeks back in again. And yes, the worst part of it was that I lost thirty-two pounds and became a walking skeleton. The doctors looked concerned and recommended that I take three milkshakes a day. I was being fed intravenously with glucose —pure sugar. Then they brought in a liquid solution of beef fat, milk and glucose. They wanted me to drink four of those every day. Well, I went for it and started gaining the weight back again, but of course it wasn't the right kind of weight to gain back. So unfortunately I listened to them in the beginning, something I'll never do again. There's a front and back to everything. Some five weeks later I started seeing Kaposi's sarcoma spots all over my torso. These have since disappeared—not completely but they've gotten much lighter. For the lesions, I make a paste out of umeboshi plum, ginger, and burnt daikon leaves, mixed together and applied every day as a plaster. It doesn't hurt . . . and it works!

But getting back to the hospital experience, I must say I got quite frightened and thought I was really on the way out. The second time in the hospital I listened to a lot of relaxation tapes, read the Simonton book, and did visualizations every day. Then, when the doctors took me back for another brain scan, they found that the four cancerous masses had disappeared. Now they were in total shock because they had no idea how that happened.

Mark: Did the doctors say whether they had ever seen that before?

Alan: They see it on rare occasions in other cancer patients. The tumors just disappear. Spontaneous remission is one label they give it. I think it was mostly due to the visualizations I was doing several times daily, which really strengthened me internally.

I had one other terrible thing happen while in the hospital. The doctors had taken me off the sulfa drug I was on for meningitis and they put me on another antibiotic. I had an allergic reaction to it, which was the worst thing I've never had in my life. My whole body turned orange and red, and was lumpy like pickles, and itched terribly. The soles of my feet still itch to this day, six weeks later. They told me it would probably last in my system for ten weeks before it would completely disappear. I still go to bed every night scratching like crazy, and it often drives me up the wall. But it should go away eventually. I am taking a home remedy for that.

As soon as I left the hospital, I had one more non-macrobiotic meal, and then started on macrobiotics again. The doctors still had me on all the steroid drugs, which was an euphoric experience, and when I started going off them, I experienced the worst depression ever. I really came close a couple of times to just ending the whole thing. Crying on weekends, crying at work—I was a total mess.

That's when I looked into Michio's spiritual training seminar. I thought that it might teach me about my place on this planet, where I came from, where I stand, and where I'm going.

Mark: Can you describe what happens in the spiritual seminar and how it affected you.

Alan: A lot of people can't really talk about the spiritual seminar. It's something you can only know through personal experience. It's transformational at a very deep level. There were about thirty people, and none of us knew each other. We all ended up crying heavily through much of it. Not out of pain or anything, just out of letting go, you know, where you get rid of the delusions and the judgments you've been holding toward others. We got in touch with our common spiritual nature, with our love of life.

Another event I loved was the chanting, which is something I've kept doing every day ever since the seminar. I do the heart sutra and about four other traditional chants, including "Aum." My favorite one seems to harmonize with my entire being. It gets everything rolling inside. When I don't have the luxury of doing it, I feel cheated and regret that I didn't have the time to do it. It's a superb preparation for the day.

Mark: When you were in the hospital on all the medication, did you feel guilty that you couldn't eat the food?

Alan: No. It was OK with me. My friend was really driving me crazy about it, though, as he's very strongly into macrobiotics whereas I tend to go off it more frequently. Like today it was very hot so I had some watermelon. Now, maybe I shouldn't have been eating the stuff, but it seemed to balance the hot weather. I guess one shouldn't feel guilty about making balance. And this brings up another part of macrobiotics in which you listen to your body. There are important messages there, signals that help us learn about balance and moderation in our lives. I wouldn't sit down and eat a lot of stuff that I intuitively knew would be harmful to me. Heeding my body's messages is often the only way I can really know what's appropriate and what isn't.

Mark: What kinds of alternative therapies have you tried?

Alan: I go twice a week for acupuncture—for energy more than anything else. There's an excellent acupuncturist in town named Naomi Rabinowitz. She's the most important person to me insofar as my getting better. After my second bout, I got worked on by a superb bodyworker named Jim Collins. He's also a trained Jungian psychologist. In retrospect, I feel that he helped pull me out of the whole thing. I was a mess, totally lost, and just didn't know what else to do, where to turn. Also, when I really felt lousy I'd at least manage to walk. I've always walked a lot because it helps me, both physically and psychologically. The exercise is just as important as the bodywork. And then there are days when you wake up and feel like you could rule the world.

Mark: Did you ever take vitamin supplements before macrobiotics?

Alan: Yes. I used to be a big vitamin-taker but stopped that when I became macrobiotic. The macrobiotic perspective makes sense to me— that vitamins are manmade and unnatural, and the body is programmed by evolution to take in the natural, chelated form of vitamins. The body really has to fight to handle the isolated, unchelated form of vitamin in order to maintain balance. I think people are looking for instant health, and vitamins sometimes provide the illusion of health.

Mark: If you could pick out two of the biggest problems or challenges for you in terms of the macrobiotic dietary approach, what would they be?

Alan: The first would be overeating, but I think that has a lot to do with the stress of getting rid of my business and my anxieties about maintaining the status quo. Once this business transition is completed I think I'll be on more solid ground. But I also know that this can be an excuse for overeating, which is something I can transform now if my intention is strong enough. Now the second challenge would be desserts. I've developed a bad habit even though all my life I was never big on desserts. When I was young and for most of my life, I'd usually have a piece of cheese, bread and fruit for dessert. But I was never allowed sodas or ice cream or things like that as a kid. And all the years I lived in New York I never had a sweet tooth, although of course I did drink three bottles of wine a day. Candy bars were a rarity.

After beginning macrobiotics for about eight months, I finally began to understand why I was craving sweets so much. The culprit is that little by little I was using too much miso and tamari soy sauce, which creates sugar cravings. And it got really bad. I mean, I was going to the health food stores and buying cookies, and then I discovered Rice Dream. And I'm still not over it. At least I'm not eating really rich desserts and I'm not eating them frequently. On the other hand, I know it's not helping my condition one bit.

It's funny to see where desserts come into the picture for most people. The traditional orientation is that dessert is a way to celebrate the meal. Now you celebrate with sweets, with drugs, with booze, and with cigarettes. And it's all a lie. On New Year's Eve, everybody drinks champagne, but all it does is space you out, give you a headache, and make you forget when you wake up the next day. I don't think a hangover should be part of celebration. This is one reason I appreciate my friend and the way he accepts things in life, the way he accepts the diet, and most of all the great support he gives me by his presence. He has extraordinary discipline, yet he's also a very free spirit. Once in a while, he has two or three pieces of pie, but he's almost insufferable. I'm grateful for the example he sets. Our relationship is wonderful.

Mark: What do you see as the most important thing for you to work on at this point in your healing process?

Alan: I think it's probably greed or gluttony, wanting more than my share. Actually I think that's the biggest problem with everybody on this planet—wanting more than our share, always expecting and desiring more. Macrobiotics helps show us the way of humility and moderation, which are things I've never been big on my total way of living and relating to other people. I was always taught that I was in some way better or special, and so I began to identify with this image that others made of me and it became my mode of being. This is terrible misinformation on a very personal level, especially when you're trying to find harmonious balance within yourself. You can't find that balance if you're always looking for it outside of yourself, or pretending that it's out there rather than inside yourself.

Mark: How long did you dance ballet?

Alan: I danced professionally for about seven years and I really loved it. I started dancing at eighteen years old. I used to do Eddy Villanova's hair and watched him dance. It made me crazy, and I told him I'd give anything to be able to do that. So he invited me to a class and I ended up taking Company classes and getting a scholarship. It was a very beautiful part of my life.

Mark: Do you miss it?

Alan: I don't miss the pain.

Mark: How's your dancer's point?

Alan: The right foot's great, the left one needs a bit of work. But I'm dancing in my own way anyway.

Oscar—Kaposi's Sarcoma ━━━━━━━━━━━━━━━━━━━━━━━━

Mark: What brought you to macrobiotics?

Oscar: I was diagnosed with AIDS just about five years ago today. At that time the medical profession didn't offer me any hope. So through the help of a friend of a friend, I obtained some magazine articles on macrobiotics.

Mark: Do you want to mention these friends' names?

Oscar: Sure! One person, Cheryl Hilliard ended up being my guardian angel. I call her that because she went through everything I went through at the beginning. She was very patient and gave me total support—emotionally more than anything else. At this point, the doctor who had diagnosed me at Beth Israel Hospital had strongly recommended chemotherapy, basically to prevent the continuing growth of the Kaposi's sarcoma that I was also diagnosed with. The first Kaposi's lesions began on the left leg on the outside calf. At that time I went in for a checkup with my lover, who was part of a study group from Beth Israel. He too had developed AIDS though he didn't come down with any of the heavy duty symptoms—basically an ARC case. His white-blood cell count was very low. So as a side investigation, he asked the study group at Beth Israel if it would be OK for me to be part of the group. At the time, they said no, as they wanted to keep the group small, but they also wanted to keep tabs on sexual partners of the people who were involved in the group.

Mark: How's your friend now?

Oscar: I guess OK. I haven't heard from him for a long time. Let's see. Then I went in for a complete physical which was a major examination of the blood and immune system.

Mark: Did they remove one of your lesions and do a biopsy?

Oscar: They took a little. They found a lesion which I hadn't even noticed. I thought it was just a bump on my leg. They took a tiny piece for biopsy and it came out positive Kaposi's. Then they decided to go back and remove the whole lesion and send it down to the Atlanta Centers for Disease Control to have a complete study of it.

Mark: This was five years ago, so you were one of the earliest cases, weren't you?

Oscar: Yes. After the biopsy, which came out positive, I was scheduled to go into the hospital for a week's time. They were going to run a battery of tests, which basically consist of various oscopies, uppers and lowers, bone-marrow tests, and so forth. At this time, a very good friend of mine gave me a magazine article from *East West Journal* about a young man who had had cancer and gotten rid of it through macrobiotics. I was very interested, read the entire article, and wanted to investigate further. It just happened that that month *Life* magazine published the article on Dr. Sattilaro, and how he overcame cancer through macrobiotics. Going through this kind of information in the month following my diagnosis made me wonder what would be the best decision to make. At the same time I was introduced to my dear friend Cheryl Hilliard, who seemed quite knowledgeable. She suggested that I postpone checking into the hospital and also postpone the chemotherapy treatment. So I told the doctor that I had to go on a business trip for the next two or three weeks and that I was not going to be back, so could he please put all those tests on hold.

Cheryl guided me very gently, because I was still not sure that this was what I wanted to do. At the same time I wanted to know more, and a lot of things that she said made perfect sense to me. So we went down to the East West bookstore and loaded up with all kinds of books about macrobiotics, magazine articles, and what not that she thought would be enlightening for me. I went home and started reading. During that week I called her two or three times a day, just trying to get reassurance and to get questions answered. To this day I don't know how she put up with it. Then after a week of this, she came over to my house and literally cleaned my kitchen. I mean clean. We threw out about three shopping bags full of junk that she decided was not necessary for me to have around. She figured if I really wanted it bad enough I could walk out of the house, and by that time I would probably change my mind. A week or so later she mentioned the fact that maybe I should see a teacher for more information and a few days later I finally agreed.

Cheryl made an appointment for me with Michio Kushi a week or so later and I went to Boston with my friend. I got lost trying to find the house, and had lunch at the Open Sesami restaurant that I found just by coincidence. I later on found out that there is no such thing in life as coincidence. We had the most wonderful lunch. I told the waitress I was going to see Michio and she directed me to the Kushis' house. We got there early. It was an experience walking into the house itself. The tranquility, the peace, how the whole house was run. And I still was not sure what I was doing there.

Mark: Were you skeptical?

Oscar: I was more afraid than I was skeptical . . . of what I was getting myself into. It sounded right, but I was still afraid.

Mark: How much had you read by that time?

Oscar: By that time I had read *Sugar Blues*. It was the very first one that was recommended in Cheryl's list. There were three other books: *Healing Ourselves, Cooking with Care and Purpose,* and *You Are All Sanpaku.* And there was another book, *Male Practice* by Dr. Mendelsohn. Even now, five years later, I still have not read anything philosophical about macrobiotics. I still have not gotten into any of Michio's books; it was basic cookbooks that I was reading. As opposed to any kind of head food, it was more like stomach food. So anyway, we walked in, met Kushi and a group of his students at a table in his beautiful old house and sat down. The first thing out of his mouth was, "Don't worry about it." At that moment, I broke into tears because after seeing dozens of doctors, going here and going there, feeling I was walking in a labyrinth, all of a sudden someone tells me not to worry. Here I was completely devastated by the condition, not knowing which way to turn. It felt so good. It was just like somebody finally opening a door or a window or just a crack in the wall to let the light shine through from the other side. I had been blinded to that light. At that particular moment, I decided this was the way I was going to go. With that first statement, "Don't worry about it," I had the incredible feeling that I had come to the right place. That's when I decided I was going to embrace life and carry on.

Mark: How did Michio seem to you when you first saw him? How did he come across?

Oscar: As a very gentle, very kind human being. I was immediately in awe of what he was saying and I didn't want to miss a sound coming out of his mouth. The fact that he spoke with an accent made me concentrate even more on what he was saying. I tried to get it all.

Mark: Do you remember anything else that Michio said?

Oscar: Yes. His last words stick in my mind to this day. He said, "Sing a happy song every day," which at that time confused me because here I was, desperate for encouragement, and this man's telling me to sing a happy song. It was crazy. I left thinking, "What happy song do I know that I could sing?"

Mark: You couldn't think of one?

Oscar: I couldn't think of any Gloria Gaynor hits that sang about happiness. And I thought, well, Grace Jones doesn't have any either. I went through the whole repertoire of records that I had and nothing joyful came up. It was very interesting. Those are the two things that really stuck in my mind about my first meeting with Michio.

Mark: When did you notice changes in your condition?

Oscar: Well, I had night sweats, I was exhausted, I was living on five, six cups of espresso coffee a day by the time I was diagnosed and I was overworked and stressed out. With macrobiotics, all this began to change right away.

Mark: What else did you eat before macrobiotics?

Oscar: I was into sweets, croissants, café con leché, you know the self-indulgent diet—the finest restaurants, the best desserts. Cuban and French cuisine, in that order, were my favorites.

Mark: What's Cuban food like?

Oscar: White rice, black beans, some spices, white bread and beef, but I was never much of a beef eater. Although my father was a big beef lover, we also had a lot of seafood too, and pork. Lots of bread. Not American white bread, but French and Italian bread. Also lots of butter and milk.

Mark: How about sweets?

Oscar: Lots of very sweet desserts, every single day. It was heavy-duty sweets. I also had café con leché every breakfast, and usually a couple in the afternoon. On the French side, it was rich, creamy sauces, milk, coffee, white bread and cheese. I still miss it.

Mark: What was the hardest thing to give up?

Oscar: Coffee. In Cuba I had at least four espressos a day. I would start with a double espresso with milk every morning. I would wake up, go to the bathroom, brush my teeth, put the coffee on, then take a shower, and by the time I was through the coffee was ready. I was usually home for lunch so I would have one or two more cups of espresso, and more in the afternoon and at dinner.

Mark: What was the next hardest thing for you to give up?

Oscar: White flour. The bread more than anything else. It was a long time before I discovered flourless breads and things like that that could quench my desire for something of that texture.

Mark: Do you eat flour products today?

Oscar: I eat some, but it's not as important as it used to be.

Mark: How long did you avoid coffee?

Oscar: It was about two years until I took my first cup again. I now drink it once a week, or at most twice a week, sometimes with milk.

I have to tell you a little bit about my friend Cheryl, who got me into all this. Cheryl was a client of another friend of mine, Mark. That's how we met. She had slowly gotten Mark interested in macrobiotics. He was already beginning to ask for brown rice at certain restaurants that we were going to. Of course to me, that was ridiculous. Imagine asking for brown rice at the Empire Diner! Then the subject of Cheryl came up as the lady who was influencing my friend Mark on all this food, like seaweed, and from that moment on I started calling her the witch doctor. Mind you, I had already made a complete picture in my head of what this woman looked like: a long haired, straggly hippie, beads, Birkenstocks, a crystal ball in her purse, the whole story. So lo and behold, she turns out to be the woman that's going to heal me through her stuff.

We met at a coffee shop on the upper East Side for the first time. When she walked in, I felt it was her, immediately, because she was an incredibly gorgeous creature—she used to be a fashion model—very tall, slender, with beautiful hair. She was the complete opposite of the witch doctor. I was floored by the fact that she was really with it, that she did not fit my negative pictures at all, that she still had room to be glamorous and gorgeous. So I was suddenly very interested in what she had to say. That was how I met Cheryl.

I came back to New York after one more visit to Boston and made up my mind. I decided not to have my bone marrow tested, not to have chemotherapy, and not to have the other tests because I knew there was absolutely no guarantee of anything constructive from these procedures.

Mark: Did you question the doctors? Did you question them as to what the results of the tests would mean?

Oscar: I did because what they wanted was more information on what was happening, how my body was reacting to the illness. At that time, they were going to send me to another hospital to have chemotherapy done. When I declined, saying I did not want to go with their treatment, my doctor was not pushy at all. As a matter of fact he was very understanding and supportive of my decision.

Mark: How did your friend respond?

Oscar: He was convinced and he gave me an incredible amount of encouragement. He was supportive in the same way I was supportive of him. It was a wonderful experience to have him and realize it worked both ways. We both embraced the cooking and laughed about our mistakes. We'd spend two hours cooking and then go out to eat because the food was impossible to eat at first.

Mark: Did you lose weight?

Oscar: Well, yes and no. Let me explain that. When I got into the diet I was very hungry all of a sudden, constantly hungry, devouring food twenty-four hours a day. My meals were incredible! As soon as I ate it just came right out again. I was not absorbing well, but I still managed to gain about ten pounds in the first six to eight weeks. My friend lost ten pounds in the same amount of time. Then I lost those ten pounds and another ten. So I dropped twenty pounds in another two months which was very creepy. I looked awful and felt great, which of course did not go very well together. By the end of the third or fourth month, I was over the physical trauma of the change. All the heavy duty headaches, the body sores and cramps, all the physical pain disappeared.

Mark: Did you ever take vitamins before macrobiotics?

Oscar: Yes, a lot when I remember it. I would go to the kitchen and swallow handfuls of pills when I felt I needed them. Maybe my body got addicted to that stuff, just like the espresso and everything else. It could have been hypoglycemia too. But Cheryl was my saving grace. I'd say, "Cheryl, guess what I had today? I had this . . ." and she'd say, "Don't worry about it." She was wonderful. She didn't make me do anything. She treated me very much like a child. When we started out she would say "Well, today we'll stop this, and tomorrow we'll stop that, and we'll stop this later on." She didn't block everything out in one day which would have made me neurotic at that particular time.

The weekend I was to stop coffee she said "Now, you're going to go through severe cases of headaches and I don't want you to take an aspirin. Just wait for a while, go to sleep if you can or have to." It had to be the worst weekend of my life. I had terrible headaches. All I wanted to do was sleep, and it was dreadful, dreadful headaches. Fortunately, I was out in the country. After that was over, I felt great. I was bicycling for four or five hours every day in the mountains, enjoying nature.

Mark: When did you start gaining weight again?

Oscar: After about a year.

Mark: And how did people respond to you during that time?

Oscar: They thought I was crazy, and that was hard to deal with. Cheryl said to me, "If I had my way I'd have you join the circus right now and get you out of this trip. That would really clear your head. I just don't want you to deal with anything else but this process." This was just an exaggerated way of putting the picture in front of me, but it worked.

Mark: You mean, so you could get out of the negative context?

Oscar: Yes, negatives. She advised me not to visit anybody I knew in the hospital. She said "You don't have what it takes to do that, so don't even attempt to fake it, or prove yourself, because you don't have it. Just concentrate on yourself for now."

Mark: Do you think that New York is a particularly stressful place to try to recover?

Oscar: No. I really don't think so.

Mark: But you go to the country every weekend.

Oscar: Yes. It's also true that at one point in my recovery process I left New York for quite a spell. My relationship with Michael was ending at the time and he was moving out of the city because he couldn't deal with it all. I felt that I really needed to leave for a while. One thing that helped me make the decision was that so many people were getting sick in New York. I mean, the percentage of friends of mine who were coming down with the illness was so great that it was beginning to affect me. I just did not want to be faced with all that suffering. So, I went away for three years. I went to Florida, which was actually the wrong place to go. I don't know why it took me three years to realize that. I think New York has a lot to offer. There's a lot to discover here, and it's easier to talk to people here.

Mark: What about your family?

Oscar: To this day my family does not know that I'm sick. No one in my family knows. My father is a very ill person and my mother's like a nurse to him, constantly. The more I looked at their problem, the more I realized that adding another one was not going to help any of us. If anything, it's going to make my life more miserable.

Mark: Did you ever have any antibody testing done for the AIDS virus?

Oscar: No. After 1983 I stopped all medical tests. My immune system testing went on for about a year after the diagnosis in 1982. During that year, every time I went to Beth Israel to have a blood test I saw a different doctor. They just kept telling me it was incredible that my blood count was going up. One time the doctor said to me, "It's a miracle that even though you're not doing anything, your blood counts are going up." I just walked out because I knew he was not interested at all in anything I had to say.

Mark: I understand that you went to Japan and studied Zen. What did you do there?

Oscar: Well, we were in a temple and had to adhere to certain Zen rules. First we'd wake up, go to meditation for fifty minutes, then go to the other side of the temple for morning ceremony. It was a very strict, regimented structure during the day, but we never knew what we were going to be doing next. In this sense it was all spontaneous.

Mark: Did you work in the garden?

Oscar: We did everything. From cleaning toilets, to cleaning kitchens, to raking the garden and making little patterns, to clearing a river of dead wood and getting covered with leeches. It was amazing. Two months of not knowing what you were going to do from one hour to the next forces you to forget, or forces you to stop worrying about what you want to do and attend to what you are doing now. Basically, it's learning to concentrate. If I was cleaning toilets, all my concentration was on that one toilet, and I'd make sure it was the best job that I could ever do. No matter what it was that I was doing, the only purpose was to do it completely, mindfully. Not to be cooking a meal and thinking of something else. To concentrate in every activity, every moment. Not to fly everywhere, but to just be here in this moment because you cannot be in two places at the same time.

Mark: What did you feel? Did you feel joy? Did you feel peace?

Oscar: I actually felt whole. I felt in tune, that I was tapping into something vast, and it was myself. I was able to think clearer. I felt crystal clear—sensing the sounds and everything around me. I was much more in tune with what was around me, the ground underneath my feet, the building itself, the whole environment.

Mark: What happened when you left the temple to return to New York?

Oscar: Well, the day I left the temple was actually one of the most worried days of my life. I did not know how I was going to react to the world. I knew I was not meant to chant every day, just to make myself more aware. At the same time, I knew I could tap that profound experience again and feel good again. But I was mortified. The train ride to Tokyo was an atrocious eight hours—eight hours of sheer hell because I did not know how I was going to react to it all.

While in Tokyo, checking out the fashion houses, I called New York. They told me my friend was very sick, so I returned. By the time I got back he had already died, and so my first day back in New York was a funeral. Amazingly, I felt really comfortable about it. Of course, I was very sorry to see him go, but I did not feel sick by it.

Mark: You accepted it.

Oscar: Yes. Then I went back and tried to pick up my life. Or should I say . . . put my life together.

Mark: Was the funeral episode different from how you were before? I mean, would you have reacted more?

Oscar: Before, I would have gotten depressed. Before, I would have started thinking, "Oh, God, when is my turn. . . ." But it didn't enter my mind. I did not associate myself with his death in that way.

Mark: You've seen a lot of people die, friends die. Assuming one has the biological potential to heal oneself and the condition is not too progressed, do you think there's an attitude in healing that touches on one's view of life and death? You mentioned the experience of becoming more whole. Do you think such attitudes and experiences make the critical difference for certain people in carrying out their own healing?

Oscar: I think it's the only way. I don't think it's possible any other way. I think you have to be spiritually connected with life to make appropriate decisions. If you are connected or aware, then you will make the right decisions and those decisions lead you to a better life. No matter what it is you're trying to get rid of, whether it's emotional or physical pain. I see my body as a kind of television, basically because I think it's just an instrument that shows what's in the air. Before macrobiotics, my antennas were compressed down into the television and they were all rusted out. I was getting only one or two channels. Macrobiotics cleaned the antennas for me. It helped me realize or capture what it was that I was missing before that was always there.

Mark: Do you feel you're cured?

Oscar: No. I have a lot of problems to get rid of still. I still have a lot of hang-ups to resolve. I'm still too sentimental, which is a very greedy feeling.

Mark: Do you have sadness about friends who keep distance from you because of their fear of AIDS?

Oscar: I'll tell you where it's hitting me more these days. I still miss not having the time to become romantic with somebody. That feeling I used to have. I was always in a relationship. The minute I was out of one—even before I was out of that one—I was already involved with another. It was a very lusty type of trip that I was into. Physical and emotional but I would categorize that right now as sentimentality and selfishness.

Mark: Were you promiscuous?

Oscar: Oh yes, very. To me the challenge of conquest was the thrill of life.

Mark: What do you mean when you say you don't have the time for that now?

Oscar: Who has the time now? I mean, I don't have the time to do that.

Mark: Is it because you don't want to?

Oscar: No. It's a lot of things. Basically, I haven't gotten to the point of not wanting. I still want it. But those are things I want to get rid of. I'm working hard to get rid of.

Mark: You think promiscuity's wrong?

Oscar: I think it's wrong. I think it's stupid. It was a habit, something I did without the awareness I have now about my needs.

Mark: Please tell about the role of the mind in your healing.

Oscar: Well, I've always been convinced about the effects of positive and negative thinking, and always try to keep a positive outlook on life. At the same time I've made a lot of mistakes with that attitude. For instance, in thinking of something bad or ugly, as my skin lesions. By saying to myself "Don't think about it," I automatically think about it. I've learned that the mind generally does not accept negative thoughts or negative commands. For instance, if I tell you "Don't think of a green outfit" the first thing that comes to mind is a green outfit. So negation does not work with the mind. It's just not registered. So I have to think about or project the image of wholeness and wellness, clarity and cleanliness. With that attitude, it's easier to achieve positive thinking. I still make a lot of mistakes, but I'm very aware, I feel confident that I'll get it sooner or later.

Appendix A

Recommendations for Medical Scientists

With respect to future AIDS research, we recommend that more attention be directed toward the following three groups: (1) *long-term healthy carriers,* those people who have demonstrated antibodies to HIV, have evidence of the virus, and yet remain symptom-free; (2) *reversers,* these people who have HIV antibodies, but do not have evidence of the virus and are symptom-free; and (3) *reverters,* those people who once demonstrated seropositivity, but later were seronegative when examined in follow-up tests. These groups should be studied carefully with regard to diet and other life-style practices, past and present. Our hypothesis is that seropositive individuals who show AIDS/ARC symptoms early on will have certain life-style characteristics that differ considerably from those who go for a long period of time without showing symptoms.

In particular, we should strive to gather the following demographic information for these three groups utilizing the epidemiological method of retrospective evaluation of lifetime profiles such as the following:

- *Dietary patterns.* This aspect focuses on predominant or general eating patterns, for example, lactovegetarian, Seventh Day Adventist, macrobiotic, Pritikin, and the typical American diet (high in protein, fats, simple sugars, and additives). Percentage of energy provided from different macronutrients (saturated and unsaturated fats, simple and complex carbohydrates, animal and vegetable protein) could be used to distinguish between the various dietary patterns. Other factors such as cooking methods and degree of food processing could be studied as well.
- *Physiological factors.* This aspect focuses on those factors which may increase susceptibility to disease or have somehow been associated with certain disease patterns. For example, the Framingham Heart Study found that the correlation between heart disease and type A blood was higher than that found in either type O or type B. Research reported in *The Lancet* has found a correlation between type A and high cholesterol levels. Thus certain physiological factors may serve as biological markers for increased risk or disease susceptibility.

- *Infant feeding.* This aspect focuses on the source of feeding during the first two years of life, whether breast milk or cow's-milk formula or other "humanized" infant formulas. We might also consider how soon solid foods were introduced and whether dairy products were consumed during the first two years (and if so, how much on average). The mother's overall dietary pattern and drug use (illicit, recreational, prescription, and over-the-counter) during pregnancy and lactation should also be taken into account.
- *Physical activity levels.* This aspect would focus on whether an individual could be considered physically active or more sedentary and inactive. An adjunct to this question might be the presence of obesity, with intermittent dieting and weight loss and then regaining weight as part of the life-style.
- *Psychological orientation.* This aspect would focus on the following: degrees of positive or negative self-esteem; internal versus external locus of control, of the extent of responsibility for one's actions; ability to relax or cope with potentially stressful circumstances; ability to express (versus repress) anger; extent of perceived alienation from human society; and various beliefs or attitudes toward health and disease, life and death, war and peace, and so on.
- *Incidence and prevalence of infectious diseases.* This aspect focuses on which infectious diseases are most common in a given population or subpopulation and, if available, statistical data on these diseases; and the type and frequency of medical treatments used for these diseases.
- *Economic status.* This aspect focuses on differences in incidence of disease between lower-class, middle-class, and upper-class (if applicable) within a given society; other possible considerations are educational status, and type of occupation.
- *Overall extent of Western technological influence, or modernization.* This aspect focuses on the following factors, for example: frequency and types of immunization; use of radiation for both diagnostic and therapeutic purposes; other nuclear and chemotherapeutic diagnostic technologies made available over the past fifty years; and use of blood transfusions.

Such data, obtained retrospectively of course, may yield some important data and might help clarify the profile of susceptibility to AIDS and other immune-related diseases. It might be helpful to extend this basic research protocol to populations showing a low incidence of AIDS and to compare the overall profiles of high- and low-incidence populations.

Appendix B

Relationship between Nutrition and Stress

Although stress is often perceived as a capricious threat from the outside world, it may also be seen as a challenge to change within and become stronger in all areas of our life, thus promoting personal growth. The most practical first step is to develop appropriate responsiveness to controllable kinds of environmental stress. This calls for a fundamental change in our thinking about human life and our relationship to our surroundings. Inevitably, such awareness leads us to consider practical considerations such as proper dietary practice, breathing, exercise, and other aspects of balanced life-style, by which we strengthen our biological integrity and adaptability toward all forms of stress, controllable as well as noncontrollable. By striving to eliminate many of the deeper physiological stresses affecting the body, health promotion and maintenance can take place more smoothly and effectively.

Since mind and body are a functional totality, we can choose to change our condition of illness by physical means or mental means, or both. In some cases, both physical and mental health is readily restored by simply adjusting one's total orientation in daily life, beginning with dietary practice. A growing body of medical research indicates that food and environmental sensitivities (allergies) can induce fatigue, irritability, headaches, listlessness, depression, anxiety, and even psychotic behavior. Other relationships involve basic biochemical mechanisms which affect brain function.

Overconsumption of protein in the form of meats, eggs, and dairy products may promote stress by altering brain chemistry. The brain produces *serotonin*, a neurotransmitter that has a calming effect in times of stress. *Tryptophan*, an amino acid used by the brain to make serotonin, can be found in high concentrations in most animal products and legumes. The ability of serotonin-containing neurons to synthesize serotonin depends on the level of tryptophan in the brain, which in turn is ultimately determined by our daily diet. However, the extra amounts of amino acids released from high-protein digestion compete with tryptophan transport, thereby restricting the brain's ability to utilize tryptophan.[1]

By contrast, through a mechanism involving insulin secretion, low-protein, high-carbohydrate meals tend to elevate brain tryptophan and serotonin concentration.[2] Complex carboydrate-rich foods such as grains and vegetables promote more efficient uptake of tryptophan for the production of serotonin and *endorphins* (multifunctional compounds involved in the alleviation of anxiety and pain, as well as the stimulation of immune function).

Other nutrients may affect the two complementary parts of the involuntary (autonomic) nervous system: the *sympathetic* and *parasympathetic* systems. The sympathetic nervous system is balanced by the parasympathetic system, which regulates secretion, glandular activity, blood flow, and general maintenance. Excessive parasympathetic activity has been correlated with depressive states, whereas sympathetic excesses are correlated with states of anxiety.[3] Two chemical substances, *choline* and *tyrosine*, function as neurotransmitter precursors to affect the parasympathetic and sympathetic responses to stress. The major physiological chemical influencing parasympathetic functions is called *acetycholine* and is directly proportional to the amount of choline in our diet. Eggs and meats are the richest sources of choline. By stimulating the parasympathetic system, acetycholine can induce increased stomach-acid secretion, excessive bowel action and glandular responses which relate to feelings of anger and frustration.[4] Diets low in choline may thereby tend to bring on a more relaxed state, with decreased aggressive drives and a more contemplative mood.

Another amino acid, tyrosine, is found in high concentrations in red meats and dairy products, particularly aged cheese. Tyrosine supports the production of the thyroid hormone, *thyroxine*, which tends to increase the activity of the sympathetic nervous system such as adrenalin secretion. Hyperalert states, anxiety and poor digestion, may all result from high tyrosine ingestion.[5]

Besides the effects of protein-rich foods, the American diet promotes stress through its excessive inclusion of refined sugars, mostly taken in the form of white sugar, corn syrups and other sweeteners, white-flour products, processed cereals, tropical fruits and numerous junk foods. Refined carbohydrates have shown a direct adverse effect on human behavior. A 1980 study reported that people who ate excessive amounts of refined carbohydrates exhibited significantly more neurotic tendencies compared to those who ate moderate amounts of simple sugars.[6] Most pronounced among adolescents, these personality changes included oversensitivity to criticism, poor impulse control, frequent irritability, hostile behavior, and a tendency to anger easily. Other characteristic reactions were: sleep disturbances and restlessness; recurrent nightmares; insomnia and walking or talking in one's sleep; chronic debilitating fatigue; depression; recurrent fevers; abdominal and chest pains; and headaches. Nutritionally, the common denominator for subjects in this study was a subclinical deficiency of *thiamine* (vitamin B_1), presumably induced by eating the highly refined foods.

The biochemical explanation behind this deficiency and the accompanying behavioral problems is relatively simple. When cereal grains are refined, much of the B-vitamin content is lost, including vitamin B_1. This vitamin and other B vitamins are necessary to metabolize all carbohydrates. When a marginal deficiency arises by eating too many refined carbohydrate foods, the body is forced to draw from its B_1 reserves, which include various brain tissues and the central nervous system. This leaching away of important nutrients eventually compromises the brain's functioning. Research shows that the first brain tissues to experience the reduction are the more primitive parts of the brain. This decline leads to the abnormal, irrational behavior often characterized as "functional neurosis."

Reinforcing these effects are those of hypoglycemia, or low blood sugar, which may result from the body's inability to regulate blood sugar levels properly. Since the brain depends on glucose for energy, hypoglycemia can have a pronounced effect on mental processes. Its most common manifestations are unclear thinking, depression, and irritability. Other symptoms include insomnia and erratic sleep patterns; persistent tension headaches; excessive sugar cravings; shaky or volatile temperament; and extreme swings in mood, from euphoria to depression.

The central problem with hypoglycemia, which is probably the most widespread and unrecognized ailment in the modern world, is not that the person does not consume enough glucose-contining food, but that the body does not properly utilize the type of sugar(s) it gets. Most people showing hypoglycemic tendencies eat plenty of carbohydrates of one form or another, but the metabolism is unbalanced so that the action of *insulin* (blood-sugar-lowering hormone) is normally or overly strong, and the mechanisms that oppose insulin are weakened.[7] The main cause of this altered metabolism is a diet rich in simple sugars, including honey, corn syrup, candies, soda pop, alcoholic beverages, ice cream, tropical fruits, fruit juices, pastries and other white-flour products. All of these foods are either low or devoid of fiber and complex carbohydrates —elements which help maintain normal sugar levels.

Certain imbalances of vitamins and minerals, commonly caused by the typical American dietary patterns, may also promote mental and emotional stress. These connections are extensively documented in *Nutrition and Mental Health* (U.S. Senate Select Committee on Nutrition and Human Needs, Parker House, Berkeley, Calif., 1980). Based on these and other studies, it has been theorized that some abnormal behaviors or impaired neurological functions may be linked to imbalances in certain essential nutrients, including iron, zinc, magnesium, vitamin B_6, vitamin B_1, and vitamin C.[8] Zinc deficiency, for example, effects the *hippocampus*, a brain-tissue site involved specifically in the acquisition of learning.[9] Other nutrients such as unsaturated fatty acids, calcium, potassium and other minerals also play a more subtle role in maintaining harmonious functioning of the nervous system.[10] Deficiencies may in some cases be related to dietary excesses of fats and refined carbohydrates. The rich, refined diets typical of most Americans is the ideal nutritional means for promoting psychological stress.

[1] Wurtman, R. J. and J. H. Growdon, "Diet Enhancement of Central Nervous System Neurotransmitters," in *Neuroendocrinology* (Sunderland, Mass.: Sinauer Associates, Inc., 1980), pp. 59–60.

[2] Fernstrom, J. D., "How Food Affects Your Brain," *Nutrition Action Newsletter* (December 1979), pp. 5–7.

[3] Schwartz, G., "Foodstuffs of the Brain," in *Food Power* (New York: McGraw-Hill Book Co., 1979), pp. 55–58.

[4] Benton, M., "Can a Vegetarian Diet Make You Mellow?" *Vegetarian Times* (June, 1985), pp. 17–18.

[5] Ibid.

[6] Lonsdale, D. and R. Shamberger, "Red Cell Transketolase as an Indicator of Nutritional Deficiency," *Am J Clin Nutr* (1980), 33 (2): 205–211.

[7] Kushi, M., *Macrobiotic Health Education Series: Diabetes and Hypoglycemia* (Tokyo and New York: Japan Publications, Inc., 1985).

[8] Schauss, A., *Nutrition and Behavior* (New Canaan, Conn.: Keats Publishing, Inc., 1985), p. 19.

[9] Ibid.

[10] Abrahamson, E. M. and A. W. Pezet, *Body, Mind, & Sugar* (New York: Avon Publishers, 1977), pp. 157–175.

Macrobiotic Resources

● **Macrobiotic Way of Life Seminar**
The *Macrobiotic Way of Life Seminar* is an introductory program offered by the Kushi Institute in Boston. It includes classes in macrobiotic cooking, home care, and kitchen setup, lectures on the philosophy of macrobiotics and the standard diet, and individual way of life guidance. It is presented monthly and includes introductory and intermediate level programs. Information on the *Macrobiotic Way of Life Seminar* is available from:

> The Kushi Institute
> 17 Station Street
> Brookline, Massachusetts 02147
> (617) 738–0045

● **Macrobiotic Residential Seminar**
The *Macrobiotic Residential Seminar* is an introductory program offered at the Kushi Foundation Berkshires Center in Becket, Massachusetts. It is a one week live-in program that includes hands-on training in macrobiotic cooking and home care, lectures on the philosophy and practice of macrobiotics, and meals prepared by a specially trained cooking staff. It is presented monthly and includes introductory and intermediate levels. Information on the *Macrobiotic Residential Seminar* is available from:

> Kushi Foundation Berkshires Center
> Box 7
> Becket, Massachusetts 01223
> (413) 623–5742

● **Kushi Institute Leadership Studies**
For those who wish to study further, the Kushi Institute in Boston offers instruction for individuals who wish to become trained and

certified macrobiotic teachers. Similar leadership training programs are offered at Kushi Institute affiliates in London, Amsterdam, Antwerp, Florence, as well as in Portugal and Switzerland. Information on *Leadership Studies* is available from the Kushi Institute in Boston.

● **Other Programs**

The Kushi Institute offers a variety of public programs including an annual Summer Conference in western Massachusetts, special weight-loss and natural beauty seminars, and intensive cooking and spiritual development training at the Berkshires Center. Information on these programs is available at either of the above addresses. Moreover, macrobiotic educational centers throughout the United States, Canada, and the world offer a variety of introductory and special programs. The Kushi Foundation publishes a *Worldwide Macrobiotic Directory* every year listing these centers and individuals. Please consult the *Directory* for the nearest macrobiotic center or qualified instructor.

● **Publications**

Books and publications with information on macrobiotics are available from the Kushi Foundation, or at other macrobiotic centers, natural foodstores, and bookstores. Ongoing developments are reported in the Kushi Foundation's periodicals, including the *East West Journal*, a monthly magazine begun in 1971 and now with an international readership of 200,000. The *EWJ* features regular articles on the macrobiotic approach to health and nutrition, as well as related subjects. Moreover, Michio and Aveline Kushi have authored numerous books on macrobiotic philosophy, cooking, diet, and way of life. The following titles are especially recommended for further study:

● **Books by Michio Kushi**

Health and Diet

1. *The Cancer-Prevention Diet* (with Alex Jack, St. Martin's Press, 1983)
2. *Diet for a Strong Heart* (with Alex Jack, St. Martin's Press, 1985)
3. *Natural Healing through Macrobiotics* (edited by Edward Esko and Marc Van Cauwenberghe, M.D., Japan Publications, 1979)
4. *Macrobiotic Home Remedies* (edited by Marc Van Cauwenberghe, M.D., Japan Publications, 1985)
5. *Macrobiotic Diet* (co-authored with Aveline Kushi; edited by Alex Jack, Japan Publications, 1985)

6. *Cancer and Heart Disease: The Macrobiotic Approach* (with various contributors; edited by Edward Esko, Japan Publications, 1982)

7. *Crime and Diet: The Macrobiotic Approach* (with various contributors; edited by Edward Esko, Japan Publications, 1987)

8. *Macrobiotic Health Education Series—Diabetes and Hypoglycemia; Allergies; Obesity, Weight Loss and Eating Disorder; Infertility and Reproductive Disorders; Arthritis; Stress and Hypertension* (with various editors, Japan Publications, 1985–90)

9. *How to See Your Health: The Book of Oriental Diagnosis* (Japan Publications, 1980)

10. *Your Face Never Lies* (Avery Publishing Group, 1983)

Philosophy and Way of Life

1. *One Peaceful World* (with Alex Jack, St. Martin's Press, 1986)

2. *The Book of Macrobiotics: The Universal Way of Health, Happiness, and Peace* (with Alex Jack, Japan Publications, revised edition, 1986)

3. *The Macrobiotic Way* (with Stephen Blauer, Avery Publishing Group, 1985)

4. *The Book of Dō-In* (Japan Publications, 1979)

5. *Macrobiotic Palm Healing* (with Olivia Oredson, Japan Publications, 1989)

6. *On the Greater View* (Avery Publishing Group, 1986)

● **Books by Aveline Kushi**

Cooking

1. *Aveline Kushi's Complete Guide to Macrobiotic Cooking for Health, Harmony, and Peace* (with Alex Jack, Warner Books, 1985)

2. *Aveline Kushi's Introducing Macrobiotic Cooking* (with Wendy Esko, Japan Publications, 1987)

3. *Aveline Kushi's Wonderful World of Salads* (with Wendy Esko, Japan Publications, 1989)

4. *The Changing Seasons Macrobiotic Cookbook* (with Wendy Esko, Avery Publishing Group, 1985)

5. *How to Cook with Miso* (Japan Publications, 1979)

6. *Macrobiotic Family Favorites* (with Wendy Esko, Japan Publications, 1987)

7. *The Macrobiotic Cancer Prevention Cookbook* (with Wendy Esko, Avery Publishing Group, 1988)

8. *Macrobiotic Food and Cooking Series—Diabetes and Hypoglycemia; Allergies; Obesity, Weight Loss and Eating Disorder; Infertility and Reproductive Disorders; Arthritis; Stress and Hypertension* (with various editors, Japan Publications, 1985–88)

Family Health

1. *Macrobiotic Pregnancy and Care of the Newborn* (with Michio Kushi; edited by Edward and Wendy Esko, Japan Publications, 1984)
2. *Macrobiotic Child Care and Family Health* (with Michio Kushi; edited by Edward and Wendy Esko, Japan Publications, 1986)
3. *Lessons of Night and Day* (Avery Publishing Group, 1985)

Philosophy and Way of Life

1. *Aveline: The Life and Dream of the Woman Behind Macrobiotics Today* (with Alex Jack, Japan Publications, 1988)

Glossary

Acquired: Not inherited but developed in the individual through some environmental influence or behavioral factor.

Acquired Immunodeficiency Syndrome (AIDS): An acquired syndrome of depressed immunity resulting in susceptibility to all variety of infections and certain cancers.

Acute infection: Any infection having a rapid onset, a short course, and pronounced symptoms; in the context of AIDS, a transient illness characterized by nonspecific symptoms such as headache, skin rash, fever, malaise, enlarged lymph nodes, and diarrhea. Thought to signify an initial reaction to infection with the AIDS virus.

Adrenal glands: Two endocrine glands, one located over each kidney and divided into two functional parts: an outer portion called the *adrenal cortex* (produces steroid hormones which regulate mineral balances and sex glands) and an inner portion called the *adrenal medulla* (produces adrenalin and noradrenalin).

Aduki (azuki) bean: A small, angular red bean related to the kidney bean. It is widely cultivated in Japan and, more recently, in the United States.

AIDS-related complex (ARC): A syndrome resembling AIDS but lacking the presence of opportunistic infection or Kaposi's sarcoma. ARC patients often have chronic systemic symptoms such as lymph-node enlargement, fever, diarrhea, lethargy and localized infections less severe than seen in persons with AIDS.

Amazaké: A sweet, creamy beverage made from mildly fermented sweet rice, and often used in macrobiotic desserts.

Anecdotal reports: Individual case reports without a control group.

Antibody: A protein formed by lymphocytes that has the capacity to react against foreign entities (antigens) such as bacteria, viruses, fungi, undigested milk proteins, or other foreign substances.

Antibody positivity: The state in which an individual has been found to have antibodies, and thus prior exposure, to a particular virus (in the case of AIDS, to Human Immunodeficiency Virus); also called *seropositivity*.

Antigen: Any foreign substance that, when introduced into the body, can elicit formation of antibody specific for that substance.

Antigen overload: A condition whereby the amount of antigens in the body has exceeded the immune system's protective capacities; also called "immune overload."

Antimitotic: A chemical substance that prevents cells from undergoing mitosis, or dividing, and is therefore used against rapidly proliferating cancer cells. These chemicals often do not distinguish between cancerous and normal cells and so can produce toxic side effects.

Antioxidant: A substance, such as vitamin C or E, that regulates the harmful combination of organic substances with oxygen, thus prolonging their usefulness to cells and preventing tissue damage.

Arame: A thin, wiry, black sea vegetable, often eaten as a small side dish. Like all sea vegetables, arame is a valuable source of vitamins, minerals, and other nutritive and detoxifying substances.

Asymptomatic: Showing no signs or symptoms of disease.

Autoimmune disease: A group of diseases in which antibodies react against the body's own cells, causing either localized or widespread damage.

Azidothymidine (AZT): An experimental antiviral drug widely used in the treatment of AIDS.

B-cell: One of two general classes of small lymphocytes found in the bone marrow, spleen, liver, and intestines. Upon stimulation by T-helper cells, B-cells differentiate into plasma cells whose main function is to produce antibodies.

Bacteria: Microscopic, one-celled microorganisms that are widely prevalent in nature, are members of the animal kingdom, and include many types able to cause disease in plants and animals.

Bancha tea: The twigs, stems, and leaves from mature Japanese tea bushes or the kukicha tree; also known as kukicha tea.

Barley: A whole cereal grain recommended for daily or regular intake; beneficial to liver functioning.

Barley malt: A natural sweetener made from malted barley.

Basophil: A granulocyte, or nonspecific immune cell, which ingests some foreign particles and may act as blood mast cells, releasing histamine and heparin into the blood during allergic reactions.

Benign: Noncancerous, mild, and apparently harmless.

Bisexual: Experiencing or showing a sexual attraction to both males and females.

Brown rice: Whole unpolished rice containing a superb balance of nutrients.

Buckwheat: A hardy cereal grass eaten in the form of kasha (whole groats) or soba noodles.

Burdock: A dark, hardy, bitter-tasting root vegetable that grows throughout most of the United States. Known as *gobo* in Japan, it is highly valued for its strengthening and tonifying qualities, especially for the kidneys and intestines.

Candida albicans: A fungus that is part of the normal flora of the mucous membranes in the respiratory, gastrointestinal, and female genital tracts. If unchecked by the natural intestinal flora or by natural immune mechanisms, this fungus may produce toxins and pathological conditions throughout much of the body.

Candidiasis: A condition produced by infection with Candida albicans, capable of harming skin, mucous membranes, bronchi, lungs, heart, vagina, digestive tract, brain and bloodstream, and producing severe systemic destruction in persons with AIDS.

Carrier: An infected person who shows no signs or symptoms of disease but who harbors the infecting virus or microorganism, and therefore is capable of spreading the disease.

Chemotherapy: Treatment of disease by any drug, though colloquially used most often with reference to cancer treatment, which carries toxic side effects and may worsen an already immunodeficient condition.

Co-factor: Any agent, substance, or environmental factor that furthers the action of an agent of disease or that contributes in some way to the disease process.

Compromised immunity: A condition of weakened immunity resulting from an excessive demand on the immune system (infections, toxins, etc.) concomitant with lack of essential support (nutrition, exercise, and stress management). Also may indicate immune overload.

Cryptosporidium: A class of protozoa containing several types capable of being opportunistic and producing severe inflammation of the small intestine and colon in compromised hosts.

Cryptococcus neoformans: A fungus that may infect the skin, lungs, or bones, but which has a predilection for the central nervous system, often causing meningitis. In the severely immunocompromised individual, this fungus may spread through the blood to any site in the body.

Cytomegalovirus: A virus capable of being opportunistic and causing disseminated disease in the severely immunocompromised individual.

Daikon: A long, white radish popular in Japan and said to have fat emulsifying properties.

Dementia: An acquired, progressive impairment of intellectual function with marked compromise in at least three of the following areas: language, memory, and visuospatial skills, personality, and cognition (such as calculation and abstruction).

Dulse: A red-purple sea vegetable used in soups, salads, and vegetable dishes or as a garnish. High in iron and other minerals.

Empirical: Based on observation or experience.

Endemic: Peculiar to a certain region; usually pertaining to a disease that occurs constantly in any particular region.

Endocrine gland: A gland whose cells secrete hormones directly into the bloodstream, and not through a duct. Examples include the pituitary, adrenals, thyroid, ovaries and testes.

Eosinophil: A granulocyte which can ingest foreign particles and which may be involved in allergic reactions; present in large quantities in all protective surfaces within the body.

Epidemic: A disease tending to occur in large outbreaks or in an unusually high incidence at certain times and places.

Epidemiology: The study of groups of people or populations as they experience a measured exposure to certain aspects of the environment (e.g. foods, smoke, and chemicals).

Epstein-Barr virus: A virus linked with infectious mononucleosis and suggested as capable of causing other diseases in immunocompromised persons.

Factor VIII: A chemical important for blood clotting, it is present in the blood of normal individuals but deficient in the blood of patients with hemophilia A.

Factor IX: A chemical important for blood clotting, it is present in the blood of normal individuals but deficient in the blood of patients with hemophilia B.

Fiber: The part of whole grains, vegetables and fruits that is not broken down in digestion and gives bulk to wastes, enhancing the removal of fecal matter and also toxins from the intestines.

Fu: Dried wheat gluten cakes or sheets.

Fungi: One-celled organisms, belonging to the plant kingdom, whose members contain a number of species capable of causing severe disease in immunocompromised persons.

Gamma interferon: A type of protein formed by cells in the presence of a virus that limits viral reproduction and that is capable of inducing viral resistance in noninfected cells of the same organism.

Generalized lymphadenopathy syndrome: A syndrome of generalized lymphadenopathy (enlargement of lymph nodes) seen with increasing frequency in groups for AIDS and thought to represent a condition related to infection with the AIDS virus.

Gomashio: Sesame seed salt made from dry-roasting and grinding sea salt and sesame seeds and crushing them in a *suribachi*.

Gonorrhea: A sexually transmitted disease linked with the bacterium *Neisseria gonorrhea* and characterized by inflammation of the genital tract with possible secondary involvement of other tissues, including the heart, outer lining of the brain and joints.

Granulocyte: Also called polymorphonuclear leukocyte (PMN), these are any of several white blood cells that show a granular cytoplasm when stained with special dyes in the laboratory. They may be further classified as a *neutrophil, eosinophil,* or *basophil.*

Hemophilia: A hereditary bleeding disorder caused by factor VIII or factor IX deficiency and characterized by bleeding into various parts of the body.

Hepatitis B: A viral liver disease that can be contracted through sexual transmission and by intravenous administration of blood contaminated with hepatitis B virus.

Herpes simplex virus: A virus linked with a variety of diseases notable for their persistence in a dormant state and tendency to recur at irregular intervals. Of the two main strains, *type 1* usually involves infection of the mouth, skin, eye, and brain, while *type 2* has an affinity for the genital tract.

Herpes zoster: An acute disease characterized by painful, vesicular eruptions on the skin or mucous membranes and linked with the *varicella zoster virus.*

Heterosexual: Experiencing or showing a sexual orientation toward the opposite sex.

High risk: See risk group.

Hijiki: A dark brown variety of sea vegetable which serves as an excellent source of calcium and other minerals; often cooked with root vegetables and served as a small side dish.

Histoplasmosis: Linked with the fungus *Histoplasma capsulatum*, capable of producing mild respiratory infection in most affected hosts and widespread disease of many organs in immunocompromised persons.

HIV: Human Immunodeficiency Virus, the presumed causative agent of AIDS.

Homosexual: Experiencing or showing a sexual attraction toward the same sex.

Host: An organism on or in which another microorganism lives and from which the foreign microorganism obtains nourishment during all or part of its existence.

Iatrogenic: From the Greek, meaning "doctor-induced"; those illnesses or conditions resulting from adverse effects of the medical treatments themselves, or from the conditions surrounding treatment (antibiotic-resistant bacteria, chemotherapy, unsterile hands, hospital food, lack of exercise and human contact, etc.). Many forms of iatrogenesis probably take place over years or even decades and thus go unrecognized. The unknown long-term effects of using aspirin and other over-the-counter medication are examples.

Idiopathic thrombocytopenic purpura: An autoimmune disease, often seen in people with AIDS or ARC, in which antibodies attack the blood platelets that mediate clotting, reducing their numbers and resulting in multiple bruises, tiny purple or red skin spots, and hemorrhage into the tissues. Typical treatment may involve heavy doses of cortizone, sometimes accompanied by removal of the spleen.

Immune system: A combination of specialized cells and proteins that assist the host organism's ability to repel or neutralize foreign substances, including environmental toxins, whole food proteins, cancer cells, and microorganisms such as viruses and bacteria.

Immunocompetence: The relative capacity of a living organism to resist and overcome infection or disease.

Immunodeficiency: Any deficiency of immune response, involving antibody-mediated or cell-mediated immunity only, or both, as in AIDS.

Immunoglobulin: Also called antibodies, any one of the globular proteins that, when administered to an individual following exposure to a transmissible agent such as the viruses causing herpes, hepatitis, or AIDS, may reduce or minimize the risk of acquiring the disease linked with the agent.

Incidence rate: The number of new cases of a disease that occur per population at risk, usually within a year and reported as the number of new cases per 100,000 people in a given population.

Incubation period: The period of time between infection and onset of symptoms.

Infection: Upon exposure, the successful entry of a host by microorganisms such as viruses, fungi, protozoa, or bacteria, with resultant disease. Infection does not necessarily accompany transmission or exposure.

Interferon: A protein, formed by animal cells in the presence of a virus, or other inducing agent, that prevents viral reproduction and is capable of protecting noninfected cells from viral infection.

Interleukin-2: A natural substance produced by lymphocytes, that promotes long-term proliferation of T-cells with beneficial effects of immune functioning.

Intravenous drug abusers: Individuals who inject substances into their bloodstream through a vein, typically with needles contaminated with blood from another intravenous drug abuser and capable of transmitting a variety of infectious diseases.

In vitro: A process or reaction occurring in a glass, test tube, or petri dish rather than in the human body; the opposite is *in vivo*, meaning under actual living conditions.

Jinenjo: A light brown Japanese mountain potato that grows to be several feet long and two to three inches wide.

Kanten: A jellied fruit dessert made from agar-agar (sea vegetable used as a thickening agent).

Kaposi's sarcoma: A previously rare cancer of the skin and lymph nodes, once seen mainly in older men of Mediterranean origin and patients receiving heavy chemotherapy and radiation treatment. Now seen frequently in those with AIDS, the condition often manifests itself clinically as painless purple to brown skin lesions. Its presence is regarded as evidence of AIDS, even in the absence of opportunistic infections.

Kinpira: A style of cooking root vegetables by first sautéing, then adding a little water, and seasoning with tamari soy sauce at the end of cooking.

Koi-koku: A rich, thick soup made from carp (or other slow-moving, white-meat fish), burdock, bancha tea, and miso.

Kombu: A type of sea vegetable often added to miso soup and whole bean dishes; recommended for daily consumption.

Kupffer's cell: A fixed phagocyte (cell-eater) lining the numerous small blood vessels in the liver; these cells filter bacteria and small foreign proteins from the blood and are involved in the formation of bile.

Kuzu: A white starch made from the root of a prolific wild vine and used for thickening soups, gravies, sauces, desserts, and for medicinal beverages.

LAV: Lymphadenopathy-Associated Virus, the name given the AIDS-related virus discovered by French scientist Luc Montagnier and co-workers; this was the first isolation of the virus that later became known as HIV.

Leukocyte: Any white blood cell.

Lotus root: Root of the water lily. Brown-skinned with a hollow-chambered off-white inside, used in many dishes and for medicinal preparations.

Lymph: A clear, watery, transparent fluid containing white blood cells and some red blood cells, and collected from tissues throughout the body. This fluid flows through a network of special lymph vessels (the *lymphatic system*) eventually connecting and adding to the general blood circulation.

Lymph nodes: Small masses of lymphoid tissue which filter out or remove bacteria, toxins, and certain proteins entering the lymphatic system.

Lymphadenopathy: A condition of chronically swollen or enlarged lymph nodes. This is one of the initial symptoms seen in many patients later diagnosed with AIDS.

Lymphatic system: The system of interconnected spaces, nodes, and vessels between tissues and organs through which lymph circulates in the body. The tonsils are an integral part of this system.

Lymphocyte: A type of white blood cell found in blood, lymph, and other specialized tissue such as bone marrow, appendix, and tonsils. B- and T-cells are the major classes of small lymphocyte.

Lymphoid: Tissues of the thymus, spleen, liver, intestines, and appendix, associated with the production or differentiation of small lymphocytes.

Lymphoma: Any tumor, usually malignant, of the lymphatic tissues.

Lymphotropism: The affinity of a virus or microbe for lymphocytes.

Macrobiotics: A way of life based on the largest possible or universal view; living in accord with natural laws or universal order. Maintained by traditional cultures thousands of years old, macrobiotics includes the understanding and practical application of this order to daily life, including the selection, preparation, and manner of cooking and eating, as well as the orientation of consciousness. From the ancient Greek *macro*, meaning "great" or "large," and *bios*, meaning "life."

Macrophage: Any of several large, scavenging phagocytes present, either fixed or free, in connective tissue and many major organs and tissues such as the bone marrow, lymph nodes liver (see Kupffer's cells), spleen, and central nervous system. Free macrophages in the blood are also called *monocytes.*

Mast cell: A large connective-tissue cell that contains the chemicals histamine, heparin, and serotonin and releases them during inflammation and allergic reactions.

Meningitis: Any inflammation of the membranes lining the spinal cord and brain.

Millet: A small yellow grain that can be prepared whole, added to soups, salads, and vegetable dishes.

Miso: A fermented soybean paste that should be used unpasteurized in soups and as a flavor enhancer. Recommended for daily intake in the standard macrobiotic diet to promote digestion and overall health.

Mucous membranes: The delicate mucus-producing membranes lining those cavities and canals communicating with the air, such as the mouth, intestines, and anus.

Multifactorial theory [of AIDS]: The theory that holds that AIDS is the final outcome of a disease process which involves multiple co-factors interacting in ways which depress the immune system and promote viral infection or processes occurring after infection (viral activation, poor antibody response, lack of macrophages, etc.).

Mycobacterium avium-intracellulare: A species of mycobacteria, a bacterial group, capable of causing severe lung disease in immunocompromised hosts.

National Institutes of Health: A division of the United States Department of Health, Education, and Welfare, located in Washington, D. C., that is devoted to both clinical and basic science research in public health and disease.

Natto: A fermented soybean dish with sticky, long strands and a strong taste and odor. A good source of protein and, when fermented by traditional methods, of vitamin B_{12}.

Natural foods: Whole foods that are unprocessed or minimally processed using traditional methods and not treated with preservatives or other artificial additives.

Natural killer cell: A nonspecific, *large granular lymphocyte* that forms a distinct category of white blood cells. It possesses some characteristics of small lymphoyctes and the granular cytoplasm of granulocytes. It can destroy cancer cells and certain virus-infected cells.

Neutrophil: A kind of granulocyte that ingests bacteria and removes and destroys cellular debris and solid particles (phagocytic) thus performing a major immune function independent from T- and B-cells.

Nigari: A natural sea salt coagulant, used when making tofu by traditional methods.

Nishime: Long, slow, gentle cooking style in which vegetables or other ingredients are boiled primarily in their own juices, giving a strong, peaceful energy.

Non-Hodgkins's lymphoma: A type of lymphoma.

Noradrenalin: Mainly serves as the chemical through which the nerve cells of the sympathetic nervous system communicate with each other.

Opportunistic: A quality of an organism such as a virus, bacterium, or fungus to produce diseases when infecting an immunologically compromised host or when placed in a particular body location in large numbers. Such organisms generally do not produce disease when colonizing an immunologically normal host. From an ecological viewpoint all microbes are opportunistic in varying degrees.

Opportunistic diseases: All infections or cancers which use the "opportunity" of weakened immunity to create disease. Two prominent examples in AIDS are pneumocystis carinii pneumonia and Kaposi's sarcoma.

Organic foods: Foods grown without the use of chemical fertilizers, herbicides, pesticides, or other artificial sprays.

Pandemic: Epidemic over a very large geographic area, usually considered of global significance.

Parasympathetic nervous system: A division of the autonomic nervous system that acts to protect, conserve, and restore body resources, often balancing the effects of the sympathetic nervous system. Parasympathetic activities prevail during the "relaxation response."

Peripheral nervous system: All of the nerves and *ganglia* (nerve bundles) outside the brain and spinal chord.

Phagocyte: Literally "cell-eater," any cell that can engulf and digest microorganisms and cellular debris. A phagocyte can either circulate freely in the blood (macrophages and neutrophils) or be fixed (microglia and Kupffer's cells).

Placebo: A pharmacologically inactive substance often used in studies to compare against clinical responses to the effects of pharmacologically active substances. This assumes that the patient's attitude toward the treatment could be influencing the results. Some placebos are sugar pills, however, and may not be useful in the case of AIDS experimentation.

Placenta: The blood-filled organ that connects the fetus by the umbilical cord to the uterine wall, that enables the exchange of blood between mother and fetus, thus facilitating the transport of fetal nourishment and essential immune components from the mother.

Pneumocystis carinii: A protozoan found widely in nature but causing no disease in normal individuals. It may cause debilitating disease, usually of the lungs, in immunocompromised persons; this is considered one of the most deadly conditions of AIDS.

Pneumonia: A type of inflammation of the lungs, most often associated with infection by certain bacteria or protozoa.

Polymorphonuclear leukocyte: A granulocyte. The name derives from the various forms granulocytic nuclei can assume.

Polyunsaturated fats: Essential fatty acids found in high concentration in whole grains, beans, seeds, and to a lesser extent, in fish. A concentrated source is vegetable oils, which should be unrefined, cold-pressed and used in moderation during cooking.

Prenatal: Existing or occurring before birth. Usually refers to environmental effects on the fetus during embryonic development.

Prevalence rate: Frequency of a disease in a population.

Protein: One of a group of complex organic chemicals which form the principal components of all tissues. Proteins are found in various forms in all living matter, including viruses.

Protozoan: A one-celled organism of the animal kingdom containing many species widely distributed in nature and capable of causing disease in immunocompromised persons.

Quarantine: Any limitation of movement, or isolation imposed on an individual or group of individuals to keep a contagious disease from being transmitted and spreading to the larger population.

Refined oil: Cooking oil that has been chemically or heat-processed to alter or remove its natural color, taste, and aroma. This form of oil is extremely harmful to the body.

Retrospective: Looking back on the past. In science, it refers to research drawing from data taken in the past, and conforming to the way the data was collected and organized at the time.

Retrovirus: A class of viruses containing RNA as its core nucleic acid and thought to be one of the most primitive life forms on earth. They include HIV and other viruses that promote immunodeficiency conditions in humans.

Rice syrup: A natural sweetener made from malted brown rice.

Risk group: A group of individuals sharing a common feature or set of features that places them at an increased probability for acquiring a given disease compared to the general population. Studies of risk must distinguish between transmissibility and susceptibility.

Sea salt: Salt obtained from the ocean. Unrefined sea salt is high in trace minerals, and contains no chemicals, sugar, or added iodine.

Sea vegetable: An edible plant that grows on the ocean floor, such as kombu, wakame, hijiki, arame, dulse, sea palm, nori, and many others.

Sometimes called "seaweed." Japanese scientists have found that several of these varieties have antiviral, antifungal, antibacterial, and anticancer properties. They are a notable source of rare but extremely valuable trace elements.

Seropositivity: Same as antibody positivity.

Seronegativity: Antibody negativity; the absence of seropositivity.

Serum: The cell-free fluid of the bloodstream, such as that appearing in a test tube after blood clots.

Shiitake mushrooms: A special medicinal variety of dried mushrooms, usually imported from Japan but also grown in the United States. Its active ingredient is *lentinan*, which may possess antiviral and anticancer properties.

Simian: Associated with monkeys, for example, simian AIDS virus.

Spleen: A lymphatic organ located between the stomach and diaphragm in the left side of the body and acting as a major center of white blood cell production, as a major blood-filtering (phagocytic) center, and as a blood volume regulator during severe hemorrhage.

Sympathetic nervous system: A division of the autonomic nervous system that acts to accelerate heart rate, constrict blood vessels and raise blood pressure, usually during the stress response.

Syndrome: A group of symptoms or signs, which, when considered altogether, are known or presumed to characterize a disease.

Systemic lupus erythematosus: An autoimmune disease characterized by fever, muscle and joint pains, skin rashes, anemia, leukopenia, renal failure and severe neurologic abnormalities. It involves destruction of the connective tissue in skin, blood vessels, and nervous system.

Tamari soy sauce: Natural soy sauce free of chemical preservatives and prepared by traditional Far Eastern methods.

Taro: The starchy, edible rootstock of a widely cultivated tropical plant with large leaves shaped like elephant ears.

T-cell: A small lymphocyte that, after maturation in the thymus or thymus-dependent tissue, is responsible for cell-mediated, specific immunity. There are three kinds of T-cells: helper, suppressor, and killer (or cytotoxic) T-cells. These cells have key roles in eliminating viruses and cancer cells. The T-helper cell is the main cell infected and destroyed by HIV.

Tekka: A condiment made from soy miso, sesame oil, burdock, lotus root, carrot, and gingerroot, cooked down to a black powder.

Tempeh: A pressed soybean cake originally from Indonesia, made from split soybeans, water, grains, and special bacterial cultures to allow fermentation. Traditionally processed tempeh is high in protein and one of the few vegetarian sources of vitamin B_{12}.

Thrush: A fungal infection due to Candida albicans, occurring most often in infants and characterized by small, whitish spots on the tongue and inner surface of the cheeks; commonly seen in AIDS patients.

Thymus: The primary control center of the lymphatic system, where T-cells mature before migrating to the lymph nodes and spleen. This gland produces the hormone *thymosin*, which mediates T-cell maturation.

Tofu: Fresh soybean curd made from soybeans, water, and *nigari*, a natural sea salt coagulant. It is high in protein and its calcium is more bio-available than that of cow's milk. It may be used in soups, vegetable dishes, salads, sauces, dressings, and other dishes.

Toxoplasma gondii: A protozoan widely found in nature, normally not disease-producing in healthy persons, but resulting in *toxoplasmosis*, a severe nervous-system disorder in immunocompromised persons.

Umeboshi: A salted pickled plum that has aged usually for several years. Its zesty, sour taste and salty flavor go well with many foods and it is used as a seasoning, in sauces, as a condiment, in beverages and in many medicinal preparations. (See *Macrobiotic Home Remedies* by Michio Kushi and Marc Van Cauwenberghe, M.D., for discussion of umeboshi's medicinal properties.)

United States Public Health Service: The agency concerned with the development of federal public health programs, including public health education, and the handling of most health problems within the jurisdiction of the U.S. federal government.

Vaccine: A preparation administered to induce immunity against a particular disease agent. It may involve a suspension of living or dead organisms or a solution of either pollens or viral or bacterial antigens. The vaccine is intended to induce immunity by stimulating antibody production without producing the disease against which the recipient is immunized.

Varicella zoster virus: A virus linked with chicken pox and herpes zoster infections.

Venereal: Pertaining to or resulting from sexual intercourse, for example, venereal disease.

Virus: Any of a vast group of minute structures composed of a protein coat encasing a core of DNA or RNA, or both, and capable of infecting all animals and plants including bacteria. Biologically classified as parasites, they are totally dependent upon the cells of the infected host for their ability to reproduce. They are capable of causing disease in immunocompromised persons and are not affected by antibiotics.

Wakame: A long, thin, green sea vegetable often added to miso soup, as well as salads and bean dishes. Recommended for daily consumption.

Western blot: A test designed to detect exposure to HIV by assessing the presence of HIV antibody; more accurate than the ELISA antibody test. The Western Blot is widely used to confirm the ELISA assays.

Medicinal References

Well-documented Books:
1. Gershwin, M. E. et al., eds. *Nutrition and Immunity.* Fla.: Academic Press, Inc., 1985.
2. Chandra, R. K. *Immunology of Nutritional Disorders.* Chicago: Year Book Medical Publishers, Inc., 1980.
3. Watson, R. R., ed. *Nutrition, Disease Resistance, and Immune Function.* New York: Marcel Dekker, Inc., 1984.
4. Weiner, M. A. and K. Goss. *Maximum Immunity.* Mass.: Houghton Mifflin Co., 1986.
5. National Academy of Sciences. *Diet, Nutrition, and Cancer.* Washington D. C.: National Research Council, 1982.

General Review Articles:
1. Chandra, R. K. "Symposium: Nutritional Deficiency, Immune Responses, and Infectious Illness." *Fed Proc* 39 (1980): 3086.
2. Chandra, R. K. and N. S. Scromshaw. "Immunocompetence in Nutritional Assessment." *Am J Clin Nutr* 33 (1980): 2694.
3. Chandra, R. K. "Immunocompetance as a Functional Index of Nutritional Status." *Brit Med Bul* 37 (1981): 89.
4. ———. "Nutritional Regulation of Immunity and Infection in the Gastrointestinal Tract." *J Pediatr Gastroenterol Nutr* 2 (1981): 181.
5. ———. "Immunodeficiency in Undernutrition and Overnutrition." *Nutr Rev* 39 (1981): 225.
6. Chandra, R. K. and D. H. Dayton. "Trace Element Regulation of Immunity and Infection." *Nutr Res* 2 (1982): 721.
7. Chandra R. K. "Nutrition, Immunity, and Infection: Present Knowledge and Future Directions." *The Lancet* 1 (1983): 688.
8. Gross, R. L. and P. M. Newberne. "Role of Nutrition in Immunologic Function." *Physiol Rev* 60 (1980): 188.
9. Beisel, W. R. "Single Nutrients and Immunity." *Am J Clin Nutr* 35 (1982): 417.

10. Beisel, W. R. et al. "Single-nutrient Effects on Immunologic Functions." *J Am Med Assoc.* 245 (1981): 53.
11. Watson, R. R. "Nutrition and Immunity." *Contemp Nutr* 6 (1981): 1.
12. Good, R. A. "Nutrition and Immunity." *J Clin Immunol* 1 (1981): 3.

Articles Related to Cancer, AIDS, and Immunodeficiency

1. Beach, R. S. et al. "Zinc, Copper, and Manganese in Immune Function and Experimental Oncogenesis." *Nutrition and Cancer* 3 (1982): 172.
2. Alderson, R. M. "Nutrition and Cancer: Evidence from Epidemiology." *Proc Nutr Soc* 40 (1981): 1.
3. "Dietary Carotene and the Risk of Lung Cancer." *Nutrition Review* 40 (1982): 265.
4. Chlebowski, R. T. "Significance of Altered Nutritional Status in AIDS." *Nutrition and Cancer* 7 (1 & 2) (1985): 85.
5. Jain, V. K. and R. K. Chandra. "Does Nutritional Deficiency Predispose to AIDS?" *Nutr Res* 4 (1984): 537.
6. Archer, R. L. and W. H. Glinsmann. "Intestinal Infection and Malnutrition Initiate AIDS." *Nutr Res* 5 (1985): 9.
7. Sidhu, G. S. and E. S. Wafas. "Some Thoughts on AIDS." *Nutr Res* 5 (1985): 3.
8. Cathcart, R. F. "Vitamin C in the Treatment of AIDS." *Med Hypotheses* 7 (1984): 1359.
9. Chandra, R. K. et al. "Inducer and Supressor T-cell Subsists in Protein-energy Malnutrition." *Nutr Res* 2 (1982): 21.
10. "Diarrhea and Malabsorption Associated with AIDS." *Nutr Rev* 43 (August 1985): 235.
11. Saavedra-Delgado, A. M. and D. D. Metcalfe. "Interactions between Food Antigens and the Immune System in the Pathogenesis of Gastrointestinal Diseases." *Ann Allergy* 55 (May 1985): 694.
12. Cunningham-Rundles, C. et al. "Dietary Protein Antigenemia in Hypogammaglobulinemia: Relationship to Spenomegaly." *Birth Defects* 19 (March 1983): 239.
13. ———. "Dietary Protein Antigenemia in Humoral Immunodeficiency." *Am J Med* 76 (February 1984): 181.
14. Tannir, N. et al. "Hypercalcemia, Unusual Bone Lesions, and Human T-cell Leukemia-lymphoma Virus in Adult T-cell Lymphoma." *Cancer* 55 (1985): 615.
15. Dworkin, B. et al. "Gastrointestinal Manifestations of AIDS: A Review of 22 Cases." *Am J Gastroenterol* 80 (October 1985): 774.

16. Allen, J. I. et al. "Severe Zinc Deficiency in Humans: Association with a Reversible T-lymphocyte Dysfunction." *Ann Intern Med* 95 (1981): 154.
17. Glassock, R. J. "Nutrition, Immunology, and Renal Disease." *Kidney Intern* 24 (Suppl 16) (1983): 194.
18. Burton, B. T., and G. H. Hirschman. "Current Concepts of Nutritional Therapy in Chronic Renal Failure: An Update." *J Am Diet Assoc* 82 (April 1983): 359.

Other Recommended Reading on AIDS:

1. *Mobilization against AIDS.* Institute of Medicine, National Academy of Sciences (1986).
2. *AIDS: Cause and Solution.* Kushi, M., C. Cottrell, and M. Mead (1987).

Index

490